Advances in
Gerontological Nursing

Elizabeth A. Swanson, PhD, RN, is an Associate Professor in the College of Nursing and the Associate Vice President for Health Professions Education in the Office of the Vice President for Health Sciences, The University of Iowa, in Iowa City, Iowa. Dr. Swanson received a BS degree in nursing and an MA degree from The University of Iowa College of Nursing, as well as a PhD degree from the College of Education.

Her work focuses on examining the effects of the nursing interventions of family–staff partnerships on staff, family, and residents with Alzheimer's disease. She is also involved in research projects investigating the impact of individualized music therapy and group music therapy on persons with Alzheimer's disease and dementia.

Toni Tripp-Reimer, RN, PhD, FAAN, is Professor and Director, Office for Nursing Research Development and Utilization at The University of Iowa College of Nursing in Iowa City, Iowa. She holds an MS in nursing and an MA and PhD in anthropology from The Ohio State University. She is also Director (or PI) of the NIH-funded Center for Gerontological Nursing Interventions Research (P30), the Institutional NRSA Training Program in Gerontological Nursing Research (T32), and the Iowa–Veterans Affairs Nursing Research Consortium.

She has conducted work concerned with health behaviors of ethnic elderly for the past 17 years through a series of seven funded projects. Her current work focuses on issues of medication self-care for rural elders, psychosocial issues in relocation, and assessment and management of acute confusion.

Advances in Gerontological Nursing

Volume 1
Issues For The 21st Century

Elizabeth A. Swanson, PhD, RN
Toni Tripp-Reimer, PhD, RN, FAAN
Editors

SPRINGER PUBLISHING COMPANY

Springer Publishing Company, Inc.
536 Broadway
New York, NY 10012-3955

Cover design by Tom Yabut
Production Editor: Pam Lankas

96 97 98 99 00 / 5 4 3 2 1

ISBN 0-8261-9110-X
ISSN 1083-8708

Printed in the United States of America

To
John and Charlotte Bertlshofer,
Ann I. Whidden, and
Charles and Harriett Davis Tripp —
Our foundation and inspiration.

Contents

Contributors   *ix*

National Advisory Panel   *xi*

Introduction to the Series   *xiii*

Introduction to the Volume   *xv*

1. Gerontological Nursing in the 21st Century: Is There a
   Future?   1
   Ann Whall

2. The Iowa Conceptual Model of Gerontological Nursing   11
   Orpha J. Glick and Toni Tripp-Reimer

3. Nursing of Rural Elders: Myth and Reality   57
   Clarann Weinert and Mary E. Burman

4. Health Promotion: Its Role in Enhancing the Health
   of the Elderly   81
   May Futrell and Dolores M. Alford

5. Nursing Interventions for Older Adults with Cognitive
   Impairment: Some Conceptual, Clinical, Research,
   and Policy Issues   103
   Ivo L. Abraham and Lisa L. Onega

6. The Nature of the Family Caregiving Role and Nursing
   Interventions for Caregiving Families   133
   Patricia G. Archbold and Barbara J. Stewart

7. Ethnic Elderly: Care Issues   157
      Veronica F. Rempusheski

8. Health and Experiences of Older Homeless Adults   177
      Sharon M. Wallsten and A. T. Panter

9. The Psychosocial Care of Older Persons:
      The Pioneering Work of Dr. Irene Burnside   213
      Linda J. Garand and Kathleen C. Buckwalter

10. Epilogue—Gazing Through the Crystal Ball:
      Gerontological Nursing Issues and Challenges
      for the 21st Century   237
      Meridean L. Maas and Kathleen C. Buckwalter

Index   *251*

Contributors

Ivo L. Abraham, PhD, CS, RN, FAAN
Professor
Schools of Nursing and Medicine
University of Virginia
Charlottesville, Virginia 22903
and
Catholic University of Leuven
Leuven, Belgium

Dolores M. Alford, PhD, RN, FAAN
Gerontic Nursing Consultant
Dallas, Texas 75220

Patricia G. Archbold, RN, DNSc, FAAN
Professor
School of Nursing
Oregon Health Sciences
  University
Portland, Oregon 97201
and
Adjunct Investigator at the Center
  for Health Research at Kaiser
  Permanente

Mary E. Burman, PhD, RN, CS
Assistant Professor
School of Nursing
University of Wyoming
Laramie, Wyoming 82071

Kathleen C. Buckwalter, PhD, RN, FAAN
Professor and Associate Director
Office for Nursing Research
  Development and Utilization
College of Nursing
The University of Iowa
Iowa City, Iowa 52242

May Futrell, PhD, RN, FAAN
Professor and Chair
Department of Nursing
University of Massachusetts at Lowell
Lowell, Massachusetts 01854

Linda J. Garand, RN, MS, CS
Geropsychiatric Clinical Nurse
  Specialist, and doctoral student
College of Nursing
The University of Iowa
Iowa City, Iowa 52242

Orpha J. Glick, PhD, RN
Associate Professor
College of Nursing
The University of Iowa
Iowa City, Iowa 52242

Meridean L. Maas, PhD, RN, FAAN
Professor
College of Nursing
The University of Iowa
Iowa City, Iowa 52242

Lisa L. Onega, PhD, RN
Center on Aging and Health
University of Virginia
Charlottesville, Virginia 22903

A. T. Panter, PhD
Assistant Professor
Department of Psychology
University of North Carolina
Chapel Hill, North Carolina 27599

Veronica F. Rempusheski, PhD, RN, FAAN
Associate Professor
Associate Dean for Research, and
    Director
Center for Nursing Science and
    Scholarly Practice
School of Nursing
University of Rochester
Rochester, New York 14642

Barbara J. Stewart, PhD
Professor
School of Nursing
Oregon Health Sciences University
Portland, Oregon 97201
and
Adjunct Investigator at the Center for
    Health Research at Kaiser
    Permanente

Elizabeth A. Swanson, PhD, RN
Associate Professor
College of Nursing
Associate Vice President for Health
    Professions Education
Office of the Vice President for
    Health Services
The University of Iowa
Iowa City, Iowa 52242

Toni Tripp-Reimer, PhD, RN, FAAN
Professor and Director
Office for Nursing Research
    Development and Utilization
and
Director
Gerontological Nursing Interventions
    Research Center
College of Nursing
The University of Iowa
Iowa City, Iowa 52242

Sharon M. Wallsten, RN, PhD
Assistant Clinical Professor
School of Nursing
Duke University
Durham, North Carolina 27710

Clarann Weinert, SC, PhD, RN, FAAN
Associate Professor
College of Nursing
Sherrick Hall
Montana State University
Bozeman, Montana 59717

Ann Whall, PhD, MSN, RN, FAAN
Professor
School of Nursing
and
Associate Director
The Geriatrics Center
The University of Michigan
Ann Arbor, Michigan 48109-0482

National Advisory Panel

Ivo L. Abraham, PhD, CS, RN,
  FAAN
Professor
Schools of Nursing and Medicine
University of Virginia
Charlottesville, Virginia, 22903
and
Catholic University of Leuven
Leuven, Belgium

Patricia G. Archbold, RN, DNSc,
  FAAN
Professor
School of Nursing
Oregon Health Sciences University
Portland, Oregon 97201

Cornelia M. Beck, PhD, RN,
  FAAN
Professor and Associate Dean for
  Research and Evaluation
College of Nursing
University of Arkansas for Medical
  Sciences
Little Rock, Arkansas 72205

Barbara A. Given, PhD, RN,
  FAAN
Professor and Director of Research
College of Nursing
Michigan State University
East Lansing, Michigan 48824

Virgene Kayser-Jones, PhD, RN,
  FAAN
Professor
School of Nursing
University of California–San Francisco
San Francisco, California 94143

Kathleen A. McCormick, PhD, RN,
  FAAN
Senior Science Advisor
Office of Science and Data
  Development
Agency for Health Care Policy and
  Research
Rockville, Maryland 20852

Virginia J. Neelon, PhD, RN
Associate Professor and Director
Biobehavioral Laboratory
School of Nursing
The University of North Carolina at
  Chapel Hill
Chapel Hill, North Carolina 27599

Linda R. Phillips, PhD, RN, FAAN
Professor
College of Nursing
University of Arizona
Tucson, Arizona 85721

Neville E. Strumpf, PhD, RN, C, FAAN
Associate Professor
School of Nursing
University of Pennsylvania
Philadelphia, Pennsylvania 19104

Thelma J. Wells, PhD, RN, FAAN, FRCN
Professor
School of Nursing
University of Wisconsin
Madison, Wisconsin 53792

May L. Wykle, PhD, RN, FAAN
Florence Cellar Professor and
  Chairperson of Gerontological
  Nursing
FPB School of Nursing
Case Western Reserve University
Cleveland, Ohio 44106

Introduction to the Series

Nursing recognizes its mandate to attend to the health needs of the rapidly growing gerontological population. To carry out that mandate, however, nursing must have suitable mechanisms for conveying theory, research, and practice issues to clinical nurses, educators, and researchers in a timely manner. Until recently, only a few publications, such as *Geriatric Nursing* and *The Journal of Gerontological Nursing,* have specifically provided current knowledge and information to nurses interested in gerontology. Although these publications are effective for their intended audience, the increasing number of nurses with advanced education in gerontological nursing has given rise to an increasingly sophisticated audience. That audience requires an equally sophisticated literature, one that can synthesize current knowledge in the field, explicate issues, report current research findings, critique current nursing practice, suggest innovative approaches for quality care, and pose research questions in order to foster and disseminate advances in the field.

Given the need for more "cutting edge" literature focused specifically on gerontological nursing, the gerontological nursing faculty at the University of Iowa College of Nursing have launched a new series, titled *Advances in Gerontological Nursing.* The publication will consist of a series of annual volumes, each focused on a particular topical area in gerontological nursing. Each volume will present eight to ten chapters, written by national experts, that analyze and critique the current state of knowledge on the topic, critically examine interventions to enhance the quality of nursing care, and offer recommendations for research and practice. The themes for each volume are selected in consultation with the National Advisory Panel, which is composed of 11 nationally known experts in gerontological nursing.

We anticipate that the gerontological nursing series will be of interest to many: faculty in both undergraduate and graduate courses with a gerontological component, students in graduate gerontology courses, students in graduate courses in administration with an interest in long-term care, and practicing gerontological nurses and administrators in long-term-care facilities, adult day care centers, and community programs.

All of us involved with this series, which promises to be a timely and exciting endeavor that is unique in its content and format, are pleased that you share our interest in gerontological nursing. We welcome you, new colleagues as well as old, and encourage your comments and suggestions.

Elizabeth Swanson, PhD, RN
Toni Tripp-Reimer, PhD, RN, FAAN
Co-editors

Introduction to the Volume

In this premier volume of *Advances in Gerontological Nursing* (AGN) we have sought to offer a long view of the field of gerontological nursing, to highlight several of the major issues and concepts most likely to confront us as we stand at the edge of one century of practice and try to envision the next 100 years. It is our hope that by sweeping our gaze across the landscape, pausing to focus on particularly distinctive features, each in turn, we can sharpen our understanding of what lies before us and decide how best to chart our course.

Thus, Ann Whall invites us to examine the critical issue of how well we in the nursing profession, particularly in nursing education, have positioned ourselves to respond to the needs of the growing population of elderly and how committed we are to making some recommended changes. Glick and Tripp-Reimer review theory evolution in gerontology and propose a conceptual model for gerontological nursing. Weinert and Burman turn our attention to the rural context as it relates to rural elders and rural nursing, examining the availability and accessibility of health care for rural elders and discussing issues of gerontological nursing research, practice, and education in the rural context.

Futrell and Alford handily dispel the traditional notion that health promotion and wellness programs have no place in the life of the elderly, as they share their analysis of what constitutes health and wellness in the elderly; describe the major elements of model health promotion programs for the elderly, including services, staffing needs, and costs; and discuss how nursing professionals can encourage the elderly to participate in such programs. Abraham and Onega look at another area of gerontological nursing that too often has been seen from a fatalistic perspective: nursing care for older adults who are cognitively impaired. They challenge us to reorient our thinking from traditional expectations about the kind and degree of improvements and symptom reductions to comprehensive and compassionate interventions that are appropriate to the progress of cognitive decline and that meet the patient's and family's needs.

For their part, Archbold and Stewart guide us in a closer look at the critical but understudied concept of the nature of the family caregiving role—a concept that they believe forms the foundation for current and future nursing interventions for caregiving families. Rempusheski helps us focus on the complex relationship between ethnic identity in elderly persons and care issues, presenting both a review of how ethnicity is defined, described, and differentiated in the literature and a framework for interpreting the range of care expected and received by ethnic elderly. The health and experiences of older adults who are homeless form the relevant context for Wallsten and Panter, who provide us with a historical view of homelessness in this country and a review of their investigation into the overall health and social support of homeless older adults in several study sites in North Carolina.

In the final chapter we take a few moments to glance behind us and reflect on how far we have come, particularly in the psychosocial care of older persons, as Garand and Buckwalter pay tribute to a pioneer of gerontological nursing, Dr. Irene Burnside. Finally, Maas and Buckwalter help us turn our gaze full circle, back to the future, building on Whall's introductory remarks and forecasting how projected changes in the demographics of the aged and the health care and service delivery systems will likely affect nursing care.

We are grateful to all of these distinguished authors for their outstanding contributions to this premier volume of *Advances in Gerontological Nursing*. We would like to acknowledge also all the support and encouragement we have received since we undertook this project. In particular, we thank the gerontological nursing faculty at the University of Iowa for their wise counsel and creative energies and the members of the National Advisory Panel for their enthusiastic belief in the importance of this series. We are pleased to have the sponsorship and expertise of Dr. Ursula Springer and her distinguished publishing house, especially Ruth Chasek, the nursing editor, who patiently guided us through the long and involved process of publication. Finally, we are fortunate to have the energy and talents of Mary Anders, who provided much needed background support in the enormous task of editing the manuscripts and readying them for the publisher. She also prepared the index for the volume.

We hope that the issues presented in this premier volume and in those to come will help to stimulate critical thinking about the future of gerontological nursing and help generate new ideas in the three critical areas of nursing policies, research, and practice so that we may continue our efforts toward enhancing the quality of life for older persons.

CHAPTER 1

Gerontological Nursing in the 21st Century: Is There a Future?

Ann Whall

With the year 2000 now only 5 years away, it seems appropriate—even crucial—to reflect on the future of gerontological nursing in the next 100 years. Is there, in fact, a future for gerontological nursing? How well have we prepared ourselves and our profession? I ask you to consider the following data on projected needs for health professionals who are specifically prepared to care for older adults in the 21st century and nursing's responses to those needs.

Author notes: This chapter draws on and synthesizes references reviewed by Whall for a White Paper Panel of the Bureau of Health Professions (BHP) on visions of gerontological nursing for the next century. It is not the report of BHP, however. The author acknowledges the ongoing discussions of K. Buckwalter, P. Ebersol, T. Fulmer, J. McDowell, M. Wykle, and Chair S. Klein as influencing the views expressed herein. Claire Collins' input into this manuscript is also recognized.

1

CURRENT NEEDS

Workforce

In 1993 the U.S. Department of Health and Human Services Bureau of Health Professions developed an agenda for health professions reform for the 21st century. The bureau, identifying a serious imbalance in the supply of primary health care providers, suggested that by 1995 a major objective must be to develop innovative approaches to expand the number of nurses in primary care.

A year later, the Pew Health Professions Commission (1994) also addressed the urgent need for primary care nurse practitioners, in a document titled "Primary Care Workforce 2000." The Pew Commission stated that developing and implementing a strategy to increase the numbers of nurse practitioners and to expand their roles to deliver primary care is critical for the next century. The commission called for increases in the number of practitioner programs, the number of nurse practitioners who work not only with the elderly but with the minority elderly, and the number of minority nurses prepared to work with this population.

Both the bureau agenda and the Pew report echo a similar work, published in 1987 by the National Institute on Aging (NIA) at the National Institutes of Health (NIH), titled "Personnel for Health Needs of the Elderly through the Year 2020." This report, which predicted an expansion of health care that is focused on preventive, rehabilitative, and primary care, stressed that more older adults would need to be assisted to maintain their functioning in the community. The report also asserted that better utilization of community resources would be required for this community care. In summary, the NIA report anticipated that a wide range of well-educated health professionals, from aides to medical specialists, would be needed to respond to the health care needs of the elderly in the next century. Estimating that primary care workers would typically have a case load of two thirds elderly clients, the NIA acknowledged that the current shortages of faculty who are prepared in gerontology would be a serious constraint upon meeting these future needs and the institute's recommendations. In other words, the report suggested that collaborative arrangements between academic health centers and other types of health care providers would have to be strengthened.

Members of the nursing profession have offered similar analyses regarding the need for more nursing personnel specifically trained to care for the elderly. Wells (1993) reported that by the year 2000, 46% of registered nurses (RNs) would be giving care to elders. Nurses practicing in primary care centers therefore should be prepared to give care to elders, she said, and nursing would have to support this preparation. Heine and Bahr (1993) added another dimension to the practice of gerontological nursing in the next century by contending that it would take place primarily in the community, with gerontological nurses providing primary care.

Education

Approaching the need for gerontological nursing from another perspective, the Association for Gerontology in Higher Education (Johnson & Connelly, 1990) discussed strategies for increasing gerontological nursing content within the curriculum of nursing programs. They recommended that the deans from the American Association of Colleges of Nursing agree to incorporate specific gerontological nursing content into all levels of their programs. More recently, Mezey (1995) noted that the failure to create models for interdisciplinary education for elder care, as well as the failure to produce adequate numbers of faculty to teach gerontology throughout the curriculum, had adversely affected the care of elder adults. Mezey further pointed out that undergraduate programs contain an inadequate amount of gerontology and that there are no national gerontological nursing curricula standards, so course content varies greatly from program to program.

Small (1993) discussed the need for effective teaching strategies for baccalaureate programs in order to present gerontological nursing content at all levels. She found that the proportion of content dedicated to elder care on state board examinations is inadequate in view of the percentages of the population that nurses will be dealing with in the next century. Small emphasized that gerontological nursing content must be part of all teaching and learning opportunities as well as all nursing specialties if we are to meet the needs of the elderly population of the next century. Moccia (1993) described primary care as "the hub of the wheel" of care; in other words, most geriatric care will be delivered in the community by primary care nurses.

Musil and Wykle (1995) identified the following content areas as vital ones that must be covered if the mental health needs of the elderly in the next century are to be met: cognitive disorders, psychiatric disorders, and substance abuse. The National League for Nursing (NLN) (1990), in conjunction with the Kellogg Foundation, has also developed curricular standards for all levels of the nursing curriculum as these relate to gerontological nursing content. The development of content recommendations regarding elder care in nursing is relatively new. The gerontological nursing curricula at all levels of nursing throughout the United States vary tremendously and for the most part do not meet the NLN's standards. Is it any wonder that state board examinations do not contain enough material that relates to the nursing care of our elders?

CONSEQUENCES OF PAST AND PRESENT PRACTICES ON GERONTOLOGICAL NURSING EDUCATION

There are several consequences stemming from the inadequate curricular content and inadequate preparation of nurses at all levels of elder care. Few students choose gerontological nursing at the graduate level, as either a major or a minor. Faculty do not understand the need to integrate or to have separate courses with gerontology-centered content and thus do not support curricular changes. Because few faculty are prepared in gerontological nursing, the leaders for these content areas are few. Finally, master's degree programs in gerontological nursing are not strongly supported by universities. The first master's degree program in gerontological nursing was developed at Duke University in 1965, but it was closed in the early 1970s along with other master's programs in nursing at Duke and did not reopen until 1992 (S. Wallsten, personal communication, January 31, 1995). Currently, enrollment remains a problem for master's degree programs in gerontological nursing. In the same vein, there are few doctoral and postdoctoral programs in nursing that focus on elders. Thus, with some notable exceptions, there are not many programs that produce doctorally prepared researchers who have an interest in this content area.

Another consequence of low enrollments, the lack of gerontology-centered content, and the lack of support for such content within nursing curricula is that nursing research that supports and addresses elder care is neither as well developed nor as advanced as other areas of nursing research. When Whall, Booth, and Jirovec (1989) reviewed gerontological nursing research less than a decade ago, they concluded that it usually demonstrated a somewhat less sophisticated methodology than other nursing research, there were few programs of research, and replication studies were seldom done. Although one can argue that the quality and quantity of gerontological nursing research has improved in recent years, the consequences of low enrollment and the lack of emphasis on gerontology in the curriculum, particularly at the graduate level, are still being felt.

All of these factors are interrelated. A faculty that is not prepared to address the needs of elders does not produce interested students who will pursue graduate education in gerontological nursing. Consequently, gerontological nursing research appears to be a poor stepchild when compared to nursing research that addresses other populations. As nursing shifts to postdoctoral education, the lack of postdoctoral fellowships in gerontology will make the situation even more acute.

When we review the need for more nursing personnel for the elderly and compare it to the consequences of past and present practices within nursing education, we are led to ask, "Is there a future for gerontological nursing in the 21st century?" As Ryden and Johnson (1992) have declared, "The handwriting is on the wall. The script is large enough for all to see" (p. 347). We in gerontological nursing can no longer ignore these issues. If nursing does not accept the challenge before it, there may not be a future for gerontological nursing as we now know it. In the past, when nursing failed to rise to the challenges before it, other practitioners took over areas not being addressed by nursing. A review of the health professions and the types of assistive personnel who have developed over time supports this view. These questions are before all of nursing: Will we meet the challenge, will we support gerontological nursing content across all curricular levels, will we use the curricular standards now being developed, or will we proceed along our present trajectory?

POSSIBILITIES FOR AN IMPROVED FUTURE

A few sources suggest a plan of action for nursing that addresses the challenges before us. The Bureau of Health Professions (USDHHS, 1993) has identified needed directions for the next century with regard to the elderly and others: increasing primary care education, strengthening and expanding public health education and practice, expanding the capacity of nursing and allied health professions to meet the increasing demands for service, increasing the numbers of health care providers who are pre-pared to work for minority and disadvantaged populations, promoting education strategies that will recruit and retain health care providers to underserved populations, advancing continuous quality improvement to improve the health professions' education and practice, and finally, strengthening the data, information systems, and education research.

The directions identified by the bureau are supported largely by the Pew Health Professions Commission (1994) report, mentioned earlier, which focuses on the primary care work force in the year 2000. The com-mission's report, which identifies possible new directions for nursing in the next century, recommends that the nursing profession focus more on the community and the community's view of its health care needs. It encourages nursing to update its educational approaches so that they are congruent with public demand. The Pew Commission further suggests that emerging patterns of health care systems be identified and accom-modated within all educational systems and that we prepare health care workers for these new settings, which will be primarily interdisciplinary in nature. The commission also urges that cost effectiveness be addressed within all of the approaches to care, which suggests that practitioners must apply increasingly complex technology more appropriately within their health care settings. Another recommendation of the Pew Commission is to focus health care in the next century on prevention and on the promo-tion of healthy lifestyles in all segments of the population. In addition, the commission recommends that parents and families be involved in all deci-sion-making processes related to the care of their family members. Finally, it recommends that health care workers learn to manage information and continue to learn information technology if they want to give competent care and maintain their professional competence throughout their lives.

NEW APPROACHES TO GERONTOLOGICAL NURSING EDUCATION

Reviewing the needs of the present and the future, the consequences of past practices, and the recommendations of the BHP, the Pew Commission, and the NIA, it is apparent that our approach to geronto-logical nursing education must change. We will probably never produce adequate numbers of gerontological nurse specialists for the year 2000; our past and present enrollments support this conclusion. Therefore, gerontological nursing content must be incorporated in all relevant master's degree programs in nursing. For example, primary care nursing programs have large enrollments at the present time, but the gerontological content of these programs is often insufficient.

Encouraging faculty who teach in the smaller gerontological nursing programs to work with their counterparts in the primary care nurse programs will produce primary care providers who are better prepared to meet the needs of the elderly in the next century. It is important to realize that nursing systems and administration programs must also work with gerontology-prepared faculty to design the systems needed for the next century. There is an additional consideration: the American Nurses Association merged the councils that address gerontological nurse practitioner and clinical specialist programs in gerontological nursing in 1991; therefore, merging this content at the master's level would probably decrease confusion as well as improve the course content in both areas. Moreover, such a merger would produce more versatile and thus better prepared practitioners to address the health care needs of the elderly in the next century.

An economical way to provide needed changes in course content within existing curricula would be to have the gerontological nursing faculty work with faculty unprepared in gerontology at all levels of the curriculum. Further, the sources reviewed above suggest that when faculty members work together to update each other in content areas, they begin to support the new content area—for example, gerontological nursing content (Ryden & Johnson, 1992). By utilizing an adult education mode and by focusing on preparing faculty currently on the job, we may be able to produce sufficient numbers of prepared faculty in time for the next century.

There are other aspects of undergraduate nursing education that should be addressed. First, sources such as Small (1993) suggest that when there is a free-standing gerontological nursing education course at the undergraduate level, students are better prepared to care for elders, and the gerontological nursing content tends to be incorporated at the graduate level. For this reason, if at all possible, a separate course in elder care should be provided in all undergraduate nursing programs.

There are, however, some educational objections to offering a separate elder care course in the undergraduate program. Our current popular curricular structure within nursing (i.e., focusing on the three sections of acute and chronic care, health promotion and disease prevention, and nursing system) does not lend itself to the type of arrangement described above. But the issue is that we have arrived at the present state of our nursing education specifically because we have *not* focused on populations across the life span. We are now able to identify needed nursing content for the life span and must therefore use it as a thread or a theme across the curriculum. Such content needs to be included if we are to meet the needs of the future.

The current practice of putting gerontological nursing content only within the chronic care division of nursing curricula has adversely affected our ability to care for elders; gerontological nursing is seen as separate from the other divisions of the curricula and as competitive rather than integral to other content. This is one reason faculty tend not to support it.

If we are to meet the needs of the future and of ourselves as an aging population of nurses, we must take a cooperative stance versus a competitive one. Gerontological nursing content should be seen as everyone's business, not as just that of a small group of faculty members. We must use gerontology-prepared faculty as resource persons across all levels of curricula and as teachers of faculty who are not prepared in this area. Team teaching can provide this kind of relationship. In addition, a gerontological curricular thread—either a gerontology minor, a gerontology major, or some other arrangement—should be incorporated across all levels of the curriculum if we are to address the recommendations put forward by groups such as the BHP, the NIA, and the Pew Commission.

Finally, one way in which we can change nursing now to meet the needs of the future is to work within the system to increase the number of questions that address elder care on state board examinations. Rather than seeing elder care as a competitor with child care, for example, we should see it as a phase of the continuum of life. As population shifts occur, the proportion of questions on state boards addressing population groups should change accordingly. However, this shift is not likely to happen unless gerontological nursing faculty members make themselves available to state board agencies within each state. Again, a cooperative approach rather than a confrontational one is needed.

CONCLUSIONS

Major recommendations from prestigious agencies, as well as from knowledgeable sources within nursing, have been put before the nursing discipline, and the question remains: Will nursing address them? Unless a large proportion of the recommendations are accommodated, there may not be a future for elder care within nursing. And if that happens, nursing will, in effect, have abandoned a whole population group for the first time in nursing history.

REFERENCES

Heine, C., & Bahr, R. T. (1993). New practice models in long term care. In M. Burke & S. Sherman (Eds.), *Gerontological nursing: Issues and opportunities for the twenty-first century* (Publication No. 14-2510, pp. 27–36). New York: National League for Nursing.

Johnson, M. A., & Connelly, J. R. (1990). *Strategies for increasing gerontology content in nursing education.* Washington, DC: Association for Gerontology in Higher Education.

Mezey, M. (1995). Why good ideas have not gone far enough: Improving gerontological nursing education. In T. Fulmer & M. A. Matzo (Eds.), *Strengthening gerontological nursing education* (pp. 3–19). New York: Springer Publishing Co.

Moccia, P. (1993). About anger and power. In M. Burke & S. Sherman (Eds.), *Gerontological nursing: Issues and opportunities for the twenty-first century* (Publication No. 14-2510, pp. 69–80). New York: National League for Nursing.

National Institute on Aging. (1987). *Personnel for health needs of the elderly through the year 2020.* Bethesda, MD: U.S. Department of Health and Human Services, Public Health Service.

National League for Nursing, The Community College–Nursing Home Partnership. (1990, October). *Report from national invitational consensus conference to identify gerontological nursing competencies for baccalaureate graduates.* Georgetown University, Washington, DC.

Pew Health Professions Commission. (1994). *Primary care workforce 2000: Federal policy paper.* San Francisco: Pew Charitable Trust/UCSF Center for Health Professions.

Ryden, M. B., & Johnson, J. A. (1992). We need to know more: Nurse educators' interest and expertise in gerontology. *Journal of Nursing Education, 31*(8), 347–351.

Small, N. R. (1993). Facilitating student learning: Effective teaching strategies for baccalaureate education. In M. Burke & S. Sherman (Eds.), *Gerontological nursing: Issues and opportunities for the twenty-first century* (Publication No. 14-2510, pp. 61–68). New York: National League for Nursing.

U.S. Department of Health and Human Services, Bureau of Health Professions. (1993). *An agenda for health professions reform.* Washington, DC: USDHHS, Public Health Service.

Wells, T. J. (1993). Setting the agenda for gerontological education. In C. Heine (Ed.), *Determining the future of gerontological nursing education: Partnerships between education and practice* (Publication No. 14-2508, pp. 6–16). New York: National League for Nursing.

Whall, A., Booth, D., & Jirovec, M. (1989). Statistics and quantitative methods in gerontological nursing research. In I. L. Abraham, J. J. Fitzpatrick, & D. M. Nadzam (Eds.), *Statistics and quantitative methods in nursing* (pp. 136–146). Orlando, FL: W. B. Saunders.

Wykle, M., & Musil, C. (1995). Psychogeriatric mental health content for gerontologic nursing education. In T. Fulmer & M. A. Matzo (Eds.), *Strengthening gerontological nursing education* (pp. 37–47). New York: Springer Publishing Co.

CHAPTER 2

The Iowa Conceptual Model of Gerontological Nursing

Orpha J. Glick and Toni Tripp-Reimer

G erontology, the study of human aging, is a broad field of study that crosses several disciplines. Within each discipline, multiple theories have evolved to both inform and shape gerontological research. As each field views human aging through its own disciplinary lens, different constructs, foci, and methods are employed. As a result, there is a large mass of disparate perspectives. Although these theories are not necessarily contradictory, they do not form a cohesive unit. No unified theory of aging has yet been established, and even the desirability of such a formulation is debated (Achenbaum & Bengtson, 1994; Marshall, 1994). In part, the lack of a unified theory stems from the multiple competing theoretical orientations within each discipline. A summary of the major discrete gerontological theories is provided in Table 2.1.

The limited theory development and theory-based research in gerontological nursing have been consistently noted (Bahr, 1992; Basson, 1967;

Author notes: Address correspondence to Orpha J. Glick, PhD, RN, 306 NB, College of Nursing, The University of Iowa, Iowa City, Iowa 52242. The authors thank Steven Warner for his assistance in developing the graphic representation of the model.

11

TABLE 2.1 Major Theoretical Perspectives in Gerontology

Discipline	Theory	Key Elements	Proponents/ Citations
Philosophy			
	Dialectical gerontology	Acknowledges contradictory features of aging and locates those contradictions within a developmental or historical framework.	Wershow (1981)
	Hermeneutic gerontology	Emphasizes understanding over explanation of sciences as well as for aging individuals.	Prado (1983)
	Critical gerontology	Emancipation from domination is goal.	Moody (1988)
Sociology–Anthropology Sociocultural			
	Age-grading	Cultural system of group organization based on structural (not chronological) age.	Bernardi (1985)
	Subculture	Aged form own subculture in American society.	Rose (1964)
	Exchange	Rational economic model; elders have less power because they control fewer resources and make fewer exchanges.	Dowd (1975)
	Modernization	Status of the aged is inversely related to level of societal industrialization.	Cowgill & Holmes (1972)

TABLE 2.1 *(continued)*

	Status: reciprocity	Elder status related to control over knowledge, economic resources, prior achievements.	Press & McCool (1972)
	Double jeopardy hypothesis	Minority group elders face discrimination from ethnicity and age.	Jackson (1980)
	Social networks	Networks of elders decrease with role loss.	Sokolovsky (1986)
	Social support: formal/ informal	As age increases, reliance on formal support systems increases and on informal systems decreases.	Cantor & Little (1985)
Social psychology			
	Activity theory	Importance of active role participation for positive adjustment.	Havighurst & Albrecht (1953); Havighurst, Neugarten, & Tobin (1963)
	Disengagement	Mutual withdrawal between elder and society.	Cumming & Henry (1961)
	Social competence/ breakdown	Breakdowns in social competence occur with crises (losses) of aging; downward spiral can be reversed through social reconstruction syndrome.	Kuypers & Bengtson (1973)
	Person–environment fit	Physical, cognitive, social model; competent individuals tolerate more change.	Lawton & Nahemow (1973)
		Optimal fit model: congruence between individual and environment.	Kahana (1982)

13

TABLE 2.1 Major Theoretical Perspectives in Gerontology *(continued)*

Discipline	Theory	Key Elements	Proponents/ Citations
		Four-factor model: individual and environmental characteristics; mediators and behavior change.	Parr (1980)
		Field fit (field theory): interaction between individual and psychological environment.	Schaie (1962)
	Life course	Aging as a lifelong process; biopsychosocial integration; cohort affected by social change (history); new patterns of aging can cause social change.	Clausen (1972); Riley (1979); Hagestad & Neugarten (1985)
	Age stratification	Unique movement and experience of social cohorts (cohort flow).	Riley (1971); Foner (1974)
Psychology Personality development	Analytic	Aging: time of reflection and introversion.	Jung (1933, 1960)
	Neo-Freudian social theorists	Aging issue: ego integrity vs. ego despair.	Erikson (1963)
		Ego differentiation *vs.* work role preoccupation; body and ego transcendence *vs.* preoccupation.	Peck (1968)
		Dialectical operations: fifth period of cognitive development.	Riegel (1973)

TABLE 2.1 *(continued)*

Life-span transitions	Developmental tasks: adjustment to changes in health, work, social roles, physical living arrangements.	Havighurst (1972)
	Developmental tasks: physical adjustments, new roles, life acceptance, death view.	Newman & Newman (1984)
	Changes in cognitive and functional ability result in increased attention to aging and mortality.	Levinson (1978)
Moral reasoning	Life crises produce moral dilemmas that result in patterning of moral decisions.	Kohlberg (1973)
Continuity	Pattern of personality traits (established early) become more pronounced in response to stresses.	Neugarten (1973); McCrae & Costa (1982); Schaie & Parham (1976); Atchley (1989),
Script	Elders order the script in the scenes of their lives to maintain sense of continuity.	Carlson (1981)
Personality dimensions		
Traits	Sense of coherence.	Sagy & Antonovsky (1990)
	Stability vs. change.	Bengston, Reedy, & Gordon (1985); McCrae & Costa (1982)
	Locus of control.	Rodin (1986)

15

TABLE 2.1 Major Theoretical Perspectives in Gerontology (*continued*)

Discipline	Theory	Proponents/Key Elements	Citations
		Rigidity vs. flexibility.	Riley & Foner (1968); Butler (1974)
	Types	Four personality types (integrated, armored-defended, passive-dependent, unintegrated) related to satisfaction.	Neugarten, Havighurst, & Tobin (1968)
		Five subtypes (mature, rocking chair, armored, angry, self-haters).	Reichard, Levson, & Peterson (1962)
Cognitive psychology	Generalized slowing hypothesis	Age deficits distributed throughout information processing system; not localized in particular stages.	Salthouse (1985)
	Schema–neural network theory	Cognition occurs on neural network rather than staged succession of information processing.	
	Crystallized vs. fluid intelligence	Crystallized (accumulation) intelligence remains stable or increases; flexible (novel) intelligence declines.	Horn (1982)
	Information loss model	Task complexity retards process times; slowing results from information loss.	Hale, Myerson, & Wagstaff (1987)

TABLE 2.1 *(continued)*

Single-peak creativity model	Creativity peaks in early 30s or 40s, followed by gradual decline.	Lehman (1953)
Divergent thinking decline	Attributed to CNS slowing, decreased motivation, and cohort effect.	Kogan (1987)
Levels of processing model	Depth of processing is dependent on meaning to elder; elders encode less deeply.	Craik (1977)
Processing deficit model		Eysenck (1974)
Signal detection theory	Separate indicators for ability to detect, discriminate, and remember target events vs. predispositional biases.	Botwinick (1973)
Terminal drop	Decline in cognitive functioning immediately prior to death.	Kleemeier (1962)
Expert schema theory	Expert's domain-specific knowledge and performance remain stable.	Perlmutter (1983)
Compensatory skill acquisition	Expert's increased skills compensate for decreased speed.	Charness (1985;
Biology System-level		
Neuroendocrine	Homeostatic mechanisms decline; pathologic stress responses increase.	Shock (1979); Timiras, Hudson, & Segall (1984)

17

TABLE 2.1 Major Theoretical Perspectives in Gerontology (*continued*)

Discipline	Theory	Key Elements	Proponents/Citations
	Immunologic	Decreased immune efficacy and accuracy result in increased infections and autoimmune processes.	Zatz & Goldstein (1985)
Cellular	Wear and tear (rate of living)	Internal (basal metabolic rate) and external (temperature, altitude) affect life span.	Sacher (1980)
	Free-radical accumulation	Oxidants (free radicals) directly damage cell membrane and cytoplasm.	Harman (1956)
	Lipofuscin (age pigment) accumulation	Increasing lipofuscin deposits in aging cells result in decreased mitochondria, cytoplasm, and endoplasmic reticulum.	Sohal (1981)
	Cross-linking	Protein (collagen) molecules form bonds over time, resulting in decreased elasticity and function.	Verzar (1963)
Molecular/genetic	Codon fidelity	Inability to decode mRNA triple codons (base-pairs) impairs accuracy of mRNA message.	Agris et al. (1985)
	Somatic mutation	Radiation exposure increases mutations, resulting in fewer functional genes.	Sziland (1959); Curtis & Miller (1971)

TABLE 2.1 *(continued)*

Error (catastrophe)	Increased RNA errors result in accumulation of protein abnormalities.	Orgel (1963); Medvedev (1972)
Hayflick limit (genetic clock)	Finite number of cell divisions programmed in DNA (species-specific).	Hayflick (1965)
Dysdifferentiation	Accumulation of molecular damage impairs gene activity.	Cutler (1975)
Antagonistic pleiotropy	Delayed expression of deleterious genes.	Williams (1957); Medawar (1957)

Brimmer, 1979; Kayser-Jones, 1981; Knowles, 1983; Martinson, 1985; Murphy & Freston, 1991; Reed, 1989, 1991b; Wolanin, 1983). However, when theory-based research has been conducted, it generally employs one of the models shown in Table 2.1. The focus of gerontological nursing differs, depending on the theoretical perspective employed. Practitioners may select various discrete theories, depending on the particular clinical situation, the nature of the patient, the health issue, the environmental context, and the therapeutic goal. An integrative approach could assist gerontological nurses to provide more comprehensive and contextually relevant care. Conceptually delineating the scope of gerontological nursing is a first step in understanding the nature of gerontological phenomena and the ways in which nursing promotes health and facilitates transitions for older adults.

The purpose of the chapter is to describe a conceptual model depicting the scope of gerontological nursing (Figure 2.1). In this model, gerontological nursing encompasses three spheres: elder, environment, and nursing. The elder sphere emphasizes the centrality of developmental and health processes in late life; developmental and health processes occur in a physical, social, cultural, and spiritual context—that is, environment, which constitutes a second sphere; nursing, the third sphere, emphasizes interventions based on accurate diagnosis of responses to personal, environmental, or person–environment phenomena toward the outcome (goal) of optimum health.

The focus on developmental processes is grounded in the belief that, phenomenologically, the life course is an evolving interpretation of bio-psychosociocultural phenomena. In this model, late-life events reflect life transitions that evoke responses affecting the level of health, which is phenomenologically experienced as well-being and is composed of the elements of functional status, health behavior, and life satisfaction. The gerontological phenomena of concern to nursing incorporate the nature of late-life transitions, the responses to these events, the environmental context, and the consequent functional health and well-being of older adults. Nursing interventions assist older adults in identifying and integrating effects of late-life transitions and support the developmental responses toward higher levels of well-being. These assistive actions are directed toward the individual, as well as the surrounding micro- and macro-environmental systems that affect the health of adults in later life.

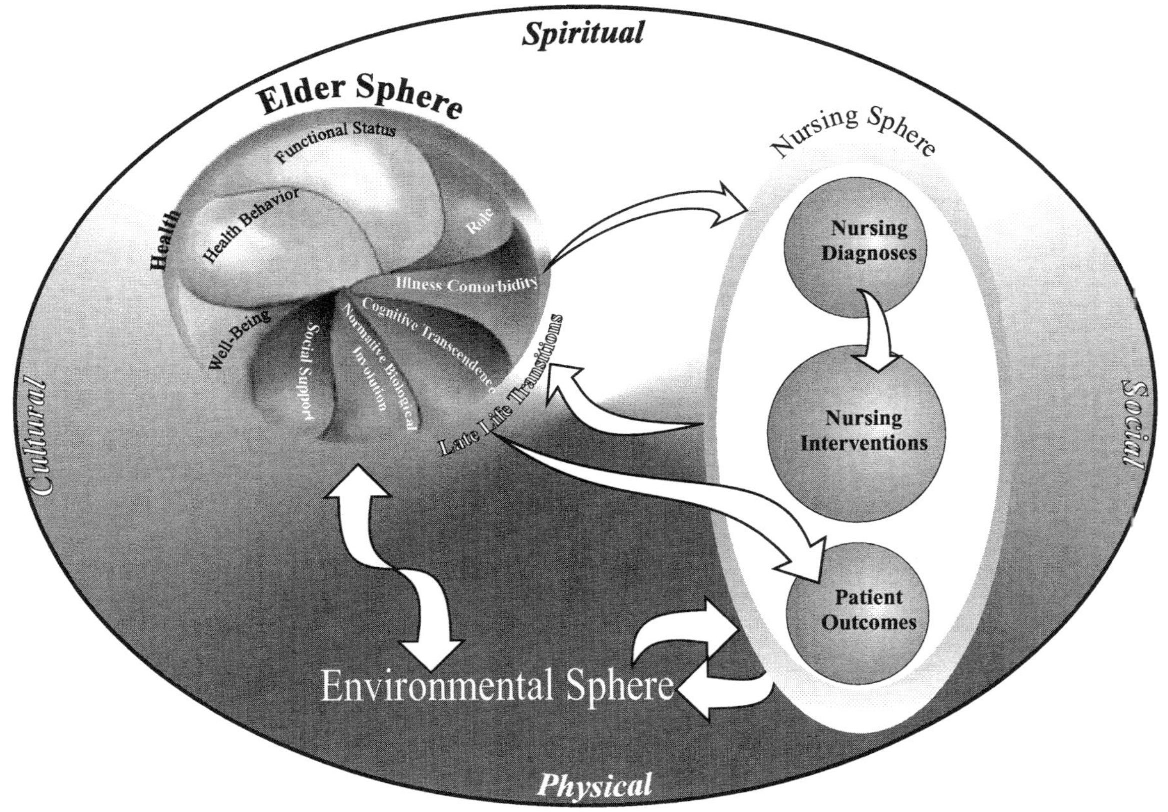

FIGURE 2.1 Model of gerontological nursing.

21

ELDER SPHERE

Late-Life Transitions

The life course is characterized by many events that represent temporary or relatively permanent transitions from one pattern of being to another. A transition is "a passage from one life phase, condition or state to another" (Meleis & Trangenstein, 1994, p. 256). Transition phenomena are internal processes that encompass change but go beyond the notion of change to incorporate complex person–environment interactions in which new or different identities, roles, relationships, and patterns of behavior emerge. Transitions take place over time, during which the individual experiences a certain disconnectedness from support systems, a loss of familiar reference points, emergence of new needs, and an incongruence between old sets of expectations and the new situation (Meleis, 1986). Transitions occur along a developmental–situational continuum and may emphasize biological, physiological, sociocultural, or environmental phenomena. Further, in late life the transitions may overlap, be concurrent and reciprocal, with both positive and negative valences.

Aging may be viewed as both positive and negative. The "biomedicalization of aging" describes a social phenomenon in which aging is viewed as inevitably pathological or abnormal (Estes & Binney, 1989, p. 588). From this perspective, aging processes are viewed negatively, that is, as deterrents or threats to well-being. In contrast, late-life transitions can be viewed as positive avenues for personal growth and ultimately as advancing development and health (Jones & Meleis, 1993). Illness events may be viewed as a means of expanding human potential, as accelerating personal growth through a heightened awareness and transformational change, rather than as the "enemy" (Moch, 1989). Similarly, late-life events can be viewed as transitions in which older adults transcend biological, psychological, social, and environmental changes and develop new perspectives of the self. This latter conceptualization draws on both the perspective of Buddhist philosophy and transpersonal/transcendent psychology (Reed, 1991a; Tornstam, 1989, 1992).

As depicted in Figure 2.1, there are five major categories of aging-related transitions in late life: (a) normative biological involution, (b) late-life illness and comorbidity, (c) cognitive developmental transitions, (d) social role transitions, and (e) social support transitions. Although individual elders experience specific personal environmental transitions, the surrounding physical, social, cultural, and spiritual environments are the "ground," or context, within which the personal and social transitions experienced by older adults take place. Thus, the construct of environment encompasses transitions in personal physical space as well as sociopolitical, economic, and cultural forces. These five categories of aging-related transitions are neither mutually exclusive nor independent transitions. Rather, they are mutual, reciprocal, interactive processes resulting in health responses that are more complex and more profound. A discussion of each category follows.

Normative Biological Involution

Involution refers to retrogressive change (Miller & Keane, 1983) in vital biological structures and processes. Normative biological involution, the "reduction in size or vital power of an organ" (Thomas, 1989, p. 939), is a universal, naturally occurring late-life transition that may have profound consequences for function and well-being. The changes in biological structures and processes can occur in a particular organ or tissue or in the whole body. They may occur from disuse after the function of the organ has been fulfilled (e.g., the uterus or thymus gland) or from disuse associated with insufficient exercise or movement (e.g., in neuromusculoskeletal systems). However, it is difficult to distinguish physical changes that occur with biological aging from those that occur because of decreased physical activity, level of motivation, influence of societal expectations, or cumulative effects of disease (Fiatarone & Evans, 1993; Kane, 1993; Spirduso & MacRae, 1990).

Aging-related biological involution encompasses major changes in all organ systems, thus altering functional capacity in all dimensions (Pendergast, Fisher, & Calkins, 1993). However, many older adults can integrate profound decrements in physical capacity without affecting the ability to function under normal conditions (Arking, 1991). What is actually compromised is functional reserve, that is, the degree of plasticity one sees in younger adults.

Although biological involution is a universal, aging-related phenomenon, the rate of biological aging is highly individual. Differences in rate of biological aging occur within organ systems of the same individual as well as among individuals in a global sense (Borkan & Norris, 1980). This variance contributes to the heterogeneity that characterizes the older adult population and has become the impetus for identifying and studying biological markers as indicators of aging rather than chronological age (Arking, 1991; Borkan, 1978; Borkan & Norris, 1980). Baker and Sprott (1988) define biomarkers "as biological parameters . . . that either alone or in some multivariate composite will in the absence of disease better predict functional capability at some late age than will chronological age" (p. 223).

The premise underlying the study of biological markers of aging is the finding that chronological age is not consistently valid in predicting functional (physiological) capacity particularly in later life (Baker & Sprott, 1988). There is also the need to distinguish aging-related changes from pathology. Although biological age is an interesting concept, it is unclear to what extent it could or will be used to shape ideologies and social policy in a way that contributes to function and life satisfaction in late life.

Late-Life Illness and Comorbidity

Late life is also characterized by prevalence of disease, illness, and comorbidity (multiple chronicities). Although the frequency of acute conditions declines with advancing age, it has been estimated that approximately 90% of older adults have chronic medical conditions (Young & Olson, 1991) that can adversely affect their function. The major chronic conditions experienced by older adults are ischemic heart disease, hypertension, vision impairment, hearing impairment, musculoskeletal impairment, and diabetes (Van Nostrand, Furner, & Suzman, 1993). Disease states often reduce physiological capacity and consequently increase functional dependency. Further, during acute episodes of illness many elders lose functional ability because they have limited reserves or are unable to mobilize reserves to regain their premorbid performance levels (Svanborg, 1993). On the other hand, a number of investigations failed to show significant relationships between some measures of comorbidity, such as number of diseases or number of hospitalizations, and self-perceived health (Mor-Barak, Scharlach, Birba, & Sokolov, 1992) or functional status (Mor et al., 1989). However, an examination of the effects of specific medical conditions showed that cerebrovascular disease and arthritis were significant predictors of functional limitations 4 years postbaseline (Boult, Kane, Thomas, Boult, & McCaffrey, 1994).

There also are primary and secondary mental health problems that compromise function and quality of life. For example, an older person's interpretation of an impairment may generate mental health responses that limit cognitive, affective, or physical capacities. The net effect is reduced physical and social activity. For example, one group of inactive, socially isolated older adults living at home was found to be more "tired," to give lower perceived health ratings, and to visit physicians and use sedatives more often than elders who weren't experiencing social isolation (Svanborg, 1993). Thus, the psychological representation of and response to actual or potential disability, as well as the social context in which it occurs, are important determinants of actual function (Schultz & Williamson, 1993).

Cognitive Developmental Transitions

In nursing, health has been linked to developmental issues throughout the life span (Reed, 1989, 1991b), but late-life adult developmental phenomena have not been well defined (Kogan, 1990; Stevenson, 1977). Jung (1933), Erikson (1963), and Peck (1968) conducted pioneering work in psychology, describing issues in ego development in late life. Although Erikson identified "integrity vs. despair" as a developmental task specific to late adulthood, Peck contended that Erikson's stage applied generally to postmiddle-age development and was not specific to late life. Jung, however, pioneered the notion of ego transcendence as a late-life phenomenon.

Developmental psychologists expanded upon the classic notions of ego development and identified several tasks specific to development beyond 70 years of age (Havighurst, 1972; Newman & Newman, 1984). They identified major developmental tasks as adjustments to changes in physical status, roles, work, living arrangements, and mortality. The ego theorists, however, emphasized acceptance of existence that transcends the mortal body.

Tornstam (1989) called for a shift in social perspectives from a positivist view of responses to aging as "disengagement" to a more phenomenological view or approach to understanding the experience of aging. He described a phenomenon called gerotranscendence, a culture-free, intrinsic process that is generated by everyday living. The process of gerotranscendence brings about a shift in perspective held by the individual that usually is followed by an increase in life satisfaction. For example, transcendence is manifested by a redefinition of time, space, and objects, an increase in a feeling of affiliation with past and future generations, and a decreased interest in superfluous social interaction, material things, and self-centeredness. Tornstam also suggested that there are degrees of gerotranscendence and that the process can be hindered or facilitated by environmental and social forces.

Similarly, Reed (1991b) formulated a theory of self-transcendence using a synthesis of life-span-development concepts specific to social-cognitive and transpersonal development and Rogers's (1990) principles of homeodynamics. According to Reed, self-transcendence is a developmental process that occurs in response to end-of-life experiences regardless of age. She defined development as a lifelong, nonlinear process of transforming the old and integrating the new. Moreover, she postulated that the well-being of an individual is related to the level of transcendence that occurs. Although a definition of well-being was not given, Reed (1989) defined transcendence as "activities and perspectives older adults characteristically engage in to expand their personal boundaries and orient themselves towards purposes greater than the self" (p. 149).

Reed (1991a) identified four categories (patterns) of self-transcendence from data obtained by asking those aged 80 to 97 to describe views and behaviors that promoted their sense of well-being at this time in their lives. The following patterns were identified:

- ◆ Introjectivity: using environmental resources to focus on inner-directed activities (e.g., travel, hobbies, housework).
- ◆ Generativity: altruistic activities (e.g., visiting, volunteering, teaching).
- ◆ Temporal integration: participants' views (active, passive, or lacking) of their past, present, and future.
- ◆ Body transcendence: an integration of aging- or illness-related physical changes.

Reed (1991b) summarized the phenomenon of self-transcendence as a process of expanding the self-boundary in three ways: (a) inwardly, as in introspection; (b) outwardly, through reaching out; and (c) temporally, by merging past and future into a perspective on the present. She notes that these processes go beyond self-identity as a goal to an "interdependent self-definition based on a strengthened sense of identity with the greater environment" (p. 67).

The developmental perspective on aging, as posited by theories of gero- and self-transcendence, offers a positive view of aging. Rather than emphasizing decrements in physical capacity for function, developmental theory provides for continued growth in dimensions such as spirituality, generativity, and inner strength in the context of aging-related transitions in late life (Ebersole & Hess, 1994). The phenomenon of gerotranscendence may also explain aging-related differences in coping with changes in health status and residence (Meeks, Carstensen, Tamsky, Wright, & Pellegrini, 1989).

Social Role Transitions

There are several major aging-related social role transitions that potentially alter personal and social identity (George, 1990). There is also evidence that there may be profound gender differences in aging-related role experiences (Theriault, 1994). Two of the major transitions, retirement and changes in family roles, are described here.

The transition from a paid work role to a pattern of living in retirement that may be less structured and purposeful can lead to alterations in self-concept. Retirement is frequently characterized as a stressful life event that may bring psychological, social, and economic uncertainty (Midanik, Soghikian, Ransom, & Tekawa, 1995). Theriault (1994) maintained that retirement is a major life transition, during which there is an internal reorganization of perceptions, expectations, and goals. She conceptualized the transition as a "work-to-retirement" process and compared anxiety levels and life satisfaction 6 months before (preretirement), at the time of retirement (intraretirement), and 6 to 12 months after retiring (postretirement). She found that anxiety levels were highest during the preretirement period and that they declined in a linear pattern at the intra- and postretirement periods. These findings suggest that internal responses to the event begin before the event actually occurs. Similarly, the high levels of preretirement anxiety support the notion that retirement introduces uncertainty even in circumstances in which it may be welcomed.

Midanik et al. (1995) compared self-reported mental health and health behaviors of recent retirees with a matched group of employees who did not retire. They found no significant differences between groups on self-reported mental health, coping, alcohol consumption, depression, and smoking; they also found that retired employees were more likely to report lower stress levels and engage in regular exercise. These investigators concluded that there are positive effects of retirement and that further study is needed to determine the stability of these findings. They also noted that, although there was an overall reduction in stress for retirees, the difference was not significant for retired women in this study.

Karp (1988) suggested that men may be more ready to disengage from work lives than women are. Cessation of a structured work life allows men to experience the freedom to participate in activities unavailable to them while working. Women, on the other hand, more frequently increased their search for occupational activity because family responsibilities had previously restricted career development. Thus, although both men and women had a "drive" to activity, it was expressed in different life spheres.

The responses to retirement may also be compounded by changes in social status and social network(s) that are associated with one's work. Mor-Barak et al. (1992) found that employment was significantly related to size of social network even after controlling for age, gender, education, and number of health problems and that the relationship between working and social network affected self-reported health. Further analyses of the effects of employment on specific social network dimensions (family network, friends network, and confidant relationships) showed that employment was significantly related to friends' network but not to family or confidant relationships.

The amount of time spent in retirement has shifted and has increased the amount of discretionary time for many elders. According to Hagestad (1990), the time spent in retirement increased from 7% in 1940 to 23% in 1979. The extent to which this trend will continue is uncertain. Increases in life span and major shifts in economic trends confound efforts to project future retirement patterns. However, because leisure activity provides a source of identity in late life, it should receive as careful planning as the work life (Bevil, O'Connor, & Mattoon, 1993).

A second group of aging-related role transitions consists of changes in family roles. These changes are brought about by events such as retirement, death of a spouse, or death of one's parents (Hagestad, 1990). Role accumulation may also occur (Ebersole & Hess, 1994). For example, parental roles extend into grandparenting roles while undergoing qualitative differences specific to relationships with children who are now parents with their own children. The timing of these events is critical to integrating the new roles. For example, persons who become grandparents too early in life may not have the peer support that often eases the impact of these changes (Hagestad, 1990). Similar phenomena occur in a social trend in which grandparents increasingly find themselves being called on to "raise" one or more grandchildren because the parent (often a single mother) has been killed or incarcerated (Dressel & Barnhill, 1994).

Barer (1994) noted that men and women often experience certain life events that alter social or family roles at different ages. For example, women may experience more role continuity in late life because they have lived more passive lives and their major domestic role continues postretirement until functional incapacity or death. In contrast, values such as competency, activity, and productivity are associated with male social roles; consequently, men often experience less postretirement role continuity. Men also may not experience relocation, widowhood, or a caregiver role until later in life than women do. That is, if a man survives past age 85, he is more likely to experience a caregiver role at a time when his own resources and energy levels are declining.

Social Support Transitions

Social support and interest in its relationship to health emerged in the 1970s at a time when social isolation and low levels of social integration were associated with negative health consequences (Hogue, 1985; Norbeck, 1988). Most of the research in social support conceptualizes social support as a buffer to stress, which, in turn, advances health. However, other investigators hypothesize that social support has a direct effect on stress and on health (Norbeck, 1988). More recently, the negative effects of social support (or its "burden") have been proposed (Kraus & Jay, 1991).

Kahn (1979) characterized social support as an "interpersonal trans-action" (p. 85) that includes expressions of positive affect toward another; affirmation of another's behavior, perception, or expressed view; and the giving of symbolic or material aid. Hogue (1985) described social support in a more reciprocal global sense, as a dynamic interactional process in which there is a "flow of emotional energy between people" (p. 65).

Isreal (1982) and later Antonucci (1990) commented on the lack of conceptual clarity in social support research, noting that terms such as emotional support, social support, and social network are used inter-changeably. Isreal (1982) developed a concept of social network and dif-ferentiated network characteristics from support characteristics. She defined social network as "person-centered" and as "structure-linkages" (p. 65) that function to provide affective support, tangible aid, and services. Isreal described both quantitative and qualitative dimensions of network. Quantitative dimensions include structural properties (i.e., size and density) and interactional properties (i.e., frequency of interaction, homogeneity of members, geographic proximity of members, and stability of relation-ships). Qualitative dimensions of network include the meaning and inten-sity of the relationship and reciprocity (i.e., giving and receiving).

Isreal and Antonucci (1987) examined the relationship between social network characteristics and psychological well-being in a sample of men and women aged 50 to 95. They found that most of the network characteristics were not significantly related to psychological well-being. However, the qualitative dimensions of affective support and reciprocal affective support were strongly associated with psychological well-being. In a later study, Connidis and McMullin (1993) confirmed the importance of the qualitative aspect of social support. They found that having children enhanced the well-being of older adults only if the parents viewed their relationship as "close." These investigators concluded that having a small network or fewer social contacts is not necessarily detrimental to well-being in older adults.

In a review of literature examining relationships between social supports, health/illness, and aging, Ryan and Austin (1989) concluded that establishing a relationship between social support and health is progressing. Yet there remains a great deal of variability in conceptualizing and measuring social support. These authors suggest that a combination of qualitative and quantitative research methods should be used to reach a better understanding of the complexities of the social support–health relationships. They also maintained that the availability of social support affects recovery from illness, duration of hospitalization, and discharge to home. Transitions in network characteristics brought about by loss, separation, or illness may affect the quality of support that is available and place an older adult in a vulnerable position. Ryan and Austin (1989) point out that the informal network may be changing at a time when the needs for affective and instrumental aid become more critical. Using cross-sectional data, Mor-Barak et al. (1992) found a significant relationship between social network and self-reported health. Moreover, age was negatively related to family network but had a positive relationship to friends network. These investigators suggested that older adults may compensate for loss of family by expanding friendship networks and that employment may become an important source of establishing a network in late life.

Health

A second major construct in the model of the elder sphere is health. In this model, health is viewed as being in process and as an outcome of developmental responses to late-life transitions. That is, health as an outcome is not simply a state of being; rather, it is a process of becoming in the context of late-life transitions. In this context, definitions of health for older adults focus on objective functional status (Wells, 1993), health behaviors, and subjective qualitative indicators such as well-being (Burgener & Chiverton, 1992) and life satisfaction (George, 1990).

Functional Status

Functional health is defined as the extent to which a person has the ability to independently carry out personal care, home management, and social functions in everyday life in a way that has meaning and purpose. It is frequently measured by assessing an individual's ability to perform basic and instrumental activities of daily living (ADLs). Tasks concerning fundamental daily activities, such as personal care or basic mobility, are classified as basic activities of daily living (BADLs). The more complex tasks associated with independent community living, such as home management and shopping, are considered instrumental ADLs, or IADLs (Guccione & Jette, 1988).

Originally, functional status was used as a measure of disability. More recently, it has been used as a measure of health in older adults (Kane, 1993) and to predict living arrangement (Bishop, 1986), admission to a nursing home (Branch & Jette, 1982), utilization of hospital and physician services (Wan & Odell, 1981), and use of paid home care (Soldo & Manton, 1985). In addition, functional status measures such as BADLs and IADLs have been used as predictors of quality of life (Katz & Stroud, 1989; Spitzer, 1987). Although enhancing quality of late life is an important goal, Branch et al. (1991) point out that it is unclear what dimensions of function actually represent an unacceptable quality of life. For example, does the functional standard for quality of life reside in the capacities for BADLs or IADLs?

Functional status is influenced by many intrinsic and extrinsic factors. Intrinsic factors include biological and behavioral characteristics; extrinsic factors include the amount and type of health care provided as well as supportive physical and social environments (Kane, 1993; Schulz & Williamson, 1993).

Estimates of the prevalence of functional dependency vary across surveys. In general, however, it has been shown that difficulty in performing ADLs increases with advancing age and that there are significantly higher rates of dependency for women than men, particularly for women who live alone (Guralnik & Simonsick, 1993; Van Nostrand, Furner, & Suzman, 1993). Guralnik and Simonsick (1993) address the difficulty in determining the distribution and determinants of functional dependency, particularly in community-dwelling elders. According to these authors, the prevalence of a condition is related to incidence and duration of that condition. Duration of functional dependency in community-dwelling elders may be influenced by survival and by outmigration. Moreover, functional status is dynamic; that is, it can improve, depending on the cause, treatment, social support, or natural course of an illness (Branch et al., 1991; Branch & Ku, 1989; Katz et al., 1983).

Health Behavior

Health behaviors, or health self-care, include all actions performed by persons to promote their own health, prevent disease, limit illness, and restore health (Dean, 1992; Levin & Idler, 1984). This broad definition places emphasis on the individual sphere rather than on that of the professional. As a result, health activities, including utilization of professional health care and adherence to therapeutic regimens, are viewed as options under the control of the person rather than professional dicta.

Considerable recent attention has been focused on the health self-care of elders (Cox, 1986; Hickey, Dean, & Holstein, 1986; Jirovec & Kasno, 1990; Kart & Dunkle, 1989; Lenihan, 1988; Vickery, Golaszewski, Wright, & Kalmer, 1988). Most of this research has been concerned with the utilization of traditional professional health services. This body of literature consistently shows that older adults are the largest single group of consumers of formal or professional health services. However, health utilization is disproportionately spread over this group: a relatively small proportion use a relatively large proportion of both inpatient and outpatient services (Kraus, 1990).

Older people engage in a variety of activities to promote their own health and to maintain a sense of well-being. However, the scope of these self-determined behaviors and their efficacy has not been fully explored (Sokolovsky & Vesperi, 1991; Tripp-Reimer & Cohen, 1987). Rather, professional standards are generally applied to assess elders' level of activity in predetermined categories of health promotion and illness prevention (Brown & McCreedy, 1986; Duffy, 1993; Rakowski, 1992; Walker, Volken, Sechrist, & Pender, 1988). Current programs to promote healthy lifestyles for the elderly include the Healthy Lifestyles for Seniors Program (Santa Monica, CA) and the New Mexico Health Promotion with Elders project (state of New Mexico). These programs generally include components of exercise, nutrition, health screening, and health habits (Alford & Futrell, 1992). However, the degree to which they build on the established practices and beliefs of the elderly has not yet been assessed.

Elders' response to symptoms and illness is patterned by both their representation of the health problem and their past experience. Illness representation is the way an individual conceptualizes and makes sense of an illness. Two kinds of illness representations are the common sense model (CSM), which is derived from psychology (Meyer, Leventhal, & Gutman, 1985), and the explanatory model (EM), which is derived from anthropology (Kleinman, 1980). The CSM emphasizes the symptom experience and its interpretation and meaning for health action for elders. In contrast, the EM emphasizes variation between patient and practitioner models of illness. Both models, however, begin with the identification of the diagnosis or illness label, the etiology, probable consequences, and treatment issues (Cohen, Tripp-Reimer, Sorofman, Lauer, & Lively, 1994).

Elders respond to both everyday symptoms and more acute or dramatic incidences. Despite evidence that self-care is the predominant form of treatment in most illness episodes, little has been known until recently about the types of daily symptoms experienced or the range of self-care options employed to treat them (Sorofman, Tripp-Reimer, Lauer, & Martin, 1990; Stoller, 1993). Self-management of symptoms related to specific chronic problems, such as arthritis (Lorig, 1993; Lorig & Holman, 1993) or functional status limitations (Norburn et al., 1995), has recently begun to be explored. However, factors that influence elders' choice of self-care treatments are yet to be determined. Further, triggers for illness behaviors in which elders seek the help and advice of others, in either the lay sector (Strain, 1990) or the professional health sector (Bausell, 1986; Mazur & Merz, 1993; Rakowski, Rice, & McHorney, 1992), have also recently been the focus of attention.

Well-Being

Health and well-being are terms frequently used in tandem to denote a goal or standard for preventive and therapeutic intervention. Health is associated with absence of diagnosed disease, whereas well-being represents qualitative, subjective judgments about quality of life. A primary goal in gerontology is to find ways to enhance the quality of life of older adults. However, quality of life is a global construct that encompasses a broad range of personal, environmental, and social variables. Moreover, there is no definition of quality of life that is universally accepted. The most frequent measures of quality of life are life satisfaction, morale, and happiness, three constructs that are highly correlated (George, 1990). However, these quality-of-life indicators may not be measurable in segments of older adult populations. Three problems have been identified in applying quality-of-life indicators to demented elderly adults. First, many of the variables used as indicators of quality of life require subjective evaluations by the individual, which may or may not be feasible when cognitive impairments are present. Second, the broad domains of quality of life are not relevant for older adults who have little or no control over where they live. Finally, a network of family and friends may not exist, and even if family and friends are present, persons with cognitive impairments may not be able to relate to them (Burgener & Chiverton, 1992).

In contrast to quality of life, the concept of well-being offers an alternative qualitative health standard. Well-being may convey a global meaning, as in Webster's definition, which describes it as "a state of being happy, healthy or prosperous." Similarly, Isreal and Antonucci (1987) defined well-being as the "extent to which positive feelings outweigh negative feelings" (p. 465), whereas George (1990) viewed it as "an individual's perceptions of overall life quality" (p. 190). Burgener and Chiverton (1992), on the other hand, conceptualized well-being as having two major components: affect and life satisfaction. Affect may be positive (e.g., happy) or negative (e.g., depressed), and it is an indicator of the emotional component of well-being. Life satisfaction is a cognitive-judgmental aspect that requires a subjective evaluation by the respondent. In a study of the effects of having children on older adults' well-being, Connidis and McMullin (1993) added "happiness" to the life satisfaction and affective indices.

Burgener and Chiverton (1992) suggested that positive and negative affects may be valid indicators of well-being in persons with cognitive impairments because they are usually reflected as behavior that can be assessed by objective observers. For example, it is thought that facial expression communicates inner experience and that it communicates more information about affective states than other body language.

Positive and negative affects also represent emotional states that are independent of one another; thus, they could be used as separate variables. It should be noted, however, that interpretations of behavior associated with affect must be made with caution because it is very easy to invoke one's own biases regarding the meaning of an individual's behavior.

ENVIRONMENTAL SPHERE

The impact of environment on health has been identified as a major concern throughout nursing's history (Williams, 1988). Early studies of environment examined it as a source of stress and disease. Several reviews have shown that nursing theory and research on environmental issues focused more on the immediate physical environment than on larger societal influences embedded in social, political, and economic structures (Chopoorian, 1986; Kleffel, 1991; Stevens, 1989). Kleffel (1991), for example, found that of 53 articles reviewed, only one study addressed the effects of social, political, and economic contexts of the environment. Although it is not possible to distinguish precise dimensional boundaries, the environmental sphere of the conceptual model (see Figure 2.1) specifies four dimensions: social, cultural, physical, and spiritual.

Social Dimension

Kim (1983) proposed a broader conceptualization of environment: as a spatial construct; a milieu for functioning; an object of human control; a source of stress, stimulation, and adaptation; and a symbiotic, interdependent system. Although identifying an ecological perspective, Kim's conception emphasizes the impact of environment on the individual in that lifestyle, activities, and habits are patterned by physical elements of the environment. Chopoorian (1986), on the other hand, proposed a conception of environment that bridges personal and societal dimensions. She proposed three major components: (a) sociopolitical structures, (b) human social relations, and (c) everyday life. In this schema, everyday life is defined as personal habits and routine activities.

Chopoorian (1986) believed that individuals interpret from everyday experience. Moreover, she argued that in the United States, social structures such as government, private industry, health care, and educational institutions operate within highly stratified, hierarchical power systems, which, in turn, filter downward to micro social systems such as the family and work groups in ways that actually reproduce organizational life in everyday life. Of particular concern to the well-being of elders is the fact that the power relations that characterize these organizational systems generate ideologies such as ageism, sexism, and classism, all of which limit alternatives open to individuals and populations. This view is consistent with the notion that policy decisions actually shape life trajectories (Hagestad, 1990) and that the sociopolitical and economic environment is often the origin of clients' most serious problems (Kleffel, 1991). Inducing sociopolitical change to equalize the distribution of power and resources at all levels of social exchange, as well as to change ideologies that characterize elders as socioeconomic liabilities, requires the concerted efforts of elders themselves as well as professional and social groups concerned with enhancing late-life development and well-being.

Cultural Dimension

The cultural dimension of elder–environment interaction (values, beliefs, and patterns of behavior) is based on ethnic affiliation (race, national origin, religion, language) and is closely related to social structures and processes in its influence on the experience of aging (Jackson, Antonucci, & Gibson, 1990; Keith, 1990; Tripp-Reimer, Johnson, & Rios, 1995). Keith (1990) noted that the influence of cultural values and traditional behaviors on older adults' experiences is mediated by an exchange between the traditions and changing social contexts as experienced by new generations and also by older people's attempts to blend traditional resources with social change. Thus, identifying cultural affiliation provides a context from which nurses may anticipate individual differences in values, religions, family structures, lines of authority, and other life patterns (Tripp-Reimer et al., 1995). Understanding and accepting individual differences that arise from cultural variation enhances the ability to facilitate late-life development in a culturally sensitive manner. This, in turn, preserves the personhood of the older individual; that is, it "accords a complete and normal identity" (Keith, 1990, p. 100).

Tripp-Reimer et al. (1995) identified several reasons for considering the cultural dimension in gerontological nursing. First, the definition and status of the elderly is largely determined by cultural factors. Second, an older person's beliefs, values, and behaviors are established through a history of enculturation, through which individual pattern and meaning are derived. Thus, although cultural heritage is a significant context for planning care, it does not predict behavior at an individual level. For example, ethnic elders do not experience the same patterns of eligibility, access, and use of health care services as do their younger counterparts.

Clearly, a person's subjective sense of aging arises from a larger sociopolitical and cultural context as well as through communication from those in the immediate family and work environment. In the United States, values such as independence and productivity can lead to guilt if older adults become more introspective and less socially integrated (Tornstam, 1989). Examining the ways in which changes in social structure effect change in cultural meanings may be an effective way to document the effects of social structure on individual behavior and attitude (George, 1995). Thus, it is imperative that nurses assist in raising consciousness about environmental forces that constrain or obstruct the processes of gerotranscendence and the development of positive self-concept as well as functional capacity and well-being.

Physical Dimension

The model of person–environment fit has provided a theoretical basis for examining the effects of personal (physical) environment on function and well-being in late life (Parmalee & Lawton, 1990). One of the major issues in addressing living space for late life is housing and the proximity of "home" to social resources such as church, community centers, shopping, health care, and related social services. Although the majority of elders live in their own homes (Czaja, Weber, & Nair, 1993), housing options that reduce or eliminate many of the functional demands of home management have been designed and continue to be studied and developed. However, as in other late-life social transitions, relocating to smaller and more protective housing may be welcomed by some and fiercely resisted by others.

There is evidence that attachment to place enhances well-being. O'Bryant (1982) found that older persons actually reported higher levels of housing satisfaction than other age groups, even when structural conditions of the homes were taken into account. O'Bryant also identified four factors that were associated with valuing and being satisfied with home: (a) personal competence and emotional security, which contributed to self-esteem; (b) having a traditional family orientation and memory; (c) the status of home ownership; and (d) the cost-versus-comfort trade-off.

The desire for elders to remain in their own homes is often met with family and societal judgments of being emotional, sentimental, and irrational. Similarly, the subjective value of home is often weighed against objective measures of housing quality, such as size and structural conditions and adequacy of utilities (e.g., plumbing and heating). Parmalee and Lawton (1990) describe the tension between the need for autonomy and the need for security when designing physical environments for older adults. Autonomy refers to a state in which elders feel or are capable of managing daily life and pursuing goals using their own resources. It implies a freedom of choice and action—the regulation of one's own life and life space. Central to the idea of facilitating autonomy is the issue of control and individual differences in the desire for control. Security, on the other hand, refers to the dependability of physical, social, and interpersonal resources for managing daily life. It addresses physical safety as well as psychological comfort (i.e., peace of mind) (Parmalee & Lawton, 1990). Balancing autonomy and security extends beyond the immediate living space to the neighborhood, where developing a sense of community contributes to physical safety and emotional security.

Another area of research designed to address person–environment transactions is the match between functional capacity, functional task demand, and spatial design characteristics that limit or enhance function. For example, the human-factors method has been used to examine relationships between aging-related changes in functional capacity and biomechanical demands of performing ADLs, as well as the interaction between ergonomic design and reduced functional capacity, which predisposes the older person to injury and/or limited independence (Czaja et al., 1993). Although the study of human factors in elder–environmental design has only recently begun, the work holds promise for developing environments that enable older adults to maintain functional independence and remain in their own homes.

Although more is being learned about aging and functional abilities, some effects of environment are difficult to isolate. Systematic study of physical and social environments that support or disadvantage older adults is needed (Birren & Birren, 1990). Efforts should also be made to measure social change and examine its effects on older individuals as well as on the aging process itself (George, 1995).

Spiritual Dimension

Despite the fact that spirituality has been addressed for centuries from a wide variety of perspectives, scientists have been reluctant to approach this topic directly. Levin (1994), for example, described the "collective amnesia" (p. xvi) of scientists regarding the significance of spiritual issues and religion for health and aging. However, the spiritual dimension is a key element in the lived experience of elderly people.

Spirituality emerges as humans address the eternal mythic questions of life: the purpose and meaning of life, truth, love, desire, evil, suffering, and death. It may be viewed as the life principle that pervades and integrates a person's entire being. Moberg (1974) defined spirituality as pertaining "to the inner resources of people, their ultimate concern around which all other values are focused, their central philosophy in life (whether designated as religious or nonreligious) which guides their conduct, and all the supernatural and non-material dimensions of human nature" (p. 259).

In the Western, classical sense, spirituality includes the transcendent (or that which exists apart from the material world—beyond basic human knowledge). More recently, however, the idea of spirituality has come to incorporate the humanistic perspective, which may exclude ideas of transcendence. Humanistic (Third Force) psychologists such as Carl Rogers and Rollo May have their roots in the existential (phenomenological) movement in European philosophy. They propose that insight into our own mortality forms the impetus to shift from the ordinary state of human existence to a higher state: from an ontic to an ontological mode. The ontic mode is characterized by forgetfulness of being, treating self and other as object ("inauthentic"). The ontological mode, on the other hand, is characterized by mindfulness of being, treating self and other as subject ("authentic") (Tiryakian, 1968; Yallom, 1980). The humanists suggest that the main purpose of life is to find meaning and that this can be accomplished through creations (or accomplishments), experiences in the world, and attitude toward suffering (Frankl, 1963). Here spirituality is the mystery in striving to be in unity with others.

In nursing, spirituality is recognized as a basic quality, inherent in all humans. The spiritual perspective has been identified as having three critical attributes: (a) connectedness (with other humans, nature, universal forces, or God), (b) belief in powers or forces beyond the self and a faith that affirms life, and (c) a creative energy. Further, the spiritual perspective provides a path for the quest for the meaning of life, organizes and guides human values and motivations, and results in self-transcendence (Haase, Britt, Coward, Leidy, & Penn, 1992; Reed, 1992).

Although spirituality is "internal" and individual-based, it may be aided or guided in its development through religion. Religion is a component of the environment external to the person and provides "options" for engaging the sacred. Religion is a universal social institution that generally is composed of three major elements: (a) a set of organized beliefs about the nature of the nonmaterial (supernatural) world, often, but not always, including concepts of a god or deities; (b) myths or sacred stories about the history and actions of the supernatural powers, beings, or forces; and (c) rituals involving symbolic acts or objects that mediate between the human and the suprahuman spheres (Campbell, 1986; Moore, 1992).

NURSING SPHERE

The nursing sphere in the conceptual model (see Figure 2.1) incorporates three nursing knowledge domains: diagnoses, interventions, and outcomes (Iowa Intervention Project, 1992). Diagnoses and outcomes represent client phenomena; the intervention domain represents nursing therapeutics that are carried out to achieve health outcomes (Iowa Intervention Project, 1996). Meleis and Trangenstein (1994) proposed that in transition processes nursing is concerned with the experience of individuals, families, and communities undergoing transitions, where health and perceived well-being are the outcomes.

Nursing Diagnoses

Nursing diagnoses are clinical judgments about individual, family, or community responses to actual or potential health problems and life processes. Three categories of nursing diagnoses have been developed: (a) actual diagnoses, which describe client responses that are specific to existing health states or conditions; (b) risk diagnoses, which describe responses that might develop in clients who are vulnerable because of increased risk factors; and (c) wellness diagnoses, which describe responses that move the client to higher levels of wellness. Diagnoses provide the basis for interventions to achieve outcomes for which the nurse is accountable (North American Nursing Diagnosis Association, 1994).

In the context of late-life transitions, diagnoses take into account the timing of the transition and where the elder is in the transition(s) process. Diagnoses also reflect emotional, attitudinal, and functional responses to the challenge(s) posed by developmental, situational, or health–illness transitions. As described earlier, change introduces uncertainty and is stressful; thus, readiness for the transition is another major focus for diagnosis and is assessed by exploring the meanings that a particular life change has for the elder. Similarly, diagnosis involves identifying what knowledge and skills are required to develop a new identity and manage changing roles and physical capacities (Schumacher & Meleis, 1994). Ebersole and Hess (1994) suggest that late-life transitions require different adaptive capacities from those of earlier stages of the life course. In late life, existential issues such as experiencing losses, redefining meanings in existence, and living in the present become the standard, replacing the performance and future orientation that characterize earlier adulthood.

In addition to individual responses, assessment and diagnosis include the physical, social, cultural, and spiritual environmental resources for and barriers to achieving optimum health behavior, functional status, and well-being. As previously shown, environmental phenomena are critical to enhancing developmental and functional capacities in late life.

The extent to which the current taxonomy of the North American Nursing Diagnosis Association represents the phenomena of aging-related late-life transitions and the environments in which they occur should be examined. Work is under way to identify relevant diagnoses in the current taxonomy and to develop needed diagnoses.

Nursing Interventions

Nursing interventions focus on assisting elders to achieve health outcomes when experiencing aging-related transitions. Meleis and Trangenstein (1994) argued that the process of facilitating transitions to enhance a sense of well-being gives nursing a unique perspective. Interventions target personal and environmental resources and barriers to achieving health outcomes. It is not feasible to include a detailed description of relevant interventions in this chapter. However, several areas for intervention are included here for purposes of illustration.

One area is assisting elderly persons to prepare for transition(s) by providing information about internal developmental processes, sources of social support, and opportunities for personal growth and role supplementation (Schumacher & Meleis, 1994). According to Ebersole and Hess (1994), individuals have very little preparation for major life transitions and do not perceive planning for changes such as retirement as a health concern (Bevil et al., 1993). As we learn more about late-life transition experiences, we will be better equipped to facilitate elders, families, and communities in their development.

Another major focus of intervention is lifestyle. As with all life stages, health promotion and primary and secondary prevention have become national and local strategies for improving health (USDHHS, 1990). Life-style interventions such as exercise promotion and nutrition counseling are particularly important in late life, when there is a tendency to slow down and become more sedentary. Moreover, lack of exercise was shown to be as predictive of functional decline as several medical conditions and variables such as visual impairment (Mor et al., 1989). For example, muscle function appears to be the most important aging-related physical change in that it interferes with ADL function as well as endurance. Studies have shown that muscle strength can be improved with resistance exercise that targets specific muscle groups used in functional tasks such as lifting, grasping, and locomotion (Hughes, Dunlop, Edelman, Chang, & Singer, 1994). Similarly, joint flexibility can be maintained or improved even in the presence of musculoskeletal disease. Hughes and associates (1994) suggested that, because of its high prevalence among older adults, musculoskeletal disease is often ignored although, in fact, any joint impairment should be considered a risk factor for functional dependence. This suggestion has implications for interventions of health screening, risk appraisal, and risk reduction.

A third major area for intervention is the facilitation of role supplementation and role enhancement. Adelmann (1994) found that elders who occupied multiple roles experienced higher levels of psychological well-being than did those with fewer roles. Ebersole and Hess (1994) also suggest that the elderly can be assisted in developing ways to enhance the exchange process through reciprocal activities and interpersonal reliance. Similarly, developmental processes such as gerotranscendence can be facilitated by engaging elders in life review (reminiscence therapy).

A fourth area of nursing intervention is management of the environment. Although safety is a priority, interventions directed to the environment go beyond physical safety to include use of sociopolitical processes to bring about change in constraining social processes and structures. Facilitating the use of social structures and processes can be done through individual efforts, such as assisting older adults to perceive and describe their own environments in a way that helps them recognize constraints on their health and freedom to participate (Kleffel, 1991). It can also be done through sociopolitical processes (Kleffel, 1991; Stevens, 1989). Although nursing has a tradition of managing the immediate physical environment to reduce its negative impact on function and well-being, Kleffel (1991) suggested that nurses' lack of awareness about the impact of the social, economic, and political environment on function and well-being has contributed to the peripheral role nursing has had in influencing change in these systems.

Enhancing health self-care capability is another major area for nursing intervention. Many chronic symptoms and illnesses require major self-care efforts to maintain health and to obtain optimal benefit from treatment and rehabilitation (Kart & Engler, 1994). One mechanism for this purpose is client education designed in accordance with characteristics of the elderly and the requisite knowledge (Dellasega, Clark, McCreary, Helmuth, & Schan, 1994). Client education focusing on self-monitoring for early detection of disease is also an important dimension of health self-care. For example, instruction in breast cancer self-examination has been shown to be effective in increasing the frequency, proficiency, and perceived skill in conducting breast self-examination (Lierman, Young, Powell-Cope, Georgiadou, & Benoliel, 1994).

Nursing-Sensitive Client Outcomes

The third component of the nursing sphere in the conceptual model is the development and evaluation of desired health outcomes. As shown in the elder sphere of the model, health outcomes in late life include functional status, health behavior, and well-being. A nursing-sensitive client outcome refers to a variable client (or patient) state, condition, or perception largely influenced by and sensitive to nursing intervention (Iowa Nursing-Sensitive Patient Outcomes Research Team, 1993). Late-life transitions are complex processes that have many contexts. Similarly, treatment is multidimensional and often interdisciplinary. Consequently, health outcomes are difficult to classify because they are influenced by multiple inputs, including the client's.

In general, the desired effect of interventions is successful management of late-life transitions and meaningful living. Indicators of successful management include but are not limited to emotional well-being, mastery of new skills and roles, meaningful relationships, functional ability, and personal transformation. As previously noted, transitions take place over time; thus, outcomes occur throughout the process and are not universally associated with a defined end point (Meleis & Trangenstein, 1994). Again, work is under way to develop observable outcome indicators that can be used to examine the effects of nursing intervention in practice and research.

SUMMARY

The conceptual model of gerontological nursing presented in this chapter delineates major life transitions experienced by adults in late life and postulates that developmental processes mediate the effects of late-life transitions moving toward higher levels of function and well-being. This model casts late life as a period in which life changes are biologically regressive yet offer opportunity for advanced development. Numerous theorists, investigators, and clinicians testify to the wide variance in personal and health characteristics of older adults. Bahr (1992) described this phenomenon as the person becoming "more who he or she is" (p. 3). Clearly, there are declining physical and social resources, yet a vast majority of older adults report higher levels of life satisfaction than do younger adults (Tornstam, 1989). The challenge for the development of gerontological nursing science is to examine the relevant diagnoses and to identify and test nursing interventions in the context of aging-related transitions and developmental processes. In addition, sensitive measures to evaluate intervention outcomes should be developed so that increments in late-life health indicators can be identified.

REFERENCES

Achenbaum, W. A., & Bengtson, V. L. (1994). Re-engaging the disengagement theory of aging: On the history and assessment of theory in gerontology. *The Gerontologist, 34,* 756–763.
Adelmann, P. K. (1994). Multiple roles and psychological well-being in a national

sample of older adults. *Journals of Gerontology: Social Sciences, 49*(6), S277–S285.

Agris, P. F., Boak, A., Basler, J. W., Voorn, C., Smith, C., & Reichlin, M. (1985). Analysis of cellular senescence through detection and assessment of RNAs and proteins important to gene expression: Transfer RNAs and autoimmune antigens. *Advances in Experimental Medicine and Biology, 190,* 509–539.

Alford, D., & Futrell, M. (1992). Wellness and health promotion of the elderly. *Nursing Outlook, 40,* 221–226.

Antonucci, T. C. (1990). Social supports and social relationships. In R. H. Binstock & L. K. George (Eds.), *Handbook of aging and the social sciences* (3rd ed., pp. 205–226). San Diego, CA: Academic Press.

Arking, R. (1991). Modifying the aging process. In R. F. Young & E. A. Olson (Eds.), *Health, illness and disability in later life* (pp. 11–24). Newbury Park, CA: Sage.

Atchley, R. C. (1989). A continuity theory of normal aging. *The Gerontologist, 29,* 183–190.

Bahr, R. T., Sr. (1992). Personhood: A theory for gerontological nursing. *Holistic Nursing Practice, 7*(1), 1–6.

Baker, G. T., & Sprott, R. L. (1988). Biomarkers of aging. *Experimental Gerontology, 23,* 223–239.

Barer, B. M. (1994). Men and women aging differently. *International Journal of Aging and Human Development, 38*(1), 29–40.

Basson, P. (1967). The gerontological nursing literature. *Nursing Research, 16*(3), 267–272.

Bausell, R. B. (1986). Health seeking behavior among the elderly. *The Gerontologist, 26,* 556–559.

Bengtson, V. L., Reedy, M., & Gordon, C. (1985). Aging and self-conceptions: Personality processes and social contexts. In J. E. Birren & K. W. Schaie (Eds.), *Handbook of the psychology of aging* (2nd ed., pp. 544–593). New York: Van Nostrand Reinhold.

Bernardi, B. (1985). *Age class systems: Social institutions and politics based on age.* London: Cambridge.

Bevil, C. A., O'Connor, P. C., & Mattoon, P. M. (1993). Leisure activity, life satisfaction and perceived health status in older adults. *Gerontology and Geriatrics Education, 14*(2), 3–17.

Birren, J. E., & Birren, B. A. (1990). The concepts, models, and history of the psychology of aging. In J. E. Birren & K. W. Schaie (Eds.), *Handbook of the psychology of aging* (3rd ed., pp. 3–20). San Diego, CA: Academic Press.

Bishop, C. (1986). Living arrangement choices of elderly singles. *Health Care Financing Review, 7,* 65–73.

Borkan, G. A. (1978). The assessment of biological age during adulthood (Doctoral dissertation, University of Michigan, 1978). *Dissertation Abstracts International, 3682-A,* 7822861.

Borkan, G. A., & Norris, A. H. (1980). Assessment of biological age using a profile of physical parameters. *Journals of Gerontology, 35*(22), 177–184.

Botwinick, J. (1973). *Aging and behavior.* New York: Springer Publishing Co.

Boult, C., Kane, R., Thomas, T., Boult, L., & McCaffrey, D. (1994). Chronic conditions that lead to functional limitation in the elderly. *Journals of Gerontology, 49*(1), M28–M36.

Branch, L., Guralnik, J., Foley, D., Kohout, F., Wetle, T., Ostfeld, A., & Katz, S. (1991). Active life expectancy for 10,000 Caucasian men and women in three communities. *Journals of Gerontology: Medical Sciences, 46*(4), M145–150.

Branch, L., & Ku, L. (1989). Transition probabilities to dependency, institutionalization, and death among elderly over a decade. *Journal of Aging and Health, 1*(3), 370–408.

Branch, L. G., & Jette, M. A. (1982). A prospective study of long-term care institutionalization among the aged. *American Journal of Public Health, 72,* 1373–1379.

Brimmer, P. F. (1979). Past, present and future in gerontological nursing research. *Journal of Gerontological Nursing, 5*(6), 27–34.

Brown, J., & McCreedy, M. (1986). The hale elderly: Health behavior and its correlates. *Research in Nursing and Health, 9,* 317–329.

Burgener, S. C., & Chiverton, P. (1992). Conceptualizing psychological well-being in cognitively-impaired older persons. *Image, 24*(2), 209–213.

Butler, R. N. (1974). Successful aging. *Mental Health, 58*(3), 7–12.

Campbell, J. (1986). *The inner reaches of outer space: Metaphor as myth and religion.* Toronto: St. James Press.

Cantor, M., & Little, V. (1985). Aging and social care. In R. H. Binstock & E. Shanas (Eds.), *Handbook of aging and the social sciences* (2nd ed., pp. 745–781). New York: Van Nostrand Reinhold.

Carlson, R. (1981). Studies in script theory. Adult analogs of a childhood nuclear scene. *Journal of Personality and Social Psychology, 40,* 501–510.

Charness, R. (1985). Aging and problem solving performance. In R. Charness (Ed.), *Aging and human performance* (pp. 225–260). New York: Wiley.

Chopoorian, T. J. (1986). Reconceptualizing the environment. In P. Moccia (Ed.), *New approaches to theory development* (pp. 39–54). New York: NLN Press.

Clausen, J. A. (1972). The life course of individuals. In M. W. Riley, M. Johnson, & A. Foner (Eds.), *Aging and society: 3. A sociology of age stratification* (pp. 457–515). New York: Russell Sage.

Cohen, M. Z., Tripp-Reimer, T., Sorofman, B., Lauer, G., & Lively, S. (1994). Explanatory models of diabetes. *Social Science and Medicine, 38*(1), 59–66.

Connidis, I. A., & McMullin, J. A. (1993). To have or have not: Parent status and the subjective well-being of older men and women. *Gerontologist, 33*(5), 630–636.

Cowgill, D. O., & Holmes, L. D. (Eds.). (1972). *Aging and modernization.* New York: Appleton-Century-Crofts.

Cox, C. (1986). The interaction model of client health behavior: Application to the study of community based elders. *Advances in Nursing Science, 9,* 40–57.

Craik, F. I. (1977). Age differences in human memory. In J. E. Birren & K. W. Schaie (Eds.), *Handbook of the psychology of aging* (pp. 384–420). New York: Van Nostrand Reinhold.

Cumming, I. M., & Henry, W. E. (1961). *Growing old: The process of disengagement.* New York: Basic Books.

Curtis, H. J., & Miller, K. (1971). Chromosome aberrations in liver cells of guinea pigs. *Journals of Gerontology, 26,* 292–293.

Cutler, R. G. (1975). Evolution of human longevity and the genetic complexity governing aging rate. *Proceedings of the National Academy of Sciences, USA, 72,* 4664–4668.

Czaja, S. J., Weber, R. A., & Nair, S. N. (1993). A human factors analysis of ADL activities: A capability-demand approach. *Journals of Gerontology, 48,* 44–48.

Dean, K. (1992). Health related behavior: Concepts and methods. In M. G. Ory, R. P. Abeles, & P. D. Lipman (Eds.), *Aging, health, and behavior* (pp. 27–56). Newbury Park, CA: Sage.

Dellasega, C., Clark, D., McCreary, D., Helmuth, A., & Schan, P. (1994). Nursing process: Teaching elderly clients. *Journal of Gerontological Nursing, 20*(1), 31–38.

Dowd, J. J. (1975). Aging as exchange: A preface to theory. *Journals of Gerontology, 30,* 584–594.

Dressel, P. L., & Barnhill, S. K. (1994). Reframing gerontological thought and practice: The case of grandmothers with daughters in prison. *The Gerontologist, 34*(5), 685–691.

Duffy, M. E. (1993). Determinants of health-promotion lifestyles in older people. *Image, 25,* 23–28.

Ebersole, P., & Hess, P. (1994). *Toward health aging* (4th ed.). St. Louis: C. V. Mosby.

Erikson, E. H. (1963). *Childhood and society.* New York: Norton.

Estes, C., & Binney, E. A. (1989). The biomedicalization of aging: Dangers and dilemmas. *The Gerontologist, 29*(5), 587–596.

Eysenck, M. W. (1974). Age differences in incidental learning. *Developmental Psychology, 10,* 936–941.

Fiatarone, M. A., & Evans, W. J. (1993). The etiology and reversibility of muscle dysfunction in the aged. *Journals of Gerontology, 48,* 77–83.

Foner, A. (1974). Age stratification and age conflict in political life. *American Sociological Review, 39,* 1081–1104.

Frankl, V. (1963). *Man's search for meaning: An introduction to logotherapy.* New York: Pocket Books.

George, L. (1990). Social structure, social processes and social-psychological states. In R. H. Binstock & L. K. George (Eds.), *Handbook of aging and the social sciences* (3rd ed., pp. 186–204). San Diego, CA: Academic Press.

George, L. K. (1995). The last half-century of aging research—and thoughts for the future. *Journals of Gerontology: Sociology, 50B*(1), S1–S3.

Guccione, A. A., & Jette, M. A. (1988). Assessing limitations in physical function in patients with arthritis. *Arthritis Care and Research, 1*(3), 170–176.

Guralnik, J., & Simonsick, E. (1993). Physical disability in older Americans. *Journals of Gerontology, 48,* 84–88.

Haase, J. E., Britt, T., Coward, D. O., Leidy, N. K., & Penn, P. E. (1992).

Simultaneous concept analysis of spiritual perspective, hope, acceptance and self-transcendence. *Image, 24,* 141–147.

Hagestad, G. O. (1990). Social perspectives on the life course. In R. H. Binstock & L. K. George (Eds.), *Handbook of aging and the social sciences* (3rd ed., pp. 151–168). San Diego, CA: Academic Press.

Hagestad, G. O., & Neugarten, B. L. (1985). Age and the life course. In R. H. Binstock & E. Shanas (Eds.), *Handbook of aging and the social sciences* (2nd ed., pp. 35–61). New York: Van Nostrand Reinhold.

Hale, S., Myerson, J., & Wagstaff, D. (1987). General slowing of nonverbal information processing: Evidence for a power law. *Journals of Gerontology, 42,* 131–136.

Harman, D. (1956). Aging: A theory based on free radical and radiation chemistry. *Journals of Gerontology, 11,* 298–300.

Havighurst, R. J. (1972). *Developmental tasks and education.* New York: McKay.

Havighurst, R. J., & Albrecht, R. (1953). *Older people.* New York: Longmans, Green.

Havighurst, R. J., Neugarten, B. L., & Tobin, S. S. (1963). Disengagement, personality and life satisfaction in the later years. In P. Hansen (Ed.), *Age with a future* (pp. 419–425). Copenhagen: Munksgård.

Hayflick, L. (1965). The limited in vitro lifetime of human diploid cell strains. *Experimental Cell Research, 57,* 614–636.

Hickey, T., Dean, K., & Holstein, B. E. (1986). Emerging trends in gerontology and geriatrics. *Social Science and Medicine, 23,* 1363–1369.

Hogue, C. C. (1985). Social support. In J. E. Hall & B. R. Weaver (Eds.), *Distributive nursing practice: A systems approach to community health* (2nd ed., pp. 58–81). Philadelphia: J. B. Lippincott.

Horn, J. L. (1982). The theory of fluid and crystallized intelligence in relation to concepts of cognitive psychology and aging in adulthood. In F. M. Craik & S. Trehub (Eds.), *Aging and cognitive processes* (pp. 237–278). New York: Plenum.

Hughes, S. L., Dunlop, D., Edelman, P., Chang, R. W., & Singer, R. H. (1994). Impact of joint impairment on longitudinal disability in elderly persons. *Journals of Gerontology: Social Sciences, 49*(6), S291–S300.

Iowa Intervention Project—McCloskey, J. C., & Bulechek, G. M. (Eds.). (1992). *Nursing interventions classification (NIC).* St. Louis: Mosby-Year Book.

Iowa Intervention Project—McCloskey, J. C., & Bulechek, G. M. (Eds.). (1996). *Nursing interventions classification (NIC)* (2nd ed.). St. Louis: Mosby-Year Book.

Iowa Nursing-Sensitive Patient Outcomes Research Team. (1993). *Nursing sensitive outcomes classification.* Unpublished report.

Isreal, B. A. (1982). Social networks and health status: Linking theory, research and practice. *Patient Counseling and Health Education, 4*(2), 65–79.

Isreal, B. A., & Antonucci, T. C. (1987). Social network characteristics and psychological well-being: A replication and extension. *Health Education Quarterly, 14*(4), 461–481.

Jackson, J. J. (1980). *Minorities and aging.* Belmont, CA: Wadsworth.

Jackson, J. S., Antonucci, T. C., & Gibson, R. C. (1990). Social support and health. In J. E. Birren & K. W. Schaie (Eds.), *Handbook of the psychology of aging* (3rd ed., pp. 103–123). San Diego, CA: Academic Press.

Jirovec, M., & Kasno, J. (1990). Self-care agency as a function of patient–environment factors among nursing home residents. *Research in Nursing and Health, 13,* 303–309.

Jones, P. S., & Meleis, A. I. (1993). Health is empowerment. *Advances in Nursing Services, 15*(3), 1–14.

Jung, C. G. (1933). *Modern man in search of a soul.* New York: Harcourt, Brace.

Jung, C. G. (1960). The stages of life. In *Collected works: 8. Structure and dynamics of the psyche.* New York: Pantheon.

Kahana, E. A. (1982). A congruence model of person–environment interaction. In M. P. Lawton, P. G. Windley, & T. O. Byerts (Eds.), *Aging and the environment: Theoretical approaches* (pp. 97–121). New York: Springer Publishing Co.

Kahn, R. L. (1979). Aging and social support. In M. W. Riley (Ed.), *Aging from birth to death: Interdisciplinary perspectives* (pp. 77–91). Boulder, CO: Westview Press.

Kane, R. L. (1993). The implications of assessment. *Journals of Gerontology, 48,* 27–31.

Karp, D. A. (1988). A decade of reminders: Changing age consciousness between fifty and sixty years old. *The Gerontologist, 28*(6), 727–738.

Kart, C., & Dunkle, R. (1989). Assessing capacity for self-care among the aged. *Journal of Aging and Health, 1,* 430–450.

Kart, C. S., & Engler, C. A. (1994). Predisposition to self-health care: Who does what for themselves and why? *Journals of Gerontology: Social Science, 49*(6), S301–S308.

Katz, S., Branch, L., Branson, M., Papsidero, S., Beck, J., & Greer, D. (1983). Active life expectancy. *New England Journal of Medicine, 309*(20), 1218–1224.

Katz, S., & Stroud, M. W. (1989). Functional assessment in geriatrics. A review of progress and directions. *Journal of the American Geriatrics Society, 37,* 267–271.

Kayser-Jones, J. S. (1981). Gerontological nursing research revisited. *Journal of Gerontological Nursing, 7,* 217–223.

Keith, J. (1990). Age in social and cultural context: Anthropological perspectives. In R. H. Binstock & L. K. George (Eds.), *Handbook of aging and the social sciences* (3rd ed., pp. 91–111). San Diego, CA: Academic Press.

Kim, H. S. (1983). *The nature of theoretical thinking in nursing.* Norwalk, CT: Appleton-Century-Crofts.

Kleemeier, R. W. (1962). Intellectual changes in the senium. *Proceedings of the American Statistical Association, 1,* 181–190.

Kleffel, D. (1991). Rethinking the environment as a domain of nursing knowledge. *Advances in Nursing Science, 14*(1), 40–51.

Kleinman, A. (1980). *Patients and healers in the context of culture.* Berkeley: University of California Press.

Knowles, L. (1983). Gerontological nursing '82. *International Journal of Nursing Studies, 20*(1), 45–54.

Kogan, N. (1987). Creativity. In G. L. Maddox (Ed.), *Encyclopedia of aging* (pp. 153–155). New York: Springer Publishing Co.

Kogan, N. (1990). Personality and aging. In J. E. Birren & K. W. Schaie (Eds.), *Handbook of the psychology of aging* (3rd ed., pp. 330–346). San Diego, CA: Academic Press.

Kohlberg, L. (1973). Continuities in childhood and adult moral development revisited. In P. Boltes & K. W. Schaie (Eds.), *Life span developmental psychology: Personality and socialization* (pp. 179–204). New York: Academic Press.

Kraus, N. (1990). Illness behavior in late life. In R. H. Binstock & L. K. George (Eds.), *Handbook of aging and the social sciences* (3rd ed., pp. 227–244). San Diego, CA: Academic Press.

Kraus, N., & Jay, G. (1991). Stress, social support, and negative interaction in later life. *Research on Aging, 13,* 333–363.

Kuypers, J. A., & Bengtson, V. L. (1973). Social breakdown and competence: A model of normal aging. *Human Development, 16,* 181–201.

Lawton, M. P., & Nahemow, L. (1973). Ecology and the aging process. In C. Eisdorfer & M. P. Lawton (Eds.), *Psychology of adult development and aging* (pp. 619–674). Washington, DC: American Psychological Association.

Lehman, H. C. (1953). *Age and achievement.* Princeton, NJ: Princeton University Press.

Lenihan, A. A. (1988). Identification of self-care behaviors in the elderly. *Journal of Professional Nursing, 4,* 285–288.

Levin, J. S. (1994). *Religion in aging and health.* Newbury Park, CA: Sage.

Levin, L., & Idler, E. (1984). Self-care in health. *Annual Review of Public Health, 4,* 181–201.

Levinson, D. J. (1978). *The seasons of a man's life.* New York: Knopf.

Lierman, L. M., Young, H. M., Powell-Cope, G., Georgiadou, F., & Benoliel, J. Q. (1994). Effects of education and support on breast self-examination in older women. *Nursing Research, 43*(3), 158–163.

Lorig, K. (1993). Self-management of chronic illness: A model for the future. *Generations, 17*(3), 11–14.

Lorig, K., & Holman, H. R. (1993). Arthritis self-management studies: A twelve-year review. *Health Education Quarterly, 20,* 17–28.

Marshall, V. W. (1994). Sociology, psychology, and the theoretical legacy of the Kansas City Studies. *The Gerontologist, 34,* 768–774.

Martinson, I. (1985). Gerontology comes of age. *Journal of Gerontological Nursing, 10*(7), 8–17.

Mazur, D., & Merz, J. (1993). How the manner of presentation of data influences older patients in determining their treatment preferences. *Journal of the American Geriatrics Society, 41,* 223–228.

McCrae, R. R., & Costa, P. T. (1982). Self-concept and the stability of personality: Cross-sectional comparisons of self-reports and ratings. *Journal of Personality and Social Psychology, 43,* 1282–1292.

Medawar, P. B. (1957). *The uniqueness of the individual.* London: Methuen.

Medvedev, Z. A. (1972). Repetition of molecular-genetic information as a possible factor in evolutionary changes of life-span. *Experimental Gerontology, 7,* 227–234.

Meeks, S., Carstensen, L. L., Tamsky, B., Wright, T. L., & Pellegrini, D. (1989). Age differences in coping: Does less mean worse? *International Journal of Aging and Human Development, 28*(2), 127–140.

Meleis, A. (1986). Theory development and domain concepts. In P. Moccia (Ed.), *New approaches to theory development* (Publication No. 15-1992, pp. 3–21). New York: National League for Nursing.

Meleis, A., & Trangenstein, P. (1994). Facilitating transitions: Redefinition of the nursing mission. *Nursing Outlook, 42,* 255–259.

Meyer, D., Leventhal, H., & Gutmann, M. (1985). The common-sense model of illness: The example of hypertension. *Health Psychology, 4,* 115–135.

Midanik, L., Soghikan, K., Ransom, L., & Tekawa, I. (1995). The effect of retirement on mental health and health behaviors: The Kaiser Permanente retirement study. *Journals of Gerontology: Social Sciences, 50B*(1), 559-561.

Miller, B. E., & Keane, C. B. (1983). *Encyclopedia and dictionary of medicine, nursing and allied health* (3rd ed., p. 601). Philadelphia: W. B. Saunders.

Moberg, D. O. (1974). Spiritual well-being in late life. In J. F. Gubrium (Ed.), *Late life communities and environmental policy* (pp. 256–279). Springfield, IL: Charles C Thomas.

Moch, S. D. (1989). Health within illness: Conceptual evolution and practice possibilities. *Advances in Nursing Science, 11*(4), 23–31.

Moody, H. R. (1988). Toward a critical gerontology: The contribution of the humanities to theories of aging. In J. E. Birren & V. L. Bengtson (Eds.), *Emergent theories of aging* (pp. 19–40). New York: Springer Publishing Co.

Moore, T. (1992). *Care of the soul: A guide for cultivating depth and sacredness in everyday life.* New York: HarperCollins.

Mor, V., Murphy, J., Masterson-Allen, S., Willey, C., Razmpour, A., Jackson, M. E., Greer, D., & Katz, S. (1989). Risk of functional decline among well elderly. *Journal of Clinical Epidemiology, 42*(9), 895–904.

Mor-Barak, M. E., Scharlach, A. E., Birba, L., & Sokolov, J. (1992). Employment, social networks and health in retirement years. *International Journal of Aging and Human Development, 35*(2), 145–159.

Murphy, E., & Freston, M. S. (1991). An analysis of theory-research linkages in published gerontological nursing studies, 1983–1989. *Advances in Nursing Science, 13*(4), 1–13.

Neugarten, B. L. (1973). Personality changes in late life: A developmental perspective. In C. Eisdorfer & M. P. Lawton (Eds.), *The psychology of adult development and aging* (pp. 311–338). Washington, DC: American Psychological Association.

Neugarten, B. L., Havighurst, R. J., & Tobin, S. S. (1968). Personality and patterns of aging. In B. L. Neugarten (Ed.), *Middle age and aging* (pp. 173–180). Chicago: University of Chicago Press.

Newman, B. M., & Newman, P. R. (1984). *Development through life: A psychosocial approach.* Homewood, IL: Dorsey.

Norbeck, J. (1988). Social support. In J. J. Fitzpatrick & J. S. Stevenson (Eds.), *Annual review of nursing research, Vol. 6* (pp. 85–109). New York: Springer Publishing Co.

Norburn, J. E., Bernard, S. L., Konrad, T. R., Woomert, A., DeFriese, G. H., Kalsbeek, W. D., Koch, G. G., & Ory, M. G. (1995). Self-care and assistance from others in coping with functional status limitations among a national sample of older adults. *Journals of Gerontology: Social Sciences, 50B,* S101–S109.

North American Nursing Diagnosis Association. (1994). *Nursing diagnoses: Definitions and classification.* Philadelphia: Author.

O'Bryant, I. (1982). The value of home to older persons. *Research on Aging, 4*(3), 349–363.

Orgel, L. E. (1963). The maintenance of the accuracy of protein synthesis and its relevance to aging. *Proceedings of the National Academy of Sciences, USA, 49,* 517–521.

Parmelee, P., & Lawton, M. (1990). The design of special environments for the aged. In J. E. Birren & K. W. Schaie (Eds.), *Handbook of the psychology of aging* (3rd ed., pp. 465–488). San Diego, CA: Academic Press.

Parr, J. (1980). The interaction of persons and living environments. In L. W. Poon (Ed.), *Aging in the 1980s* (pp. 393–406). Washington, DC: American Psychological Association.

Peck, R. C. (1968). Psychological developments in the second half of life. In B. Neugarten (Ed.), *Middle age and aging* (pp. 88–92). Chicago: University of Chicago Press.

Pendergast, D. R., Fisher, N. M., & Calkins, E. (1993). Cardiovascular, neuromuscular, and metabolic alterations with age leading to frailty. *Journals of Gerontology, 48,* 61–67.

Perlmutter, M. (1988). Cognitive potential through life. In J. E. Birren & V. L. Bengtson (Eds.), *Emergent theories of aging* (pp. 247–268). New York: Springer Publishing Co.

Prado, C. G. (1983). Aging and narrative. *International Journal of Applied Philosophy, 1,* 1–14.

Press, I., & McKool, M. (1972). Social structure and status of the aged: Toward some valid cross-cultural generalizations. *Aging and Human Development, 3,* 279–306.

Rakowski, W. (1992). Disease prevention and health promotion with older adults. In M. G. Ory, R. P. Abeles, & P. D. Lipman (Eds,), *Aging, health, and behavior* (pp. 239–275). Newbury Park, CA: Sage.

Rakowski, W., Rice, C., & McHorney, C. (1992). Information seeking about health among older adults. *Behavior, Health and Aging, 2,* 181–198.

Reed, P. (1989). Mental health of older adults. *Western Journal of Nursing Research, 11*(2), 143–163.

Reed, P. G. (1991a). Self-transcendence and mental health in oldest-old adults. *Nursing Research, 40*(1), 1–11.

Reed, P. G. (1991b). Toward a nursing theory of self-transcendence: Deductive reformulation using developmental theories. *Advances in Nursing Science, 13*(4), 64–77.

Reed, P. G. (1992). An emerging paradigm for the investigation of spirituality in nursing. *Research in Nursing and Health, 15,* 349–357.

Reichard, S., Levson, F., & Peterson, P. G. (1962). *Aging and personality.* New York: Wiley.

Reigel, K. F. (1973). Dialectical operations: The final period of cognitive development. *Human Development, 16,* 346–370.

Riley, M. W. (1971). Social gerontology and the age stratification of society. *The Gerontologist, 11,* 79–87.

Riley, M. W. (1979). Life-course perspectives. In M. W. Riley (Ed.), *Aging from birth to death: Interdisciplinary perspectives* (pp. 3–13). Washington, DC: Westview.

Riley, M. W., & Foner, A. (Eds.). (1968). *Aging and society.* New York: Russell Sage.

Rodin, J. (1986). Aging and health: Effects of the sense of control. *Science, 233,* 1271–1276.

Rogers, M. (1990). Nursing: Science of unitary, irreducible human beings: Update 1990. In E. A. M. Barrett (Ed.), *Visions of Rogers' science-based nursing* (pp. 5–12). New York: NLN Press.

Rose, A. M. (1964). A current theoretical issue in social gerontology. *The Gerontologist, 4,* 46–50.

Ryan, M. C., & Austin, A. G. (1989). Social supports and social networks in the aged. *Image, 21*(3), 176–180.

Sacher, G. A. (1980). Theory in gerontology. *Annual Review of Gerontology and Geriatrics, 1,* 3–24.

Sagy, S., & Antonovsky, A. (1990). Explaining life satisfaction in later life: The sense of coherence model and activity theory. *Behavior, Health and Aging, 1*(1), 11–25.

Salthouse, T. A. (1985). *A theory of cognitive aging.* Amsterdam: North-Holland.

Schaie, K. W. (1962). A field-theory approach to age changes in cognitive behavior. *Vita Humana, 5,* 129–141.

Schaie, K. W., & Parham, I. (1976). Stability of adult personality traits: Fact or fable? *Journal of Personality and Social Psychology, 34,* 146–158.

Schulz, R., & Williamson, G. M. (1993). Psychosocial and behavioral dimensions of physical frailty. *Journals of Gerontology, 48,* 39–43.

Schumacher, K. D., & Meleis, A. (1994). Transitions: A central concept in nursing. *Image, 26*(2), 119–127.

Shock, N. W. (1979). Systems physiology and aging. *Federal Proceedings, 38,* 161–169.

Sohal, R. S. (1981). *Age pigments.* Amsterdam: Elsevier.

Sokolovsky, J. (1986). Network methodologies in the study of aging. In C. L. Fry & J. Keith (Eds.), *New methods for old age research* (pp. 231–262). South Hadley, MA: Bergin & Garvey.

Sokolovsky, J., & Vesperi, M. D. (1991, Winter). The cultural context of well-being in old age. *Generations,* pp. 21–24.

Soldo, B., & Manton, G. K. (1985). Health status and service needs of the oldest old: Current patterns and future trends. *Milbank Quarterly, 63,* 286–323.

Sorofman, B., Tripp-Reimer, T., Lauer, G., & Martin, M. (1990). Symptom self-care. *Holistic Nursing Practice, 4*(2), 45–55.

Spirduso, W., & MacRae, P. G. (1990). Motor performance and aging. In J. E.

Birren & K. W. Schaie (Eds.), *Handbook of the psychology of aging* (3rd ed., pp. 184–200). San Diego, CA: Academic Press.

Spitzer, W. O. (1987). State of science 1986: Quality of life and functional status as target variables for research. *Journal of Chronic Disease, 40,* 465–471.

Stevens, P. (1989). A critical reconceptualization of environment in nursing: Implications for methodology. *Advances in Nursing Science, 11*(4), 56–68.

Stevenson, J. S. (1977). *Issues and crises during middlescence.* New York: Appleton-Century-Crofts.

Stoller, E. P. (1993). Interpretations of symptoms by older people: A health diary study. *Journal of Aging and Health, 5,* 58–81.

Strain, L. (1990). Lay consultation among the elderly. *Journal of Aging and Health, 2,* 103–122.

Svanborg, A. (1993). A medical-social intervention in a 70-year-old Swedish population: Is it possible to postpone functional decline in aging? *Journals of Gerontology, 48,* 84–88.

Sziland, L. (1959). On the nature of the aging process. *Proceedings of the National Academy of Sciences, USA, 45,* 30–45.

Theriault, J. (1994). Retirement as a psychosocial transition: Process of adaptation to change. *International Journal of Aging and Human Development, 38*(2), 153–170.

Thomas, C. L. (Ed.). (1989). *Taber's cyclopedic medical dictionary* (16th ed., p. 939). Philadelphia: F. A. Davis.

Timiras, P. S., Hudson, D. B., & Segall, P. E. (1984). Lifetime brain serotonin: Regional effects of age and precursor availability. *Neurobiology of Aging, 5*(3), 235–242.

Tiryakian, E. A. (1968). The existential self and the person. In C. Gordon & K. J. Gergen, *The self in social interaction* (pp. 75–86). New York: Wiley.

Tornstam, L. (1989). Gerotranscendence: A reformulation of the disengagement theory. *Aging, 1,* 55–63.

Tornstam, L. (1992). The quo vadis of gerontology: On the scientific paradigm of gerontology. *The Gerontologist, 32*(3), 318–326.

Tripp-Reimer, T., & Cohen, M. (1987). Using phenomenology in health promotion research. In M. J. Duffy & N. J. Pender (Eds.), *Conceptual issues in health promotion research* (pp. 121–127). Indianapolis: Sigma Theta Tau.

Tripp-Reimer, T., Johnson, R., & Rios, H. (1995). Cultural dimensions in gerontological nursing. In M. Stanley & P. Gauntlett Beare (Eds.), *Gerontological nursing.* Philadelphia: F. A. Davis.

U.S. Department of Health and Human Services. (1990). *Healthy people 2000.* Washington, DC: USDHHS, Public Health Department.

Van Nostrand, J., Furner, S., & Suzman, R. (Eds.). (1993). Health data on older Americans: United States, 1992. *Vital Health Statistics, 3,* 27.

Verzar, F. (1963). *Lectures on experimental gerontology.* Springfield, IL: C. C Thomas.

Vickery, D., Golaszewski, T., Wright, E., & Kalmer, H. (1988). Effect of self-care interventions on the use of medical service within a Medicare population. *Medical Care, 26,* 580–588.

Walker, S., Volken, K., Sechrist, K., & Pender, N. (1988). Health promoting life styles of older adults. *Advances in Nursing Science, 11*(1), 76–90.

Wan, H. T., & Odell, G. B. (1981). Factors affecting the use of social and health services for the elderly. *Aging and Society, 1,* 95–115.

Wells, T. (1993). Setting the agenda for gerontological nursing education. In C. Heine (Ed.), *Determining the future of gerontological nursing education.* New York: NLN Press.

Wershow, H. J. (1981). *Controversial issues in gerontology.* New York: Springer Publishing Co.

Williams, G. C. (1957). Pleiotropy, natural selection, and the evolution of senescence. *Evolution, 11,* 398–411.

Williams, M. A. (1988). The physical environment and patient care. In J. J. Fitzpatrick & J. S. Stevenson (Eds.), *Annual review of nursing research, Vol. 6* (pp. 61–83). New York: Springer Publishing Co.

Wolanin, M. O. (1983). Clinical geriatric nursing research. In J. J. Fitzpatrick & J. S. Stevenson (Eds.), *Annual review of nursing research, Vol. 1* (pp. 77–79). New York: Springer Publishing Co.

Yallom, I. D. (1980). *Existential psychotherapy.* New York: Basic Books.

Young, R. F., & Olson, E. A. (1991). Overview of health and disease in later life. In R. F. Young & E. A. Olson (Eds.), *Health, illness and disability in later life* (pp. 1–7). Newbury Park, CA: Sage.

Zatz, M. M., & Goldstein, A. L. (1985). Thymosins, lymphokines, and the immunology of aging. *Gerontology, 31,* 263–277.

CHAPTER 3

Nursing of Rural Elders: Myth and Reality

Clarann Weinert and Mary E. Burman

Interest in rural issues has grown dramatically in the past decade, with increasing attention to the life circumstances and needs of rural dwellers. Because large numbers of this population are elderly, the problems of older persons who live on farms or in rural communities have become the focus of special attention (Dwyer, Lee, & Coward, 1990). Moreover, the impact of social and physical environments on the aging process and the lifestyle of elders is increasingly recognized (Coward, McLaughlin, Duncan, & Bull, 1994). Nursing also has intensified its concern with the health and health care of rural dwellers. This concern is evidenced by an emerging theory of rural nursing (Long & Weinert, 1989), publications devoted to rural nursing (Anderson, 1993; Bushy, 1991a, 1991b; Weinert & Burman, 1994; Winstead-Fry, Tiffany, & Shippee-Rice, 1992), and organizational efforts such as the establishment of the American Nurses Association Rural/Frontier Health Task Force and the American Academy of Nursing Expert Panel on Rural Populations.

Author notes: Send correspondence to Clarann Weinert, SC, PhD, RN, FAAN, College of Nursing, Sherrick Hall, Montana State University, Bozeman, Montana, 59717, telephone (406) 994-6036.

Heightened interest in rural health and rural nursing is timely, given the momentum for health care changes in the United States. Nurses are at the forefront as the country stands poised to undertake dramatic changes in the way health care is delivered. A shift away from illness and cure to a focus on wellness and care is called for in *Nursing's Agenda for Health Care Reform* (American Nurses Association [ANA], 1991). A restructured system would enhance consumer access to primary care by delivering services in a variety of community-based settings that are accessible, convenient, and familiar. Populations considered vulnerable because of inadequate access to basic health services, such as the rural elderly, would be targeted with special programs. The restructured health care system described in *Nursing's Agenda* is well suited to meet the needs of the rural elderly. Nurses have a rich history of delivering services in convenient and familiar rural sites and maximizing the use of local settings, including schools, homes, workplaces, and community facilities (ANA, 1991).

The purposes of this chapter are the following: (a) to describe the rural context, specifically related to rural elders and rural nursing; (b) to examine the availability and accessibility of health care for rural elders; and (c) to discuss issues for gerontological nursing related to research, practice, and education. The intent of this chapter is not to re-create the "wheel of rural elderly health and health services"; landmark publications are available for those who desire to explore health services and community-based services for the rural elderly (Coward, Bull, Kukulka, & Galliher, 1994; Krout, 1994b). Rather, the focus of this chapter will be on nursing issues in the provision of rural elder care.

RURAL CONTEXT

Definition of *Rural*

Policymakers and researchers have debated for many years what constitutes "rural" (Coward, McLaughlin et al., 1994). There has been widespread concern regarding a health care crisis in rural areas but little agreement as to what rural areas are (Hewitt, 1992). Two dichotomous definitions based on population size are widely used: the urban and rural categorization (U.S. Bureau of the Census, 1987) and the metropolitan and nonmetropolitan classification (Office of Management and Budget,

1983). The simplicity of these definitions is misleading. Rural America is much too diverse to be separated into distinct parts. Regional variation is manifested by the rural poor in the South, Hispanic dwellers in the Southwest, farmers and ranchers in the West and Great Plains, and the Pennsylvania Amish. Consequently, as much within-group variance as between-group variance may occur when using dichotomous classifications (Coward, McLaughlin et al., 1994). Recent effort has been focused on examining *rural* as a continuum that incorporates population, economic, occupational, and access factors (Cordes, 1987; Coward, McLaughlin et al., 1994; Ide, 1992; Krout, 1994a). Likewise, a new interval-level research measure has recently been introduced: the Montana State University Rurality Index, which is designed to assign a degree of rurality based on county population and distance to emergency care (Weinert & Boik, 1995).

As noted by Coward and colleagues (Coward, McLaughlin et al., 1994), debate over rural definition and measurement is hardly an obscure academic exercise, and conceptual and measurement issues are not trivial. Inability to define *rural* adequately thwarts researchers' and policymakers' attempts to articulate rural health needs clearly, inhibits allocation of health care resources, and deters the development of a theory base on which to deliver rural health care. Given that resolution of the definition debate is not immediately forthcoming, interpretations of the literature and research involving rural populations must be done with caution. The lens though which rural issues and the rural elderly are to be viewed must be tinted with the reality that rural America overall is not homogeneous and that rural elders are a very heterogeneous group.

Demographics

One in four older Americans (8.2 million) lives in a nonmetropolitan area (National Center for Health Statistics [NCHS], 1993). In 1990, 15% of the nonmetropolitan population was elderly, compared to 12% of the metropolitan population (NCHS, 1993). In 1990, 12% of the rural population was 65 years and older, whereas in 1960 only 9% of the rural population was elderly (Profile of the Rural U.S., 1993). The fastest-growing segment of the population is the oldest-old (age 85 or older) (Fischer, 1993). *Rural* is not synonymous with farming, as only 10% of rural elderly live on farms (Krout, 1994a). In 1980, 33% of rural elderly lived in the South, 24% in the Northeast, 26% in the Midwest, and only 17% in the

West (Office of Technology Assessment, 1990). Despite the fact that 33% of all rural elderly live in the South, the proportion of elderly is not greater in the nonmetropolitan South than in other regions (NCHS, 1993). At the beginning and the end of the 1980s, there was a net positive exchange of elderly persons into nonmetropolitan areas from metropolitan areas (Clifford & Lilley, 1993).

Typically, older rural residents have lower incomes than do older urban residents and are more likely to live in poverty. Nearly half of all older Americans with poverty-level incomes live in rural areas and small towns (Glasgow & Beale, 1985). The educational level of nonmetropolitan elders is lower than that of metropolitan elders (U.S. Senate, 1988). Rural elders are more likely to own their own homes; however, their housing tends to be in poorer condition than that of their urban counterparts (Clark, B., 1992). The oldest-old in rural areas are strikingly different from the young-old (Fischer, 1993). They are more likely to be poor, widowed women living alone, with less formal education, more limitations in daily functioning, and fewer social contacts. Limited public transportation has been a problem for rural elders (Rosenbloom, 1988). Reported frequency of contact with their children indicates that they do not have particularly strong family ties (Krout, 1988). Further, impaired rural elderly are less likely than impaired urban elderly to live with a child (Lee, Dwyer, & Coward, 1990).

Health Profile

Coward, McLaughlin, Duncan, and Bull (1994) concluded that the health profile of rural elders is different from that of their urban counterparts. On some health dimensions rural elderly do not differ from urban elderly, on some they rate lower, and on others they rate higher. In general, rural elders experience more health problems, have more functional limitations, and rate their health poorer than do urban elders. Within rural populations, diversity in factors such as occupation, age, and race results in significant differences in health status. Older rural farmers tend to have the best health profiles; nonfarm rural elders have the worst. Nonfarm rural elders report the most health problems and have the lowest functional ability in comparison to all other residential categories. Lee (1993a) found that older farmers and ranchers perceive their physical health less positively than do younger farmers and ranchers. Rural black elderly persons rate their health less positively than do their urban counterparts (NCHS, 1993).

The mental health profile of rural elderly is not clearly described. Incidence of depression in older rural adults is low, and major depressive disorders are fewer in rural areas than in urban areas (Blazer et al., 1985; O'Hara, Kohout, & Wallace, 1985). However, Johnson et al. (1988) found no difference in depression scores between urban and rural older adults. Thorson and Powell (1993) challenged the myth of urban versus rural differences as anecdotal and noted that conventional stereotypes of the health status of the rural elderly lack empirical support.

Johnson (1991) reported that positive health practices related to nutrition, sleep, exercise, and safe driving are practiced infrequently and inconsistently. For some health practices, such as complying with high-fiber and low-fat diets, maintaining appropriate weight, and refraining from heavy smoking and drinking, rural and urban differences are small (NCHS, 1993). However, rural older adults are less likely to have routine examinations, such as annual dental checkups, clinical breast screening exams, and mammograms (Mansfield, Preston, & Crawford, 1989; NCHS, 1993).

Although it is possible to construct a general profile of the health status and health-seeking behaviors of the rural elderly, care must be taken not to stereotype. The caveat that the rural elderly are a heterogeneous group is compounded by the fact that studies are not consistent or of even quality. The lack of a consistent definition of *rural,* failure to use comparison groups, lack of control for key demographic variables, and other methodological flaws are a strong signal to use the existing literature discriminatingly.

Rural Nursing

The diversity and complexity of rural areas are reflected in rural nursing practice. As Bigbee (1993) noted, rural nursing is not just a diluted or less sophisticated brand of urban nursing. A strong generalist role is combined with multiple expectations for those practicing nursing in rural settings (Bigbee, 1993; Lassiter, 1985; Rolshoven, 1982; Scharff, 1987). In the United States, nurses have historically played a central role in rural health care delivery. Today rural nursing has emerged as a strong entity in the health care delivery market (Bigbee, 1993). An understanding of subcultural values, beliefs, and norms that play a key role in how rural people define health and from whom they seek care is critical to rural nursing practice (Weinert, 1994). As noted by Long (1993), health care planning demands a knowledge of and respect for the ways in which rural dwellers conceptualize health. An effort has begun to develop a rural nursing theory on which to base nursing practice (Long & Weinert, 1989; Weinert & Long, 1990). Although rural nursing research has many limitations, a slowly growing cadre of nurse scientists is being prepared to engage in sophisticated studies of rural health and health care (Weinert & Burman, 1994).

The challenges of the "subspeciality" of rural nursing are not trivial. To address these theory, research, and practice issues, nurse researchers must have an adequate profile of nurses living and practicing in rural settings. An understanding of the characteristics of rural nurses can assist researchers and policymakers in finding ways to advocate for programs at federal and state levels, facilitate professional development of nurses, enhance the access of registered nurses (RNs) to upward-mobility programs, facilitate networking among rural nurses, and enable nurses to become better advocates for the rural elderly. However, just as it is difficult to get an accurate profile of rural elderly, so too it is difficult to describe rural nurses accurately. Information is lacking, and data bases are often not comparable because of inconsistencies in the definition of *rural.*

Approximately 1.9 million RNs are in practice today in the United States. Approximately 140,000 of these work in counties of fewer than 50,000 residents. In rural America there are only 384 RNs per 100,000 people, whereas in the United States in general there are 675 RNs per 100,000 population. This ratio varies widely by geographic location, with a high of 749 RNs per 100,000 in the mid-Atlantic states to a low of 254 RNs per 100,000 in the East South Central states (C. Wasem, personal communication, January 26, 1994).

Overall, the education level of rural RNs is lower than that of RNs practicing in urban settings. In urban areas, 36.1% of RNs have diplomas; 27.2%, associate degrees; and 29.5%, baccalaureate degrees, as the highest level of education. In rural areas, 41.2% have diplomas; 36.2%, associate degrees; and only 20.1%, BSN preparation. Rural nurses are older than urban nurses, and collectively, the oldest group of nurses comprises those working in the smallest rural counties (C. Wasem, personal communication, January 26, 1994).

The settings in which rural nurses practice reflect the rural health care system. Almost one fifth (19.9%) work in nursing homes, and 53% work in hospitals. This situation contrasts with the picture of urban nursing, where 68.9% work in hospitals and only 6.6% in nursing homes (C. Wasem, personal communication, January 26, 1994). This pattern is most likely associated with the fact that many small rural counties do not have hospitals, yet may have nursing homes. With hospital closures and restructuring, some acute care facilities in rural areas have been converted to provide nursing home services to meet the needs of the large elderly population.

The public health infrastructure has traditionally been a mainstay in rural health care delivery. More rural than urban nurses are employed in public health nursing (11.8% and 6.3%, respectively). In the smallest counties, 14.4% of RNs are employed in public health. In a recent survey of 10 states, 50% or more of the public health nurses were prepared at less than a BSN level (C. Wasem, personal communication, January 26, 1994). Dunkin (1993) reported that, nationwide, rural public health nurses are less likely to be prepared at the BSN level and much less likely to be prepared at the master's or doctoral level. Finally, the percentage of nurses working in school health in rural counties of between 10,000 and 25,000 residents is 4.3%, whereas in large counties and in urban areas only 2.9% are working in school health.

Nurse practitioners (NPs) play a valuable role in providing primary care in rural areas. NPs practice in all 50 states, and family nurse practitioners constitute the majority of rural nurse practitioners (American Academy of Nurse Practitioners [AANP], 1988; Towers, 1988). Seventy percent of rural NPs provide care to the elderly (AANP, 1988). Since 1984 the percentage of NPs has decreased in rural areas, from 18% to 15.8%. Health care reform plans, by both President Clinton and the American Nurses Association, call for expanded roles and increased use of advanced practice nurses (APNs). However, this call may provide yet another challenge to rural nursing and actually decrease the number of APNs available to practice in rural areas. The incentives to work in large urban systems that offer more varied work environments and higher salaries could provide greater recruiting power. In addition, physician assistants and clinical nurse specialists will be used to "back-fill" the positions left in hospitals when medical residents shift from subspeciality fields to primary care and from inpatient settings to ambulatory care settings (Physicians Payment Review Commission, 1993). Currently, other advanced practice nurses, such as certified registered nurse anesthetists (CRNAs), also play a critical role in rural health care.

In summary, rural elders and rural nurses are very heterogeneous groups. In general, rural elders are increasing as a proportion of the population. Older adults in rural areas are better off on some health measures, poorer on some, and equal on others, compared to urban elders. Rural nurses tend to be older, to have less education, and to work in noninstitutional settings.

AVAILABILITY AND ACCESSIBILITY OF HEALTH CARE

Crisis in Rural Health Care

Health care for all rural dwellers has been characterized as in a crisis (Straub & Walzer, 1992b). Decreased population bases for many rural areas, inequities between rural and urban areas in governmental reimbursement for health care, expensive advances in technology with resulting shifts in patient care to urban centers, and continued increased demands for health care because of the growing number of rural elders have led to this crisis (Straub & Walzer, 1992a). Many rural health organizations are small, serve large areas, and may lack the capacity to change rapidly as health care in general changes (Burman, Steffes, & Weinert, 1994; Krout, 1991). Geographic isolation, economic deprivation, lack of rural human service infrastructure, and lack of a trained labor pool further inhibit the ability of rural health care organizations to respond to changes in the system (Bull, Howard, & Bane, 1991).

Amundson (1993) argued forcefully that external forces are not the only cause of the current crisis in rural health care; communities have been unable to identify and respond effectively to the health needs and expectancies of local constituencies. He asserted that rural areas are characterized by an outmigration of residents to urban centers for care, ineffective community leadership, poor quality of care, and inadequate performance of health care providers. Amundson's assertions may be supported in part by another study examining long-term-care development in rural communities, which showed that the factors related to effective long-term-care services in communities include good leadership, broad horizontal networking among local constituencies and providers, connections with central decision makers in the larger political arena, and values and attitudes that support the development of these services (Kaiser, Camp, & Gibbons, 1987).

In general, rural elders have access to fewer health care services and a more restricted range than do urban elders (Hassinger, Hicks, & Godino, 1993; Krout, 1994a, 1994c). However, Salmon, Nelson, and Rous (1993) argued that the notion that rural areas have fewer services is simplistic and that a more accurate representation is that rural areas have greater variability or an uneven development of health care for elders. This variability within rural areas is evident in the distribution of physicians, nurses, and dentists (Coward, McLaughlin et al., 1994; NCHS, 1993). Wallace and Colsher (1994) noted that lowered availability of providers results in lowered utilization rates for rural elders. An additional problem is longer waiting and traveling times for health care (NCHS, 1993). In Montana, round-trip mileage for cancer treatment for those living in isolated rural areas averages 214 miles (Bender, Weinert, Faulkner, & Quimby, 1991). Rural elders differ in their perception of acceptability of local health care resources; some elect to travel considerable distances for medical care and hospitalization, and others stay within the local community for care (Magilvy, Congdon, & Martinez, 1994).

Long-Term-Care Continuum

Health care for elders, whether rural or urban, has been described as a continuum of care, ranging from community-based services and in-home services to institutional care (Nelson & Salmon, 1993). Older adults move back and forth along this continuum of care as their needs and abilities change. Diagnostic, preventive, therapeutic, rehabilitative, supportive, and maintenance services should be available. Specific services include adult day care, respite care, in-home personal care, information and referral, congregate meals, Meals-on-Wheels, and nursing home care (Havens & Kyle, 1993). The desired outcome of these services is to allow the older adult to "age in place": to remain in his or her own home (Havens & Kyle, 1993).

Almost 80% of all elder care is provided by informal resources (Havens & Kyle, 1993); family members, usually spouses or adult children, typically provide the most assistance (Craig, 1991; Stoller & Lee, 1994). Functional and behavioral needs are met primarily by the informal network resources (Schultz, 1990). Informal sources of help are generally supplemented only when the needs of the elder exceed the abilities of available informal resources.

Rural areas generally offer few community-based services, and there is a huge variation in their availability (Krout, 1994a, 1994c). Little research has examined the availability of community-based services, such as congregate meals and adult day care, but differences between rural and urban areas have been found in the provision of senior center programs and activities (Krout, 1987). Rural Area Agencies on Aging (AAAs) serve larger, more sparsely populated areas with poorer and older elderly populations, compared to urban AAAs (Krout, 1991). Salmon, Nelson, and Rous (1993) found that specific community-based services should be examined separately. To illustrate, transportation expenditures are greater in rural areas, whereas expenditures for adult day care and protective services are greater in urban areas. Rural elders are less likely to use community-based services, with the exception of senior center programs, than are urban elders (Coward, McLaughlin et al., 1994). Lack of awareness of available community resources may lead to less use of services by rural elders (Schultz, 1990).

Rural providers and clients have described significant gaps in home-based services for the elderly (Buehler & Lee, 1992; Burman et al., 1994; Magilvy, Congdon, & Martinez, 1994; Sharp, Halpert, & Breytspraak, 1988). However, few differences in availability between urban and rural settings have been found in empirical studies (Nelson & Salmon, 1993; Redford & Severns, 1994). Other factors, such as provider characteristics and area poverty levels, have a greater influence on availability and accessibility. Despite the similarities in home health care availability in rural and urban areas (Nelson, 1994; Redford & Severns, 1994), rural elders with functional limitations are less likely to receive that care (Clark, D., 1992; NCHS, 1993). Furthermore, rural elders have more skilled care needs than do urban elders (Schultz, 1990). The urban advantage in home care use may be due to higher reimbursement ceilings, more Visiting Nurse Associations, and greater availability of support services (Kenney, 1993).

Finally, diversity also is evident in institutional care: rural areas have fewer nursing home beds, 26.9 per 1,000, than do urban areas, which have 35.1 per 1,000 (Nelson & Salmon, 1993; Salmon et al., 1993), but rural counties are overrepresented in both the highest and lowest quartiles. Dubay (1993) attributed increased access to nursing homes in some rural populations to swing beds (acute care beds that can be used for long-term care when the necessity arises). Shaughnessy (1994) found a significantly higher proportion of nursing homes combined with hospitals in rural areas than in urban areas, and rural nursing homes provide relatively more intermediate levels of care and less skilled care than do urban nursing homes. Sadly, rural elders may be institutionalized at a greater rate than urban elders (Greene, 1984; Shaughnessy, 1994).

Rural hospitals have had a rocky history, particularly since the implementation of prospective payment by Medicare. Disproportionately high rates of rural hospital closures have sparked great concern locally and nationally. Duncan (1994) described a double jeopardy for rural hospitals: the people with the greatest need for local hospital care, found in great numbers in rural areas, are those who are "least desirable" from a reimbursement standpoint. Rural hospitals tend to be small, although in the aggregate they represent a large share of the hospital sector (Duncan, 1994). Inpatient mental health services are most likely to be found in heavily urbanized areas and least likely to be found in the most rural areas (Wagenfeld, Goldsmith, Stiles, & Manderscheid, 1988). Differences between urban and rural use of hospitals are minimized, however, if age is controlled for (Hicks, 1992).

In conclusion, health care in rural areas is characterized by fewer resources and high variability. The most rural areas are likely to have the fewest resources. The sparseness and variability in rural health services for older adults may have an impact on the ability to "manage" care, whether through case management or through formal managed care systems (Parker et al., 1991). In general, rural elders tend to use health care resources to a lesser degree than their urban counterparts do. This difference may be due to lack of availability and accessibility of services; inadequate knowledge of available health care resources; confounding effects of poverty, unemployment, and lack of insurance; and a discomfort with formal resources on the part of rural populations (Dwyer et al., 1990; Hassinger et al., 1993; Hicks, 1992; Magilvy et al., 1994; Weinert & Long, 1987).

ISSUES FOR RURAL GERONTOLOGICAL NURSING

Research

The body of research on rural elders has grown phenomenally in the past decade; however, rural nursing research is limited. The knowledge base for rural gerontological nursing practice is inadequate, and many unanswered questions remain to be addressed by nurse researchers (Coward,

McLaughlin et al., 1994; Weinert & Burman, 1994). The developing theory base needs further validation within and between rural populations and in contrast with urban populations (Weinert & Burman, 1994). Further, nursing research must examine in more careful detail the health-seeking behaviors of various rural groups and the corresponding differences in health status and in the health care delivery systems.

Rural research, including that involving elderly populations, is of widely differing levels of sophistication. Studies are often divergent in content and conclusions, ranging from highly structured data-based studies to individual case studies and anecdotal reports (Weinert & Burman, 1994). As with many bodies of research, studies examining rural populations and health-related phenomena suffer from small sample sizes, cross-sectional designs, and lack of random sampling. Unique flaws also plague rural research: lack of clear or consistent definitions, limited samples (such as elders living in a particular state), and few targeted research programs (Weinert & Burman, 1994).

To enhance the rural gerontological nursing knowledge base, targeted programs of research are needed. Very few studies on rural topics address similar topic areas and little in-depth investigation and knowledge development are evident (Weinert & Burman, 1994). Buckwalter and colleagues are an exception. This team of researchers and clinicians has examined the mental health problems of rural older adults, focusing on cognitively impaired elders, and has concluded that the rural elderly have limited access to psychiatrists and are underserved by community mental health centers (Buckwalter, Abraham, Smith, & Smullen, 1993; Buckwalter, McLeran, Mitchell, & Andrews, 1988; Buckwalter, Smith, Zevenbergen, & Russell, 1991). In addition, too few health professionals are adequately prepared to meet the mental health needs of the rural elderly; general practitioners, public health nurses, social service workers, and others dealing with the rural elderly must be educated to understand mental health needs, provide basic care, and make referrals.

Establishing beginning projects, as well as developing programs of research, may be very difficult for rural nurse researchers. Those nurses in the best position to do research focused on the health and health care of rural elders often are located in environments with limited resources for research, such as small health care organizations many miles from a health services library or facility. Rapidly expanding computer communication technologies are extremely valuable, allowing linkages between isolated nurse clinicians, nurse researchers, university faculty, other health care providers, and rural health care organizations, such as Area Health Education Centers (AHECs) and the National Rural Health Association.

Students and practicing nurses must have their interest stimulated in rural health and health care issues for older adults. Recent publications on rural nursing (e.g., Bushy, 1991a, 1991b) and those on rural gerontological nursing (Johnson, 1991; Lee, 1993a, 1993b) should be helpful. Predoctoral and postdoctoral programs focusing on rural elder care issues can help nurses understand rural concepts, gerontological theories and practices, and methodologies appropriate for rural populations. In a broader sense, such programs also can help nurses gain an appreciation of the challenges and opportunities of rural research. Mentor programs could be developed between nursing faculty in isolated rural areas and successful faculty scholars at larger research institutions.

Practice

Gaps clearly exist in the delivery of adequate and appropriate care to older adults in rural areas, and nurses are in a position to address some of these unmet needs. Yet nurses should be aware of the realities. First, a general disparity exists between the availability and use of services between urban and rural areas. Are rural elderly able to obtain the services they need so that they may "age in place"? Second, the supply of rural health practitioners, particularly nurses, has been a continual problem. Finally, although this is a time of many opportunities, given the possibility of health care reform, this is also a time of fiscal conservatism. Money will not be "thrown" at rural problems.

The array of innovative models to deliver services to rural (and urban) elders is fairly extensive and follows the general notion of a continuum of care. Rural gerontological nurses are advised to use and adapt what is available. Lee (1993b), describing individual and community-level strategies for providing nursing care to rural elderly clients, recommended "multipurpose packages" that serve the elderly as well as other rural populations, using existing community systems and structures such as churches and schools as sites for care and formulating linkages between providers to increase coordination and decrease duplication of services. Nursing centers (or nurse-managed clinics) have been promoted as a means to meet the health needs of rural dwellers, including older adults (Barger, 1991; Barnett & Bigbee, 1991).

Several issues arise when adapting existing urban programs to rural areas or when taking existing programs from one rural setting to another. First, if the model has been developed in an urban setting, is it appropriate for a rural setting? Or if it was developed in one rural setting, is it appropriate for another rural setting? Program planners must recognize the limitations of rural health care delivery systems, as well as the unique features of local areas, such as environmental, social, political, and economic factors. Shippee-Rice and Mahoney (1992) described a family caregiver training program designed to "assist caregivers to meet their caretaking responsibilities with greater skill and knowledge and with less physical and emotional strain on themselves and the elderly care recipients" (p. 100). The program is based on a partnership between a nurse facilitator and rural caregivers, in which caregivers identify unique needs to be addressed in the training. With some modification this program probably would be useful in a variety of rural settings because the focus is on identifying specific and unique needs of rural caregivers.

Second, how can available local resources, people, and organizations be used in delivering programs to the elderly? To be successful, programs also need to incorporate local informal helping networks. Many programs have effectively used community volunteers to provide a variety of in-home and community-based services for elders. For example, partnerships between nurse researchers, rural communities, and rural elders with arthritis was the basis of the Arthritis Self-Care Project (Goeppinger, 1993). Community members, trained by nurses, taught others how to deal with the emotional and physical aspects of chronic arthritis. Partnerships such as the Arthritis Self-Care Project can lead to positive participant outcomes, including increased knowledge about arthritis and self-management, enhanced self-care behaviors, and decreased pain and helplessness. Reciprocity also is an important issue for rural elders and should be considered in program development (Stoller & Lee, 1994). Incorporating mechanisms, through payment or other forms of reimbursement, for elders to reciprocate for services provided may be an important factor for successful rural programs. For example, paying the wages of in-home assistants may enhance the psychological independence of rural elders and decrease feelings of dependency.

Third, a variety of mechanisms to "go to the client," rather than having the client come to the health care provider, should be considered. Outreach programs for education and ambulatory care could be very beneficial. A promising model for support of rural elders is through the use of computers (Brennan, Moore, & Smyth, 1991). ComputerLink was developed to provide electronic linkages between caregivers of Alzheimer's disease patients, the primary goal being to provide social support. In this nursing research project, computers were found to be readily accepted and used by the caregivers. For people separated by large geographic distances, electronic computer networks may become an innovative way to deliver nursing services such as providing information and giving support. However, when adapting this model to a rural setting, the area's ability to undertake such a project must be assessed. What is the level of comfort with computers of the providers and participants? Are computer technicians available to handle computer problems? What are the available capabilities for linkages with existing computer networks?

Fourth, are the resources available to implement a particular program in a rural area, given the nature of rural health care, which is characterized by fewer available resources, and of rural nursing, which is typified by older nurses and few nurses prepared at advanced levels? Although a variety of models have been described for delivery of health care resources to older adults, the challenge is to develop programs that can be sustained, given the strengths and limitations in the rural nursing resource base. For example, models that rely heavily on APNs may not be appropriate at this time in rural areas.

Education

Just as health care in general is undergoing changes, nursing education is being transformed. New models of faculty practice are being created that blend research, teaching, and clinical practice. A variety of strategies will be needed to maintain and enhance the cadre of rural gerontological nurses.

First, undergraduate and graduate nursing curricula must be carefully examined. Are the skills necessary to practice in a rural, generalist setting being provided? In addition to basic nursing skills, rural gerontological nurses also need to have skills in community assessment, development, and leadership. Successful gerontological nursing interventions involve partnerships designed to mobilize community resources. For example, the Geriatric Center at East Tennessee State University has developed a collaborative adult day care center (Turner, 1991). "Health ministers," key resource persons from the community, are trained to provide peer support to families with frail and/or cognitively impaired elders. This kind of mobilization of community resources takes specialized skills, and we must make certain nurses have these.

In addition, creative strategies must be used for delivery of both basic and continuing nursing education to facilitate the professional development of practicing rural nurses. The focus on specialization, typical of many nursing education programs, may be a deterrent to practice in rural areas. The generalist role of the rural nurse may be uncomfortable and undesirable to students and nurses coming from a strong specialization orientation. Generalist preparation, interdisciplinary orientation, and even dual preparation, such as an RN and emergency medical technician (EMT), for example, may be appropriate for rural areas. Although several schools of nursing have successfully used rural health practicums (Arlton, 1984; McDonough, Lambert, & Billue, 1992; Predhomme, 1985), there are, unfortunately, too few of them (Straub & Frels, 1992). Currently, schools of nursing have little incentive to build rural programs, given fiscal constraints, adequate student enrollments, and job opportunities in urban areas for graduating students (Weis, 1992).

For rural nurses working with older adults, continuing education and professional development can be very challenging. Continuing education programs must capitalize on available resources. What role do AHECs and agricultural extension agencies play in the continuing education of practicing nurses? Information technologies already available can provide linkages for rural nurses with on-line computer searches, data bases, and current nursing information. In addition, electronic linkages with academic and health care institutions are available to assist with clinical and research issues. For example, two-way interactive video from the Medical College of Georgia Telemedicine Project is used to provide educational programs to remote sites in the Continuing Health Professions Education Program (C. Schultz, personal communication, January 1994). In Colorado, students and health care providers can connect electronically with the University of Colorado using Denver Free-Net to access health-related information on Parkinson's disease, men's health, and school health.

The Nursing Approaches to Quality Care for the Elderly module series developed at Montana State University is one creative approach to meet the needs of practicing rural nurses interested in gerontology (Cudney, 1991). Twenty modules, each consisting of a videotape and booklet, cover all topics required for certification by the American Nurses Association as a gerontological nurse. Fifteen of the modules address common clinical problems, and the remaining five focus on leadership and management. These in-depth, comprehensive self-study modules feature interviews with and demonstrations by rural and nationally known gerontological nurse experts (S. Cudney, personal communication, February 10, 1994).

A final, very sensitive issue is that of entry into practice. Associate degree (AD) education programs have been a way to increase the supply of RNs in rural areas because these programs often target older, nontraditional students, are generally less costly than 4-year programs, and take less time than 4-ycar programs (Weis, 1992). However, the large numbers of AD graduates may be a deterrent to the professional practice of rural gerontological nursing, which calls for a generalist approach with sophisticated clinical and leadership skills.

Consequently, we need to work toward differentiation of institutional nursing practice and community/public health nursing while facilitating the return of AD/diploma nurses for completion of the BSN. Targeting students from rural areas may be one mechanism to increase the supply of rural nurses (Weis, 1992). Educational programs must be tailored to the needs of rural nurses and made more "user-friendly." Telecommunications to remote locations can play a significant role in delivering educational programs. The University of Wyoming School of Nursing is using compressed video to broadcast undergraduate nursing courses to RNs throughout Wyoming. Interactive TV is used at the University of New Mexico to broadcast nursing courses via satellite. Anyone can pick up the courses by "dish," and prerequisites can be obtained at local community colleges.

CONCLUSIONS

Disparities exist in the health and health care of urban and rural elders. Those living in rural areas tend to be in poorer health and to have access to fewer health care resources. Nursing is in a position to work toward resolution of these discrepancies in health status and health care. Indeed, rural nurses have a long history of caring and activism to address the health care needs of rural elders.

Furthermore, the ideas put forth in *Nursing's Agenda for Health Care Reform* (ANA, 1991) support enhancing access to quality services in convenient and familiar locations. These ideas should facilitate meeting the health needs of rural elders. Nurses should work toward the development of adequate in-home and community-based services for rural elders. To accomplish this, rural nurses must be able to mobilize community resources through coalition building and sensitivity to unique rural values and beliefs. Nurses working with rural older adults must confront both the myths and realities of rural life and rural health care. Rural environments are extremely varied and provide challenges in meeting the needs of the elderly. Contrary to television commercials, the lives of few elderly correspond to romantic notions of country living, with rocking chairs, rolling farm fields, and lots of grandchildren squealing with wiggly puppies. Yet rural life also can create a supportive milieu in which older Americans can thrive. Rural gerontological nurses are uniquely qualified to help elders realize this latter vision of rural America.

REFERENCES

American Academy of Nurse Practitioners (AANP). (1988). *American Academy of Nurse Practitioners National Survey.* Unpublished report.
American Nurses Association. (1991). *Nursing's agenda for health care reform.* Washington, DC: Author.
Amundson, B. (1993). Myth and reality in the rural health service crisis: Facing up to community responsibilities. *Journal of Rural Health, 8,* 176–187.
Anderson, J. (1993). Rural nursing. *Nursing Clinics of North America, 28,* 121–226.
Arlton, D. (1984). The rural nursing practicum. *Nursing Outlook, 32,* 204–206.
Barger, S. (1991). The nursing center: A model for rural nursing practice. *Nursing and Health Care, 12,* 290–294.
Barnett, J., & Bigbee, J. (1991). Nursing centers: One approach to rural health care. In A. Bushy (Ed.), *Rural nursing* (Vol. 2, pp. 166–178). Newbury Park, CA: Sage.
Bender, L., Weinert, C., Faulkner, L., & Quimby, R. (1991). *Montana families living with cancer.* Bozeman, MT: Montana State University, College of Nursing.
Bigbee, J. (1993). The uniqueness of rural nursing. *Nursing Clinics of North America, 28,* 131–144.
Blazer, D., George, L., Landerman, R., Pennyback, M., Melville, M., Woodbury, M., Manton, K., Jordon, K., & Locke, B. (1985). Psychiatric disorders: A rural/urban comparison. *Archives of General Psychiatry, 42,* 651–656.
Brennan, P., Moore, S., & Smyth, K. (1991). ComputerLink: Electronic support for the home caregiver. *Advances in Nursing Science, 13*(4), 14–27.
Buckwalter, K., Abraham, I., Smith, M., & Smullen, D. (1993). Nursing outreach to rural elderly people who are mentally ill. *Hospital and Community Psychiatry, 44,* 821–823.

Buckwalter, K., McLeran, K., Mitchell, S., & Andrews, P. (1988). Responding to mental health needs of the elderly in rural areas: A collaborative geriatric education center model. *Gerontology and Geriatrics Education, 8*(3/4), 69–80.

Buckwalter, K., Smith, M., Zevenbergen, P., & Russell, D. (1991). Mental health services of the Rural Elderly Outreach Program. *The Gerontologist, 31,* 408–412.

Buehler, J., & Lee, H. (1992). Exploration of home care resources for rural families with cancer. *Cancer Nursing, 15,* 299–308.

Bull, C., Howard, D., & Bane, S. (1991). *Challenges and solutions to the provision of programs and services to rural elders.* Kansas City: University of Missouri–Kansas City.

Burman, M., Steffes, M., & Weinert, C. (1994). Cancer care in Montana. *Home Health Care Services Quarterly, 14*(2/3), 37–52.

Bushy, A. (Ed.). (1991a). *Rural nursing* (Vol. 1). Newbury Park, CA: Sage.

Bushy, A. (Ed.). (1991b). *Rural nursing* (Vol. 2). Newbury Park, CA: Sage.

Clark, B. (1992). Housing for rural elders. In C. Bull & S. Bane (Eds.), *The future of aging in rural America* (pp. 101–115). Kansas City, MO: National Resource Center for Rural Elderly.

Clark, D. (1992). Residence differences in formal and informal long-term care. *The Gerontologist, 32,* 227–233.

Clifford, W., & Lilley, S. (1993). Rural elderly: Their demographic characteristics. In C. Bull (Ed.), *Aging in rural America* (pp. 3–16). Newbury Park, CA: Sage.

Cordes, S. (1987). The changing rural environment and the relationship between health services and rural development. *Health Services Research, 23,* 757–784.

Coward, R., Bull, C., Kukulka, G., & Galliher, J. (1994). *Health services for rural elders.* New York: Springer Publishing Co.

Coward, R., McLaughlin, D., Duncan, R., & Bull, C. (1994). An overview of health and aging in rural American. In R. Coward, N. Bull, G. Kukulka, & J. Galliher (Eds.), *Health services for rural elders* (pp. 1–32). New York: Springer Publishing Co.

Craig, C. (1991). Down home: An ethnography about community process and health of older persons in a rural setting (Doctoral dissertation, University of Colorado Health Sciences Center, 1991). *Dissertation Abstracts International, 52,* 12B.

Cudney, S. (1991). Making gerontic continuing education accessible for rural nurses. *Journal of Gerontological Nursing, 17*(7), 29–34.

Dubay, L. (1993). Explaining urban–rural differences in the use of skilled nursing facility benefit. *Medical Care, 31,* 111–129.

Duncan, R. (1994). Rural hospitals and rural elders. In R. Coward, C. Bull, G. Kukulka, & J. Galliher (Eds.), *Health services for rural elders* (pp. 127–143). New York: Springer Publishing Co.

Dunkin, J. (1993). *The state of public health nursing.* In *Proceedings of an Invitational Conference for Regions VIII and X* (pp. 11–19). Spokane, WA: Division of Nursing and Office of Rural Health Policy, Maternal and Child Health Bureau.

Dwyer, J., Lee, G., & Coward, R. (1990). The health status, health services utilization, and support networks of the rural elderly: A decade review. *Journal of Rural Health, 6,* 379–398.

Fischer, L. (1993). The oldest-old in rural Minnesota. In C. Bull (Ed.), *Aging in rural America* (pp. 30–42). Newbury Park, CA: Sage.

Glasgow, J., & Beale, C. (1985). Rural elderly in demographic perspective. *Rural Development Perspectives, 2*(1), 22–26.

Goeppinger, J. (1993). Health promotion for rural populations: Partnership interventions. *Family and Community Health, 16,* 1–10.

Greene, V. (1984). Premature institutionalization among the rural elderly in Arizona. *Public Health Reports, 99,* 58–63.

Hassinger, E., Hicks, L., & Godino, V. (1993). A literature review of health issues of the rural elderly. *Journal of Rural Health, 9,* 68–75.

Havens, B., & Kyle, B. (1993). Formal long-term care. In C. Bull (Ed.), *Aging in rural America* (pp. 173–188). Newbury Park, CA: Sage.

Hewitt, M. (1992). Defining rural areas: Impact on health care policy and research. In W. Gesler & T. Ricketts (Eds.), *Health in rural North America* (pp. 25–54). New Brunswick, NJ: Rutgers University Press.

Hicks, L. (1992). Access and utilization: Special populations—special needs. In L. Straub & N. Walzer (Eds.), *Rural health care. Innovation in a changing environment* (pp. 20–35). Westport, CT: Praeger.

Ide, B. (1992, 4th quarter). A process model of rural nursing. *Texas Journal of Rural Health,* pp. 30–34.

Johnson, J. (1991). Health-care practices of the rural aged. *Journal of Gerontological Nursing, 17,* 15–19.

Johnson, T., Hendricks, J., Turner, H., Stallones, I., Marx, M., & Garrity, T. (1988). Social networks and depression among the elderly: Metropolitan/nonmetropolitan comparisons. *Journal of Rural Health, 4,* 72–83.

Kaiser, M., Camp, H., & Gibbons, J. (1987). Services for the rural elderly: A developmental model. *Journal of Gerontological Social Work, 11*(1/2), 25–45.

Kenney, G. (1993). Is access to home health care a problem in rural areas? *American Journal of Public Health, 83,* 412–414.

Krout, J. (1987). Rural-urban differences in senior center activities and services. *The Gerontologist, 27,* 92–97.

Krout, J. (1988). Rural versus urban differences in elderly parents' contact with their children. *The Gerontologist, 28,* 198–203.

Krout, J. (1991). Rural Area Agencies on Aging: An overview of activities and policy issues. *Journal of Aging Studies, 5,* 409–424.

Krout, J. (1994a). An overview of older rural populations and community-based services. In J. Krout (Ed.), *Providing community-based services to the rural elderly* (pp. 3–18). Thousand Oaks, CA: Sage.

Krout, J. (Ed.). (1994b). *Providing community-based services to the rural elderly.* Thousand Oaks, CA: Sage.

Krout, J. (1994c). Rural aging community-based services. In R. Coward, C. Bull, G. Kukulka, & J. Galliher (Eds.), *Health services for rural elders* (pp. 84–107). New York: Springer Publishing Co.

Lassiter, P. (1985). Education for rural health professionals: Nurses. *Journal of Rural Health, 1,* 23–26.

Lee, G., Dwyer, J., & Coward, R. (1990). Residential location and proximity to children among impaired elderly parents *Rural Sociology, 55,* 579–589.

Lee, H. (1993a). Health perceptions of middle, "new middle," and older rural adults. *Family and Community Health, 16,* 19–27.

Lee, H. (1993b). Rural elderly individuals: Strategies for delivery of nursing care. *Nursing Clinics of North America, 28,* 219–230.

Long, K. (1993). The concept of health. *Nursing Clinics of North America, 28,* 123–130.

Long, K., & Weinert, C. (1989). Rural nursing: Developing the theory base. *Scholarly Inquiry for Nursing, 3,* 113–127.

Magilvy, J., Congdon, J., & Martinez, R. (1994). Circles of care: Home care and community supports for rural older adults. *Advances in Nursing Science, 16*(3), 22–33.

Mansfield, P., Preston, D., & Crawford, C. (1989). The health behaviors of rural women: Comparisons with an urban sample. *Health Values, 13*(6), 12–20.

McDonough, J., Lambert, V., & Billue, J. (1992). A rural nursing practicum: Making it work. *Nurse Educator, 17*(4), 30–34.

National Center for Health Statistics. (1993). *Common beliefs about the rural elderly: What do national data tell us?* (DHHS Publication No. PHS 93–1412). Washington, DC: U.S. Government Printing Office.

Nelson, G. (1994). In-home services for rural elders. In R. Coward, C. Bull, G. Kukulka, & J. Galliher (Eds.), *Health services for rural elders* (pp. 65–83). New York: Springer Publishing Co.

Nelson, G., & Salmon, M. (1993). Systems of home and community care. In C. Bull (Ed.), *Aging in rural America* (pp. 189–203). Newbury Park, CA: Sage.

Office of Management and Budget. (1983). *Metropolitan statistical areas.* Washington, DC: U.S. Government Printing Office. (NTIS No. PB83-218891)

Office of Technology Assessment. (1990). *Health care in rural America* (OTA Publication No. OTA-H-434). Washington, DC: U.S. Government Printing Office.

O'Hara, M., Kohout, F., & Wallace, R. (1985). Depression among the rural elderly: A study of prevalence and correlates. *Journal of Nervous and Mental Diseases, 173,* 582–589.

Parker, M., Quinn, J., Viehl, M., McKinely, A., Polich, C., Detzner, D., Hartwell, S., & Korn, K. (1991). Case management in rural areas: Definition, clients, financing, staffing, and service issues. In A. Bushy (Ed.), *Rural nursing* (Vol. 2, pp. 29–40). Newbury Park, CA: Sage.

Physicians Payment Review Commission. (1993). *Physician Payment Review Commission: Annual report to Congress.* Washington, DC: Author.

Predhomme, J. (1985). Bringing baccalaureate nursing education to the rural setting. *Journal of Nursing Education, 24,* 123–125.

Profile of the Rural U.S. (1993). *Aging, 365,* 11.

Redford, L., & Severns, A. (1994). Home health services in rural America. In J.

Krout (Ed.), *Providing community-based services to the rural elderly* (pp. 221–242). Thousand Oaks, CA: Sage.

Rolshoven, R. (1982). Rural nursing: A challenge not for everyone. *Nursing Careers, 3,* 10–15.

Rosenbloom, S. (1988). *Mobility needs of the elderly* (Special Report No. 218). Washington, DC: Transportation Research Board.

Salmon, M., Nelson, G., & Rous, S. (1993). The continuum of care revisited: A rural perspective. *The Gerontologist, 33,* 658–666.

Scharff, J. (1987). *The nature and scope of rural nursing: Distinctive characteristics.* Unpublished master's thesis, Montana State University, Bozeman.

Schultz, A. (1990). Rural/urban differences in health care needs of the elderly after discharge to home (Doctoral dissertation, Oregon Health Sciences University, 1990). *Dissertation Abstracts International, 52,* 5761B.

Sharp, T., Halpert, B., & Breytspraak, L. (1988). Impact of Medicare's prospective payment system and the farm crisis on the health care of the elderly: A case study. *Journal of Rural Health, 4*(3), 45–56.

Shaughnessy, P. (1994). Changing institutional long-term care to improve rural health care. In R. Coward, C. Bull, G. Kukulka, & J. Galliher (Eds.), *Health services for rural elders* (pp. 144–181). New York: Springer Publishing Co.

Shippee-Rice, R., & Mahoney, D. (1992). Training family caregivers of rural elderly. In P. Winstead-Fry, J. Tiffany, & R. Shippee-Rice (Eds.), *Rural health nursing* (pp. 79–126). New York: National League for Nursing Press.

Stoller, E., & Lee, G. (1994). Informal care of rural elders. In R. Coward, C. Bull, G. Kukulka, & J. Galliher (Eds.), *Health services for rural elders* (pp. 33–64). New York: Springer Publishing Co.

Straub, L., & Frels, L. (1992). The role of nursing education in preparing students for rural practice. *Journal of Rural Health, 8,* 291–297.

Straub, L., & Walzer, N. (1992a). Financing the demand for rural health care. In L. Straub & N. Walzer (Eds.), *Rural health care. Innovation in a changing environment* (pp. 3–19). Westport, CT: Praeger.

Straub, L., & Walzer, N. (Eds.). (1992b). *Rural health care. Innovation in a changing environment.* Westport, CT: Praeger.

Thorson, J., & Powell, F. (1993). The rural aged, social value, and health care. In C. Bull (Ed.), *Aging in rural America* (pp. 134–145). Newbury Park, CA: Sage.

Towers, J. (1988). *Utilization of nurse practitioners in care of the rural elderly: Testimony of the American Academy of Nurse Practitioners before the Senate Select Committee on Aging.*

Turner, T. (1991). Health promotion for rural black elderly: Community-based program development. In A. Bushy (Ed.), *Rural nursing* (Vol. 1, pp. 256–266). Newbury Park, CA: Sage.

U.S. Bureau of the Census. (1987). *Statistical abstract of the United States: 1988* (108th ed.). Washington, DC: U.S. Government Printing Office.

U.S. Senate, Special Committee on Aging. (1988). *Developments in aging: 1987* (Vol. 3). Washington, DC: U.S. Government Printing Office.

Wagenfeld, M., Goldsmith, H., Stiles, D., & Manderscheid, R. (1988). Inpatient mental health services in metropolitan and nonmetropolitan counties. *Journal of Rural Community Psychology, 9*(2), 13–28.

Wallace, R., & Colsher, R. (1994). Improving ambulatory and acute services for the rural elderly: Current solutions, research, and policy directions. In R. Coward, C. Bull, G. Kukulka, & J. Galliher (Eds.), *Health services for rural elders* (pp. 108–126). New York: Springer Publishing Co.

Weinert, C. (1994). Rural nursing: Legacy, science, trajectory. *Communicating Nursing Research, 27,* 63–77.

Weinert, C., & Boik, R. (1995). MSU rurality index: Development and evaluation. *Research in Nursing and Health, 18,* 453–464.

Weinert, C., & Burman, M. (1994). Rural health and health-seeking behaviors. In J. J. Fitzpatrick & J. S. Stevenson (Eds.), *Annual review of nursing research, Vol. 12* (pp. 65–92). New York: Springer Publishing Co.

Weinert, C., & Long, K. (1987). Understanding the health needs of rural families. *Family Relations, 36,* 450–455.

Weinert, C., & Long, K. (1990). Rural families and health care: Refining the knowledge base. *Journal of Marriage and Family Review, 15*(1&2), 57–75.

Weis, E. (1992). Preparing and recruiting nurses for innovating rural practice roles. In L. Straub & N. Walzer (Eds.), *Rural health care. Innovation in a changing environment* (pp. 90–101). Westport, CT: Praeger.

Winstead-Fry, P., Tiffany, J., & Shippee-Rice, R. (Eds.). (1992). *Rural health nursing.* New York: National League for Nursing Press.

CHAPTER 4

Health Promotion: Its Role in Enhancing the Health of the Elderly

May Futrell and Dolores M. Alford

Health promotion and disease prevention are concepts not usually associated with the older adult because aging is perceived by many as a time of poor health, sickness, and dependency. Given these images, why would health promotion strategies benefit an older person? Is there a role for health promotion after an individual has reached middle age? What does health and wellness mean at 65, 85, 100 years of age?

This chapter integrates the state of the science on the topic and identifies and discusses conflicting points of view and controversial questions as well as points of agreement. The authors offer definitions of health and wellness, discuss elements of a wellness program for older persons, and describe a wellness/health promotion model for the elderly, including the issues of costs and care delivery. The authors also comment on the difficulties faced by professionals who are responsible for older persons who do not want to be well, are not willing to expend the energy to be well, or cannot afford to be well. Finally, the chapter includes some suggestions about what research is needed in the area of health promotion and future projections for health promotion.

WELLNESS IS DIFFERENT FOR THE ELDERLY THAN FOR THE YOUNG

Changing Demographics

Demographic predictions (Spencer, 1989) anticipate startling changes in the composition of the population of the United States as the year 2000 approaches. The overall population will have grown to nearly 270 million people and will be older, with 35 million people (13%) over 65 years of age. The oldest-old (85+), the fastest-growing part of the aging group, will comprise 4.6 million (1.7%) by the year 2000. Cultural diversity will increase in proportion to the total population, with the white elderly representing a smaller portion of the total than they have in the past. Demographic projections for older persons in other racial/ethnic groups provide little data of value, even though the overall populations will increase at a greater role than the white population (Hispanics, 11.3%; blacks, 13.1%; and Indians, Alaskan Natives, and Asians, 4.3%). These changes in the composition of the U.S. population will have a profound effect on the life-style, health, and wellness of the country's different cultural and age groups.

If older persons are to be able to live satisfying, healthy lives, society must be instrumental in assisting older persons to enjoy their later years. Society must explain what it means when it uses terms like "health" and "wellness" and must explain and/or demonstrate whether health is different for older adults than it is for children, adolescents, and the middle-aged. Society also must explain the part that culture and environment play in establishing and maintaining a person's health and well-being.

Evolving Definitions of Health and Wellness

Definitions and concepts of health and wellness have evolved slowly. To be truly applicable to the elderly, a definition of health must take into account the situations and conditions experienced by the elderly in a cultural/environmental context. The World Health Organization (1948) has defined health as a state of complete physical, mental, and social well-being, and not merely the absence of disease or infirmity. Can older adults meet this definition when long-term physical and mental health problems confront them? Is the frail 90-year-old well and healthy?

Dunn (1961) defined health as "an integrated method of functioning which is oriented toward maximizing the potential of which the individual is capable within the environment where he is functioning" (pp. 4–5). Filner and Williams (1979) offered a definition that allowed for even broader interpretation: "The ability to live and function effectively in society and to exercise self-reliance and autonomy to the maximum extent feasible, but not necessarily as total freedom from disease" (p. 379).

Health for the elderly, then, becomes a part of wellness. Alford and Futrell (1992) recommend a broad definition encompassing these two terms:

> For the elderly of the next century, healthy independence will relate to the functional ability of older individuals and their needs for health promotion/protection, housing, and social services. No longer can health care itself be construed as the traditional concept of medicine, nursing, and various therapies. A comprehensive view of health—including social/environmental health in a holistic framework for the elderly—will be the model of health and wellness care in the 21st century. . . . Race and ethnicity also determine the beliefs in and use of health promotion/protection services. (p. 221)

Interestingly, the prestigious Committee on Health Promotion and Disability Prevention for the Second Fifty (Berg & Cassells, 1990) of the Institute of Medicine seemed to equate health and wellness with "quality of life" for older people but declined to define what they meant by quality of life. The committee's decision was probably wise, because the heterogeneity of the older population and the right of each older person to define his or her own "quality" do not easily lend themselves to quantification or criteria-setting.

Ebersole and Hess (1994) state: "Only now have the elderly and aging been included in considering health in a positive manner. One needs to control his or her own destiny. Behavior more than medical care is important in maintaining health" (p. 52). In an effort to promote their own health, Americans have anxiously looked at their life-styles. Haber (1989) suggests that the elderly have changed certain habits, such as smoking and diet, and younger adults have exercised. Rowe (1987) maintains that the goal for health care for the elderly should be maintaining functional capability. He feels that, in order to do this, health promotion/disease prevention ought to focus on the "maintenance of full function as nearly as possible to the end of life" (pp. 9–10).

ELEMENTS OF A HEALTH PROMOTION
PROGRAM FOR THE ELDERLY

Health promotion is defined by the 1992 *Cumulative Index to the Nursing Allied Health Literature* "as the process of fostering awareness, influencing attitudes and identifying alternatives so that individuals can make informed choices and change their behavior to achieve an optimum level of physical and mental health and improve their physical and social environment" (p. 118). This definition assumes that the individual is responsible for his or her own wellness and health. Health professionals can help by being good role models and supporting individuals in their search for control over their destiny.

Health promotion is seen by some (Walker, Sechrist, & Pender, 1987) as part of a lifestyle. It "is a multidimensional pattern of self-initiated actions and perceptions that serve to maintain or enhance the level of wellness, self-actualization and fulfillment of the individual" (p. 77). Distinguishing between health promotion and disease prevention is difficult for the elderly to conceptualize, and even more difficult to implement, because older persons often have chronic illnesses and disabilities that require both health promotion and disease prevention at the same time.

The following comments, adapted from Pender (1987), may help to clarify the differences and aid in planning strategies that will help individuals to change their lifestyles and to make decisions in favor of healthier lifestyles.

Health promotion is a combination of health education and related interventions designed to support behavior conducive to health. Activities are directed toward increasing the level of well-being and actualizing the health potential of individuals, families, communities, and society. Health promotion is *not* disease- or problem-specific, the province of prevention. Health promotion requires the person to use approach behaviors, whereas prevention uses avoidance behaviors. Health promotion seeks to expand on an individual's positive potential for health and represents *acting* on the environment, rather than just *reacting* to external influences or threats.

Healthy People 2000 (USDHHS, 1990) lists priorities for health promotion and disease prevention, with objectives for different age groups. These priorities are organized into three categories: (a) health promotion, (b) health protection, and (c) preventive services. In the "Older Adults" section, the introduction states: "The most important aspect of health promotion among older people is to maintain health and functional independence. Although it is commonly believed that health problems in old age are inevitable, many are in fact preventable or can be controlled" (p. 587).

The basis for the recommendation is to encourage older adults to improve the quality of their lives by preventing morbidity and disability and by preserving functional capacity. This statement implies that it is never too late to change certain risk behaviors that might injure health and functional ability. The document suggests improving diet and nutrition, reducing tobacco use, and controlling weight. Physical activity is suggested as the key ingredient to healthy aging. Strong social support and regular primary care services are suggested as important aspects of risk reduction for older adults.

MODELS OF HEALTH PROMOTION PROGRAMS FOR THE ELDERLY

Programs of wellness/health promotion for older adults are not new, for the real pioneering work has already been done. What is needed now is to refine the models and adapt them to meet particular group needs. There also must be a more general acceptance by the public of the value of these programs.

Probably the most famous of wellness/health promotion programs for older adults is the On Lok Senior Health Services of San Francisco, which was started to meet the needs of elders in an Asian community. This center, whose participants range in age from 58 to 105, provides health and social services, assistance with activities of daily living, and a sense of family (Der-McLeod & Hansen, 1992).

Another innovative wellness/health promotion center model is the Wallingford Wellness Project (WWP), sponsored by a grant from the Administration on Aging (FallCreek, Warner-Reitz, & Mettler, 1986). The target population of the WWP at the time of the granting period was the over-75, high-risk elderly group. The focus of the grant was to "develop and evaluate a multifaceted health promotion program, which addressed physical fitness, nutrition, stress management, and communication skills for elders living independently in the community" (FallCreek et al., 1986).

In addition to On Lok and the WWP, other models have focused on vulnerable elderly in need of improved nutrition, health promotion, and reduction of social stresses. Examples include the Healthy Lifestyles for Seniors project (Warner-Reitz & Grothe, 1981) and the Santa Monica City Senior Nutrition and Recreation Program in Santa Monica, California (FallCreek et al., 1986); the Healthwise Program in Boise, Idaho (Kemper, 1986); and the New Mexico Statewide Health Promotion with Elders project (Fallcreek et al., 1986). The inheritors of these early programs are private and government-sponsored senior centers with health promotion programs. The YWCAs and YMCAs have "Prime Time Seniors" programs that offer physical fitness and stress reduction services. Health fairs are sponsored by banks, which also offer health promotion and social/financial services to members of their "50-Plus" clubs. Local health clubs and "spas" often have programs tailored for their over-50 clients. Federally assisted senior nutrition centers often have nurses on staff to teach healthy life-styles, do screenings, and provide health maintenance services. The American Nurses Association (1992) reported that there were 250 urban and rural community nursing centers providing the elderly with health promotion/health maintenance services. Most of these centers were managed by faculty and students from local nursing schools.

PRIORITIES, SERVICES, AND COSTS

Priorities

Issues of priorities, services, and costs of health promotion programs for the elderly are complex and numerous. "The National Health Promotion and Disease Prevention Objectives," in *Healthy People 2000* (USDHHS, 1990), prioritized objectives and considerations as "primary prevention, strong social support and regular primary care services" (p. 587). Champlin (1991) was of the opinion that access to community-based services was the main priority for meeting the health needs of the elderly. Muhlenkamp and Sayles (1986) found that self-esteem and social support were crucial if positive lifestyle health practices were to occur. Schmidt (1990) stated that preventive services that are clinically effective as well as cost-effective and person-specific were crucial to a health promotion program.

No matter which among the diverse models of wellness/health promotion programs for the elderly is used, the following strategies merit consideration when planning and organizing programs and/or centers:

◆ Identify services to be delivered. The center must be able to say what it can and cannot do.

◆ Present services on a level acceptable and affordable to the target population.

◆ Know and understand the target population's demographics, health beliefs and values, and communication abilities. Pay particular attention to the ethnic diversity of older adults (Gibson, 1994; Yee & Weaver, 1994).

◆ Ensure the accessibility of the program. The target population should be able to reach the center and should be able to move about the center.

◆ Involve users of the program in center activities, such as determining calendars for health promotion programs and concomitant screenings, evaluating services, and making suggestions for new services.

◆ Make using the center enjoyable and social.

◆ Provide users of the program with information about community resources not offered at the center.

◆ Avoid taking an illness approach to wellness care. Focus on healthy life-style practices rather than on illness care.

◆ Evaluate the programs of the center yearly to determine if criteria for services are relevant, if goals have or have not been attained and why, if clients served are satisfied or not, if demographics and needs of clients are changing and why, if clients are indeed practicing positive life-style habits and if these practices are making a difference, and last but not least, if the services are cost-effective.

◆ Ensure that all care deliverers maintain their expertise and enthusiasm.

Services Offered

Health Promotion Programs

Older adults attend programs, seminars, symposia, or even have one-to-one instruction on how to feel well, change attitudes, and protect and maintain health. This health promotion learning can be considered a guide or how-to resource on helping the individual achieve as high a level of wellness as possible.

Health Screening/Health Protection Services

Although health screening and health protection services are part of a prevention program, they are often held in conjunction with health promotion programs. In fact, the availability of mammography and other screenings, such as those for vision, hearing, dental needs, or foot problems, often provides the impetus for older adults to attend the health promotion programs. Health protection services might include immunizations, vaccinations, review of all drugs in one's medicine cabinet, review of one's environment for hazards, and so on.

Health Maintenance Services

Planned, periodic monitoring of older adults' physical, psychological, and sociological status by a team of health professionals in a wellness/health promotion center falls within the area of health maintenance. Such services might include monitoring health status in relation to older clients' chronic diseases: their functional abilities, their emotional and/or psychological responses to changes in their bodies and environments, the effectiveness of any treatments and drug therapies, any changes in the pathology of their diseases, and so forth. Older persons would be evaluated for any new health problem and would be assisted to enter the "illness system" if necessary. It is hoped that during the health maintenance visits older persons would report their life-style behaviors or changes of behavior that promote wellness. Praise for making positive changes and offers of support to maintain the positive changes in life-style would serve as reinforcement of these positive behaviors.

The health maintenance services of wellness/health promotion programs include services for health promotion, early detection of problems, health maintenance, mental health, gender-specific conditions, social needs, and environment/safety concerns (see Table 4.1).

Personnel Needs

One of the most exciting career opportunities for gerontological nurses is as a nurse practitioner (GNP) or clinical specialist (GCS) in a wellness/health promotion center (Burke & Walsh, 1993). The gerontological nurse in advanced practice may be a direct provider of services or a case manager, as described in the Carondelet St. Mary's Health Maintenance Organization (HMO) of Tucson, Arizona, which is the most prominent model of such services today (Etheridge, 1991; Falk, 1991; Gerber, 1994). The advanced practice gerontological nurse (GCS or GNP) can use a vast

TABLE 4.1 Wellness Program Services

Health promotion services	Programs/presentations, live and by audiovisual
	Handouts of health promotion literature
Screening services	Comprehensive health/social history
	Physical examinations, including appropriate laboratory studies
	Cognitive function assessments
	Assessment for depression
	Functional assessments
	Social assessments
	Environmental assessments
	Life-style habits assessments
	Sensory assessments
	Medication knowledge and use, screening especially for misuse
	Nutritional assessments
	Dental assessments
Health maintenance services	Planned periodic monitoring of chronic illnesses, risk factors, ability to provide self-care
Mental health services	Counseling for emotional states, such as depression, loneliness, isolation, grief
Gender-specific services	Counseling and assistance with caregiving burdens
	Widow-to-widow programs
	Assessments and care for conditions such as osteoporosis, cancers, prostate problems, breast problems, or aspects of sexuality
Social services	Financial resources
	Housing
	Transportation
	Family dynamics
	Communicating with others
	Legal resources
	Religious/spiritual resources
Environmental safety services	Defensive driving
	Avoidance of hazards that could lead to accidents
	Neighborhood evaluation for safety
	Use of appliances
	Stop-smoking programs

amount of clinical knowledge to help bring the elderly to whatever level of wellness they can attain and/or help them maintain that level of wellness (Papenhausen, 1990). The work is exciting, challenging, and rewarding.

Depending on the physical size and complexity of services offered by the center, personnel needs might include the following:

Professional Staff

- ◆ Nurse practitioners/clinical nurse specialists in gerontological nursing and geropsychiatric nursing
- ◆ Social worker
- ◆ Gerontologist

Clinical Support Staff

- ◆ Nurse aides
- ◆ Volunteers

Office Staff

- ◆ Center manager
- ◆ Receptionist/secretary
- ◆ Insurance clerk
- ◆ Volunteers
- ◆ Driver (for van if this is part of the center offerings)

Other Personnel

- ◆ Janitorial
- ◆ Accounting/Tax
- ◆ Legal

Faculty/Students

- ◆ Nursing professors
- ◆ Undergraduate and graduate students

Costs

One key issue in health promotion and health maintenance programs lies in the question of who pays for such care and services. Incentives for being well have usually not been provided in our current reimbursement systems. Our so-called health insurance system has been for ill-health, not for "well-health." Reimbursement or payment for health promotion, health protection, and health maintenance has not been allowed under most insurance programs. Medicare itself is an illness-focused program.

Free or Low-Cost Resource Materials

Interestingly, health promotion programs can cost very little except in time and some materials. In addition, there is a plethora of excellent resource materials for the lay public that is available for the asking. For example, the federal government has numerous publications on health topics, such as *Age Pages,* which are available through the Government Printing Office. The Social Security Administration has excellent publications related to work, Social Security, and Medicare. The American Association of Retired Persons (AARP) has current literature on topics such as financial strategies, safety, social services, and health/wellness. Drug companies have selected pamphlets on managing chronic illnesses. The health-related private organizations also have excellent materials on living with chronic diseases. Consumer magazines, grocery store handouts, and newspaper articles provide excellent materials for customers. Television programs often offer viewers health-related literature from their health-oriented programs. These materials can be used in health promotion programs, where their content can be interpreted for the audience.

Guest speakers can be enticed to volunteer or can be underwritten by interested organizations. Students wanting to practice their teaching or presentation abilities are also a good resource for speakers. Drug companies often maintain a speakers' bureau that can be utilized for programs.

Professional fees for mammograms and other health screenings can often be waived or nominal. Now that Medicare is finally reimbursing for mammograms, even this once prohibitively costly diagnostic service has become affordable for most women.

For small groups, the presence of a VCR and TV monitor means that health promotion programs can be placed in reception rooms (let's not call them waiting rooms, for there should be no waiting) so that older clients can view short programs in a leisurely manner. Often such viewing provides socialization for the older clients, especially when refreshments are available.

Costs for Space and Furniture

Costs of wellness-center space will vary. Space should meet all regulatory and life-safety codes and be accessible to the elderly. Center space can be donated by apartment complexes, long-term-care facilities, universities, hospitals, physicians' offices, city governments, and the private sector.

Durable items such as furniture and office and clinic equipment do not have to be expensive. Used furniture and equipment, such as computers, typewriters, exam tables and stools, lights, and cabinets, can give long usage. Fund drives can be held to pay for other equipment and disposable items.

Staffing Costs

The biggest expense will be in personnel—that is, professional staff. Again, volunteers can be utilized as receptionists and aides if the proper preservice training and orientation are done. For the center to be reimbursed by Medicare or Medicaid and/or managed care organizations, there must be a skilled insurance clerk on staff.

In some instances, especially if the center is large, a center manager will be necessary. If the center is underwritten by charitable organizations, city governments, or universities, a board of directors will have to be appointed. Even though the directors are generally not paid for their services, there are hidden costs related to communication, insurance, meetings, and perhaps refreshments.

Insurance

Obtaining the necessary insurance—property, liability, workmen's compensation, and health insurance—will also be a major cost, as will legal and accounting consultants to the center. The usual cost of running an office must be figured into overhead. Bids may be required for certain purposes, such as furniture, telephone systems, and waste management.

Budget and Fees

To take all of these costs into consideration, a budget must be devised. Once the overhead is determined, then fees charged to the users of the center can be calculated. Even when the center's costs are underwritten, users should be encouraged to contribute a fee for each visit. For example, in one of the author's (Alford's) centers, the fee for each visit is $1. In another model, a box for contributions is placed on the receptionist's desk so that clients can voluntarily contribute whatever amount they wish. Interestingly, families of clients seen in the center often contribute large sums to express their gratitude for the care their older family members are receiving.

If a health care reform package does become a reality in this country, services (especially those delivered by nurse practitioners) that older adults receive in wellness and health promotion centers will most likely be covered (Lamb, 1994). The paperwork involved in such reimbursement will add to the costs of center administration.

Comparison to Illness-Care Costs

Providing wellness/health promotion services to older adults is not cheap, but it is a bargain compared to what illness care costs. Rogers, Supino, and Grower (1986) gave a breakdown of the cost of case finding, which included the fees of all health professionals involved, and costs of services, forms, and treatment; none was low. Vogt (1994) reported on cost-effectiveness (i.e., savings) data gleaned from studies of several prevention and early detection services, such as smoking cessation programs ($220–$13,000), mammography ($20,000–$232,000), hypertension management ($11,612–$82,600), cervical cancer screening ($6,444–$499,367), and cholesterol screening/treatment ($18–$10,000,000). Vogt cautions that the heterogeneity of the people served and the diversity of the models of care in these studies greatly influence costs. Kennie (1986) was of the opinion that "there have been few attempts to analyze the financial implications of health maintenance measures for the elderly" (p. 77). This seems to hold true for nursing, for many studies and reports make no mention of costs (Butler, 1994) or use only general phrases, such as "cost-effective" (Muhlenkamp & Sayles, 1986) and "cost controlled/ savings" (Lamb, 1994). Therefore, the issue of cost of services and reimbursement for wellness/health promotion programs, especially as it relates to health care reform, must be addressed in nursing research (Riesch, 1992).

ENCOURAGING THE ELDERLY TO USE A WELLNESS/HEALTH PROMOTION CENTER

Health promotion programs are often the key ingredient that entices older persons to use a new wellness center. By using a free program with refreshments as introductory public relations, center personnel can not only "show off" their knowledge, but have direct contact with prospective clients.

At first, center personnel might suggest and offer some of the programs. When the clients begin to feel comfortable with the staff, program advisory committees can be formed to assist in choosing programs clients want. An example of a yearly calendar of health promotion programs, with accompanying health screenings and projects, is shown in Table 4.2.

In this author's (Alford's) experience, older persons who have come to health promotion programs have not only been eager learners, but they have often taken extra handout materials to use in imparting the information to other family members. Sometimes they have even brought their younger family members to the programs with them.

Once the word gets out about the programs the center is holding, especially if the programs are creative and spark lively debate, clients begin to get more involved. Most of all, potential program presenters begin to volunteer their services.

Do the programs make a difference? Yes, they can (Schmidt, 1990). One of the best ways to evaluate the effectiveness of the programs is in the individual sessions the elderly have with the staff of the wellness center. For example, in this author's (Alford's) experience, a diabetic woman who had refused to adhere to her prescribed American Diabetes Association diet, refused to protect her feet, and often missed or overused her sulfonylurea drug, began to see the nurse practitioner in the wellness center after attending a health promotion program on foot care.

This client knew little about her disease and how to do the self-care that would keep her chronic illness under control, so the information was provided to her. Her attitudes about her health changed, and she started making her lifestyle healthier. She stopped baking and eating cakes. She ate more vegetables and fruit. She inspected her feet daily and began wearing comfortable walking shoes rather than sandals. She started a

TABLE 4.2   Example of a Yearly Calendar of Health Promotion Programs

Month	Program	Screening/Projects
January	Aging Well	Make the year's healthy life-style calendar
February	Keeping Hearts Healthy	Blood pressure/cardiac screening
March	Optimizing Vision	Vision/glaucoma screening
April	Health Roots	Making autobiographical audio/ videotapes for heirs
May	Healthy Eating	Making family recipes healthy
June	Healthy Travel	Preparing health diaries
July	Summer Protectives	Skin screening
August	Optimizing Hearing	Hearing screening
September	Look What's in My Medicine Cabinet	Review content of medicine cabinets
October	Environmental Safety	Self-screen of environment, using a checklist
November	Winter Protectives	Give flu shots
December	Surviving the Holidays	Making holiday schedules for stress reduction

daily walking program. The focus remained on lifestyle, not on her disease. With instruction and praise for her good lifestyle habits, this woman is actually healthier today than she was 10 years ago, when she first started at the center. At age 83, she takes no medication for her diabetes, which is well controlled. Her feet are in good condition. Her weight is within "normal" range. She continues to walk daily. She does all of her own activities of daily living, and she is helpful to neighbors, family, and church members.

WORKING WITH THE ELDERLY WHO DO NOT WANT TO BE WELL

A challenge to health professionals is how to work with older adults who do not want to be well, who are not willing to expend the energy to be well, and who cannot afford to be well. The efforts of professionals and policymakers to make and keep older individuals well may not be met with the same enthusiasm by the elderly themselves. Frequently, the changes in life-style that might be required to establish healthy behaviors are too expensive, time-consuming, and painful for the older person. Health professionals can present the information and make suggestions and comments, but they should not make the decision for lifestyle change for the elderly person. Davis (1991) reminds us that "we have a legal and ethical tradition that allows competent adults to make reasoned decisions about their well-being including the refusal of treatment. This tradition is grounded in the ethical privilege of autonomy" (p. 23). This right of self-determination includes the incompetent person. If it has been determined legally or by a group of caretakers that the person cannot make a rational decision in a given situation, then a surrogate decision maker is required. The decisions are then made for the client by this surrogate in the manner in which the client would have made the decision if competent (Davis, 1991).

Before giving up on an older client who is competent and does not seem interested in being well, the health professional should evaluate all the reasons for the lack of interest. What effect could an illness be having? Are there signs of depression or side effects of drugs that are causing distress? Has the individual been responsible for his or her health, or has the individual been dependent on others and never controlled his or her wellness? Perhaps this individual is using illness as an attention-getting mechanism. Health professionals can help the elderly move toward greater responsibility for their own health by encouraging them to talk about the decisions they can make to modify their behavior and improve their wellness. Support systems (family, financial, and social) play an important role in health promotion. Unfortunately, these support systems are not available for some elderly people. Perceptions of health and wellness differ among individuals, and these individuals have the right to make rational decisions, based on knowledge and personal preference, to forgo a change in lifestyle.

RESEARCH IN HEALTH PROMOTION

Health promotion research is a relatively new and evolving area. Studies have been undertaken by many disciplines, using special populations and/or focusing on specific behaviors that contribute to illness. Kulbok and Baldwin (1992) noted that nursing research conducted between 1982 and 1990 used the terms *health promotion* and *preventive health* interchangeably. Methodologies differed, as did the conceptualization of health promotion and prevention behaviors. Redland and Stuifbergen (1993), in a comprehensive review of the health promotion literature, found other disciplines tending to add maintenance of health to health promotion behaviors. These authors suggest that further study in the following areas is needed: demographic and socioeconomic characteristics, motivation, self-efficacy and relapse tendencies, and barriers and facilitators. Intervention strategies must include these factors in order to help the individual maintain healthy behavior over time. Research should be conducted on outcomes of health promotion programs, both short-term and long-term. Studies of this type pose many difficulties with measurement; however, evaluation of outcomes is necessary.

Another area that holds much promise for gerontological nursing researchers is the study of how quality of life for nursing home residents can be influenced through health promotion strategies (Robertson, 1991). Since OBRA '87 regulations require staff to promote the highest possible quality of life for nursing home residents, research is needed to investigate the benefits/outcomes of health promotion interventions in long-term care (Benner, 1985).

Studies of the health promotion efforts for the very old and the minority old should focus on those who need assistance, not only with life-style changes they can make, but in learning about types of services available, their costs, and how to procure them. Multicultural studies that describe the unique health promotion needs of the elderly who live in urban, suburban, and rural settings must also be conducted.

Marketing of health promotion strategies to various age groups is another area of viable research. Promotion of functional health is a concept new to marketing. The present marketing emphasis has been to promote fitness, especially physical fitness and exercise. Strategies are needed to promote wellness and quality-of-life issues.

SOME FUTURE DIRECTIONS IN HEALTH PROMOTION FOR OLDER ADULTS

Health promotion as a strategy to improve wellness will take on more importance as individuals realize that it is in their best interests to stay well and functioning. This will mean a better quality of life and fewer financial problems. As health care reform causes us to look at insurance, costs, and individual responsibility, programs helping individuals to stay fit across the life span will take on meaning for everyone, including the elderly. However, the biggest barrier to health care reform just might be the lack of health professionals prepared to provide wellness/health promotion services rather than the illness services that have so characterized the health professions.

Health care reform must include a review of the financing of health care and health promotion; the structure of the delivery system, including nursing homes and home care; as well as the issues of race and gender. Public policy-making must take into consideration poverty, living alone, and functional limitations that are barriers to wellness. Interventions require consideration of economics (Harrington & Estes, 1994). To make the transition easier for health professionals and to ensure that the elderly receive quality health promotion services, the development of gerontic nursing institutes has been proposed by Alford and Futrell (1992). Gerontic nursing institutes are one method of providing wellness/health promotion services to older adults. Housed in colleges of nursing at the university level, the institutes would function as regional resource centers to prepare gerontological nurses, house library resources on aging, and provide continuing education programs in gerontological nursing and cosponsorship of programs with other health professionals. The institutes would also provide or arrange for clinical practice settings for the care of older adults whether sick or well, conduct and participate in research on aging and gerontological nursing, serve as advocates for older adults, and influence health and social policy regarding older adults.

The value of the institutes would be the concentration in one location of considerable expertise that would be accessible to health professionals and consumers alike. Funding for the institutes would come from university budgets, endowments and other gifts, income generated in the practice areas, continuing education fees, publications, and research grants.

The institutes would have on staff not only academics but practitioners as well. For example, a wellness center might be managed by a GNP, but faculty members would also practice in the center as direct caregivers, as instructors to their students, and as researchers. The institutes would coordinate health team approaches to curriculum, practice, and research in the care of older adults. They would help foster collegial and contractual relationships with other professional schools at the university (e.g., medicine, pharmacy, social work, various therapies).

The institutes would be a "one-stop" resource for older adults, their families, and caregivers. Older persons would be used as cherished advisers on programs, curriculum, grants, and health policy proposals. The institutes would facilitate the change in focus from an illness-oriented society to a wellness-oriented society.

Research in health promotion is evolving, and the authors have discussed areas needing further exploration by nursing researchers as well as researchers in other disciplines. Policymakers use facts and findings from research. Therefore, research is a policy issue, and strengthening this component of policymaking is crucial. The content area of health promotion needs to be addressed. Consideration of lifestyle and its relevance to anyone other than the middle-income group might be worth investigating. Policy issues will take on importance as the role of health promotion in health care becomes clearer. The stage is set for a challenging and exciting, significant social change from illness to wellness concepts and practices in the 21st century for older persons and health professionals alike.

REFERENCES

Alford, D. M., & Futrell, M. (1992). Wellness and health promotion of the elderly. *Nursing Outlook, 40,* 221–226.

American Nurses Association. (1992). Community nursing centers gaining ground as solution to health issues. *American Journal of Nursing, 92,* 70.

Benner, P. (1985). Quality of life: A phenomenological perspective on explanation, prediction, and understanding in nursing science. *Advances in Nursing Science, 8,* 1–14.

Berg, R., & Cassells, J. (Eds.). (1990). *The second fifty years: Promoting health and preventing disability.* Washington, DC: National Academy Press.

Burke, M. M., & Walsh, M. B. (1993). New opportunities in gerontologic nursing. *Nursing, 23*(12), 40–41.

Butler, F. (1994, October). *Nurse managed clinics: Challenges and directions for health care reform.* Poster presented at the American Academy of Nursing Scientific Meeting, Phoenix, AZ.

Champlin, L. (1991). "Eldercare" goal: Integrate health, social needs. *Geriatrics, 46,* 67–70.

Cumulative index to the nursing allied health literature. (1992). Glendale, CA: CINAHL Information Systems.

Davis, A. (1991). Ethical issues in gerontological nursing. In W. Chenitz, J. Stone, & S. Salisbury (Eds.), *Clinical gerontological nursing* (pp. 15–23). Philadelphia: W. B. Saunders.

Der-McLeod, D., & Hansen, J. (1992, Summer). On Lok: The family continuum. *Generations, 18,* 71–72.

Dunn, H. L. (1961). *High level wellness.* Arlington, VA: R. L. Beatty, Ltd.

Ebersole, P., & Hess, P. (1994). *Toward healthy aging: Human needs and nursing response* (4th ed.). St. Louis: C. V. Mosby.

Etheridge, P. (1991). A nursing HMO: Carondelet St. Mary's experience. *Nursing Management, 22,* 22–27.

Falk, C. (1991). Our HMO offers more than medical care. *RN, 54,* 17–18.

FallCreek, S., Warner-Reitz, A., & Mettler, M. (1986). Designing health promotion programs for elders. In K. Dychtwald (Ed.), *Wellness and health promotion for the elderly* (pp. 219–233). Rockville, MD: Aspen.

Filner, B., & Williams, T. F. (1979). Health promotion for the elderly: Reducing functional dependency. In *Healthy people: The Surgeon General's report on health promotion and disease prevention: Background papers* (Publication No. 79-55071A, pp. 365–386). Washington, DC: U.S. Government Printing Office.

Gerber, L. (1994). Case management models—geriatric nursing prototypes for growth. *Journal of Gerontological Nursing, 20,* 18–24.

Gibson, R. (1994). The age-by-race gap in health and mortality in the older population: A social science research agenda. *The Gerontologist, 34,* 454–462.

Haber, D. (1989). *Healthy care for an aging society.* New York: Hemisphere.

Harrington, C., & Estes, C. (1994). *Health policy and nursing.* Boston: Jones and Bartlett.

Kemper, D. (1986). The healthwise program: Growing younger. In K. Dychtwald (Ed.), *Wellness and health promotion for the elderly* (pp. 263–273). Rockville, MD: Aspen.

Kennie, D. (1986). Health maintenance of the elderly. *Clinics in Geriatric Medicine, 2,* 53–83.

Kulbok, P., & Baldwin, P. (1992). From preventive health behaviors to health promotion: Advancing a positive construct of health. *Advances in Nursing Science, 14,* 501.

Lamb, G. (1994, October). *New delivery systems: The call to community.* Paper presented at the American Academy of Nursing Scientific Meeting, Phoenix, AZ.

Muhlenkamp, A., & Sayles, J. (1986). Self-esteem, social support, and positive health practices. *Nursing Research, 35,* 334–338.

Paperhausen, J. L. (1990). Case management: A model of advanced practice? *Clinical Nurse Specialist, 4*(4), 169–170.

Pender, N. (1987). *Health promotion in nursing practice.* Norwalk, CT: Appleton-Century-Crofts.

Redland, A., & Stuifbergen, A. (1993). Strategies for maintenance of health promoting behaviors. *Nursing Clinics of North America, 28,* 427–442.

Riesch, S. (1992). Nursing centers: An analysis of the anecdotal literature. *Journal of Professional Nursing, 8,* 16–25.

Robertson, J. (1991). Promoting health among institutionalized elderly. *Journal of Gerontological Nursing, 17,* 15–19.

Rogers, J., Supino, P., & Grower, R. (1986). Proposed evaluation criteria for screening programs for the elderly. *Gerontologist, 26*(5), 564–570.

Rowe, J. (1987) *Toward successful aging: A strategy for health promotion and disease prevention for older persons.* Washington, DC: Association for Gerontology in Higher Education.

Schmidt, R. (1990, November). *Outcomes of evaluating healthy aging interventions in patients over 65 in the primary care practice: Health watch of Arizona.* Paper presented at the 43rd Annual Scientific Meeting of the Gerontological Society of America, Boston.

Spencer, G. (1989). Projections of the population of the United States by age, sex, and race: 1988 to 2080. *Current population reports, population estimates and projections* (Series P-25, No. 1018). Washington, DC: U.S. Department of Commerce, Bureau of the Census.

U.S. Department of Health and Human Services. (1990). *Healthy people 2000: National health promotion and disease prevention objectives.* Washington, DC: U.S. Government Printing Office.

Vogt, T. (1994, Spring). Cost-effectiveness of prevention programs for older people. *Generations, 18,* 63–68.

Walker, S. N., Sechrist, K. R., & Pender, N. J. (1987). The health promoting lifestyle profile: Development and psychometric characteristics. *Nursing Research, 36,* 76–81.

Warner-Reitz, A., & Grothe, C. (1981). *Healthy lifestyles for seniors: An interdisciplinary approach to healthy aging.* New York: Meals for Millions/Freedom from Hunger Foundation.

World Health Organization. (1948). *Constitution of the World Health Organization.* Geneva, Switzerland: Basic Documents, WHO.

Yee, B., & Weaver, G. (1994, Spring). Ethnic minorities and health promotion: Developing a "culturally competent" agenda. *Generations, 18,* 39–44.

CHAPTER 5

Nursing Interventions for Older Adults with Cognitive Impairment: Some Conceptual, Clinical, Research, and Policy Issues

Ivo L. Abraham and Lisa L. Onega

Because the various forms of irreversible cognitive impairment cause such devastating intellectual, functional, behavioral, and emotional losses in patients, often with seemingly little opportunity for maintenance or improvement, nursing care has too often remained limited to custodial and physical care. Granted, patients with cognitive impairment have little if any chance of recovery, yet there is room to

Author notes: Supported by grants from the Division of Nursing, United States Department of Health and Human Services; the W. K. Kellogg Foundation; the John A. Hartford Foundation; and the Belgian Ministry of Public Health and the Environment.

Address correspondence to the first author at School of Nursing, University of Virginia, McLeod Hall, Charlottesville, Virginia 22903, USA. Email: iabraham@ virginia.edu.

work on delaying and slowing down the decline, maintaining status for a certain time, or, just as important, providing high quality and sensitive care as the cognitive decline progresses. The fatalistic perspective that not much can be done in terms of nursing care for the cognitively impaired, especially those in advanced stages, is both a disregard (if not neglect) of the care to which a patient is entitled and testimony to a lack of creative commitment on the part of nurses.

The source of this view about care for cognitively impaired older adults may be traditional biomedical (and nursing) thinking, which emphasizes improvement as the only indicator of quality of care. This mode of thinking should be abandoned in the care of the cognitively impaired (and care of the elderly in general). To put it graphically, pursuing an upward curve of improved capacity or a downward curve of symptom reduction, which are the traditional hallmarks of therapeutic success and quality care, ignores the reality of aging and its natural trajectories of decline as well as the reality of cognitive impairment and its inevitable graduation from mild to severe.

We need to reorient our clinical, research, and policy thinking and move away from the expectation of an upward curve of improvement or a downward curve of symptom reduction. Considering that older adults with cognitive decline are on an accelerated trajectory of decline characterized by a steep curve, effectiveness of interventions for this population can be evidenced by three situations. An effective intervention may achieve one of the following:

1. *A less steep curve of decline* (i.e., a curve with a negative coefficient that is smaller than the slope coefficient prior to intervention), indicating that the intervention slowed down the process of decline.
2. *A flattening of the curve,* indicating that the intervention was able to temporarily postpone (or perhaps even eliminate) the decline.
3. *A positive curve,* which, important from both research and clinical vantage points, would indicate not only improvement from a zero level but a "double" improvement from the declined level to the zero level and on up from that level.

Indeed, much can be done for older adults with cognitive impairment; however, it requires on the part of nurses a willingness to fundamentally rethink how, why, and to what end they provide care; how they investigate the processes and outcomes of their interventions and models of care; and how this translates into appropriate policymaking.

In this chapter we first address several conceptual issues, followed by a discussion of the role of nursing within a multidisciplinary context. Next we review areas of clinical scholarship and research related to nursing interventions for older adults with cognitive impairment. We conclude with some implications and future directions for practice, research, and policy. Note that this chapter is focused on *interventions*. The major tenet is that once cognitive impairment has been identified and assessed as to its degree and the areas of cognitive functioning affected, it is important for nurses to provide interventions that will maximize functioning, slow the progress of cognitive decline, and meet the patient's and family's needs in a comprehensive and compassionate manner.

Given the focus on interventions, cognitive assessment is not addressed in this chapter. Such assessment, as part of comprehensive nursing and multidisciplinary evaluation of the older adult with cognitive impairment, is essential to the selection and implementation of nursing interventions. However, we refer the readers to some of our other work on nursing (Abraham et al., 1990; Abraham, Smullen, & Thompson-Heisterman, 1992; Thompson-Heisterman, Smullen, & Abraham, 1992) and multidisciplinary assessment (Abraham, Holroyd et al., 1994), including the use of standardized screening instruments (Abraham, 1995; Abraham, Manning et al., 1993, 1994).

Because its purpose is not to provide an exhaustive review, this chapter is selective. The decisions as to what is included and what is not were made intuitively rather than through application of clear criteria. We chose to focus on what we believe are pertinent and urgent issues, to be presented as intervention issues within a larger conceptual context of working with the cognitively impaired. Much of our belief is based on clinical experience and (the intuition of) an intervention's promise in contributing to quality care; emerging research support for areas of intervention and the relevance to policy considerations were considered as well. We wish that more of the chapter could be grounded in research-based knowledge. Perhaps in line with the fatalistic perspective that not much can be done for older adults with cognitive impairment, nursing research in this area is still limited. Even though one might find many publications on nursing care of the cognitively impaired, many studies are methodologically or conceptually weak. We chose not to include these studies unless they were pilot studies for subsequent larger investigations. Although some of the studies thus excluded might have offered potentially interesting new insights into nursing care of older adults with cognitive impairment, the conceptual or methodological concerns cast too much doubt on the validity and replicability of the findings.

Another difficulty with the research base is that many large-scale interventions supported by significant federal or private grants are still in the implementation phases, and at best, only preliminary results are available. We chose to apply the perhaps overly stringent criterion that findings must have been published (or accepted for publication) in peer-reviewed literature or that they are being reported in manuscripts in progress or under review. Otherwise, waiting a few years until the larger-scale initiatives referenced in this chapter have been completed will prove to be a service to the studies as well as the users of the new knowledge. This applies, for instance, to studies by Buckwalter and associates (University of Iowa) on the progressively lowered stress threshold (PLST) model, and by Beck (University of Arkansas) and the late Baldwin (University of Maryland) on behavioral management. These studies undoubtedly will propel nursing knowledge about care of older adults with dementing illness forward, yet it might benefit the studies and the discipline to await the empirical findings. Finally, we do not make a distinction between the various care environments for the elderly with cognitive impairment (for an overview, see Abraham, Onega, Chalifoux, & Maes, 1994; Maas, Swanson, Specht, & Buckwalter, 1994). Even though much of the content of this chapter is based on work in long-term-care facilities, with some professional creativity much of this knowledge can be extended to other care environments, including the home. In addition, when patients change care environments, it may be necessary that interventions used in the old setting be continued in the new setting. This refers to the importance of fluidity of care, the transparent and "seamless" transitioning of all aspects of nursing and elder care from one setting to another (Abraham, 1994).

CONCEPTUAL FOUNDATIONS

Because of the need to think less in terms of improvement and more in terms of delay and maintenance, it is important to put forward some basic principles that govern nursing interventions for older adults with cognitive impairment. These principles apply to the interventions described in this chapter, but they can be extended to nursing care of elderly patients suffering from cognitive impairment in general.

Context of Nursing Care for the Cognitively Impaired

Foremost, nursing must consider the clinical needs of the cognitively impaired within the triad of the individual patient, the family, and the community. Because of the variety of potential and actual needs, nursing interventions must be integrated into the overall 24-hour delivery of care that is typically needed by older adults with cognitive impairment, regardless of the setting in which the care is provided. Nursing interventions may focus alternately on prevention, cure, or palliative care (Abraham, Chalifoux et al., 1993).

Beck and Heacock (1988) outline five critical premises governing the planning, implementation, and evaluation of nursing care for older adults with cognitive impairment:

1. The goal of nursing interventions is to help the patient . . . remain as independent as possible and to function at the highest physical, emotional, intellectual, and social level for as long as possible.
2. Cognition underlies behavior, and thus a patient's level of cognitive functioning guides the selection of nursing interventions.
3. The success of an intervention is directly related to a thorough assessment of the individual's assets and limitations in each of his or her dimensions.
4. The interventions build on the individual's remaining capacities and attempt to compensate for the individual's deficits.
5. Disabilities in one area do not reflect the degree of impairment in another area (p. 95).

Relatedly, these authors advocate a holistic approach that integrates the physical, emotional, cognitive, and social dimensions.

Hall and Buckwalter (1991) speak of "whole disease care planning" for patients with Alzheimer's disease. The choice of interventions should be determined by the stage of the disease and the lost versus remaining functional capabilities. This approach is particularly important in the confused and ambulatory dementia stages of the disease. Hall and Buckwalter prescribe interventions for both stages that are essentially similar in focus and aim but differ in terms of intensity and implementation. In the confused stage, established routines are important, but these should change to simplified routines in the ambulatory dementia stage. Self-cuing by patients using memory prosthetics should change to other-cued memory supports as the disease progresses. At the environmental level (social and physical), large-group socialization is replaced by small-group socialization, and routine stimulus environments are replaced by modified and thus controlled environmental stimuli. Break periods to permit rest and recuperation might suffice for confused patients but should be formalized into formal rest periods and naps for ambulatory dementing patients. Reminiscence is important in both stages, but it is complemented by, respectively, reality orientation efforts or validation therapy in the two stages.

Cognition

It is essential to adopt a dynamic perspective on cognition. Too often cognition is seen as a characteristic or skill in relative independence of other human characteristics or skills. However, cognition is an *interactive, mediating,* and *regulating* human function. Cognition is what enables us to plan and implement activities. It is the force that links together the praxic aspects of tasks; for instance, cognition enables us to determine the order in which we should put on clothing so as to be dressed properly. Cognition is also the mediator, if not modulator, of emotion and emotional expression; for instance, it helps us experience, interpret, and give meaning to feelings, and it assists us in finding ways of expressing these feelings. Cognition provides structure to our coping processes; for instance, we think when we appraise a stressful situation, explore options, and choose a coping approach. Cognition is critical to learning, which is more than skill acquisition and includes organization, association, and judgment of relevance. Cognitive decline, then, does not just lead to poorer cognitive status, whether measured by a simple screening test or a comprehensive neuropsychological battery. Because of the central role of cognition in the physical, functional, emotional, and social dimensions of human functioning, cognitive decline leads directly to impairment in each of these dimensions. In sum, existentially, cognitive decline is not the loss of the isolated human function called cognition; rather, it is the loss of one's mind and one's ability to mind.

A dynamic perspective on cognition influences how we describe cognitive impairment in a way that is relevant to nursing. The conventional approach is to adopt medical descriptions and classifications. However, nursing care might benefit from a nursing-specific and nursing-relevant description of the clinical phenomenology of irreversible cognitive impairment. Hall (1988) distinguishes between four symptom clusters associated with progressive dementing illness, which we summarize here:

1. Intellectual losses, specifically loss of
   ◆ memory, from memory for recent events to general memorial dysfunction
   ◆ sense of time
   ◆ ability to abstract
   ◆ ability to choose, decide, solve problems, and reason
   ◆ judgment
   ◆ perceptual ability, from changes in perceptual ability to ability to identify visual and auditory stimuli
   ◆ expressive and receptive language abilities
2. Affective or personality losses:
   ◆ loss of affect
   ◆ diminished inhibitions, such as emotional ability, loss of tact in increasingly spontaneous conversations, loss of temper control, inability to delay gratification
   ◆ confabulation and perseveration
   ◆ reduced attention span
   ◆ increased preoccupation with self
   ◆ social withdrawal, especially in an effort to avoid complex or overwhelming stimuli
   ◆ antisocial behavior
   ◆ psychotic features, especially paranoid delusions
3. Conative or planning losses, in particular,
   ◆ loss of ability to execute activities, including loss of planning ability; ability to perform voluntary activities; and ability to perform activities requiring cognition to set goals, organize, and complete tasks
   ◆ loss of function, starting with instrumental activities of daily living (ADLs) and progressing to the loss of physical ADLs
   ◆ motor apraxia
   ◆ increased fatigue and loss of energy reserve
   ◆ frustration, refusal to participate, or helplessness when losses are challenged
   ◆ preoccupation with function, which worsens performance
4. Behavioral losses:
   ◆ catastrophic behaviors
   ◆ confused or agitated night awakening
   ◆ wandering
   ◆ violence, agitation, anxiety

- ◆ withdrawal or avoidance
- ◆ noisy behavior
- ◆ purposeless behavior
- ◆ compulsive repetitive behavior
- ◆ other cognitively and socially inaccessible behaviors

In a paper on managing aggressive behavior in demented elderly, Ryden and Feldt (1992) stressed the importance of goal-directed care. Although the five goals they proposed are offered in the context of managing aggression, the goals can be extended to older adults with cognitive impairment in general: to feel safe, to feel physically comfortable, to experience a sense of control, to experience minimal stress, and to experience pleasure.

Progressively Lowered Stress Threshold

The notion of stress is an important element in care of the cognitively impaired older adult. Hall and Buckwalter (Hall, 1988, 1994a; Hall & Buckwalter, 1987) proposed the conceptual model of the PLST: specifically, that the threshold for a person's ability to manage stressful stimuli declines as the level of cognitive impairment becomes more severe. Having proposed the PLST initially as a hypothetical model, Buckwalter and associates are currently engaged in a multiyear study using the PLST model. What is particularly attractive about this model, coupled with Hall's (1988) four-dimensional conceptualization of signs and symptoms of Alzheimer's disease, is that the model offers an intrinsic nursing foundation for linking interventions with various manifestations of dementing illness.

The PLST model departs from the generally accepted perspective that all humans have a certain stress threshold. As long as stressors, individually and cumulatively, stay below this threshold, people exhibit normal (adaptive) behavior. However, as stressors intensify and get closer to the threshold, there is increased risk of anxious behavior. This behavior is still adaptive, but it forms the transition between functional and dysfunctional responses to stressors. If stressors intensify further, anxious behavior will prove to be an insufficient adaptation response, and the threshold into dysfunctional behavior will be crossed.

According to the PLST model, cognitively impaired persons have a threshold that is markedly lower than that of cognitively intact persons.

In fact, the threshold becomes lower and lower as the dementia progresses from the early to the later stages. For instance, a stressor level that is still manageable in the forgetful stage of the disease may elicit anxious bchavior in the confused stage and dysfunctional behavior in the ambulatory dementia stage. In addition, Buckwalter and associates have been able to show that the behavioral manifestations associated with PLST follow a consistent course over a 24-hour period. For instance, during the morning, patients are subjected to various environmental stimuli, such as noise associated with daily care, noise from maintenance and housekeeping, general activity level from various clinical duties, and noise from television and from other residents. Gradually, the stressor level accumulates, and the cumulative stress level tends to reach the anxious "prethreshold" level around midday. This change may explain, for instance, the prevalence of agitated behaviors during mealtimes. As the day progresses, with more stressor stimuli in the environment, the patient is likely to cycle in and out of anxious and dysfunctional behavior; such behavioral phenomena are explained as sundowning and nighttime awakening.

In addition to offering a framework for understanding patient behavior, the PLST model emphasizes the importance of managing environmental stimuli as a central part of residential care for patients with dementing illness. The goal would be to create environments in which the stressor level is controlled in such a way that patients, at most, reach the anxious behavior level but do not progress to dysfunctional behavior.

ROLE OF NURSING WITHIN MULTIDISCIPLINARY CARE

Nursing care, as an independent and interdependent part of the overall care to older adults with cognitive impairment, will be more comprehensive, more effective, and of higher quality if it is part of a multidisciplinary team effort (Frances et al., 1988). Differential but complementary and intersecting roles can be identified. The physician is primarily responsible for diagnosing, identifying causes, and planning medical treatment. The nurse is primarily responsible for patient and family education, serving as the patient and family support person, coordinating daily care, and implementing nursing-specific interventions (among others, those described in this chapter). Nurses bring to geriatric care a dual emphasis on (a) functional ability and self-care and (b) holistic and comprehensive care (Abraham, Chalifoux et al., 1993). Clinical pharmacologists provide the important functions of attuning pharmacological treatment to the patient's health and cognitive status and of addressing polypharmacy problems such as interactions, side effects, and toxicity. The dentist's role is not limited to just oral hygiene and preventive and restorative dental care but also comprises oral and mandibular functioning (including swallowing), dentures and other dental prosthetics, and taste and feeding functions. Social workers provide support functions to families while also serving as a bridge to community-based care services—assuring at least continuity but also, it is hoped, fluidity of care.

Hirst (1989) specified several roles of the geriatric clinical nurse specialist in the care of older adults with cognitive impairment. These roles go beyond the responsibilities of nursing staff; however, they highlight the professional nursing opportunities in dementia care and provide a context for thinking about advanced practice with elderly patients with cognitive impairment: role model, implementer, change agent, consultant, educator, advocate, manager, researcher, and mentor. With policy and legislative discussions about advanced practice going on around the country, it is essential that the multidimensional and "multichallenge" role of nurses be recognized if not formalized. Several of the functions described by Hirst go beyond the conventional role of nurses, even those practicing at an advanced level. As we come to recognize their increasingly pivotal role in the care of older adults with cognitive impairment, it is essential that nurses be empowered legislatively to fulfill these responsibilities and assure quality of care in home, community, and acute and long-term-care settings.

The changing role of nursing raises the question of what is good multidisciplinary care. Too often, multidisciplinary care is "vertical-parallel" care, in which several disciplines work alongside each other quite independently, with interactions limited to communication and information exchange. The *multi* in *multidisciplinary* refers more to the number of disciplines involved than to their integration across disciplinary boundaries. At the other end of the continuum is the operationalization of multidisciplinary care as the *blurring* of disciplinary boundaries (or the illusion thereof). Here the fact that multiple disciplines work together from their various vantage points and expertise is less important than that they all work together—perhaps more for the sake of working together (and worker satisfaction) than for the sake of patient care.

Good, effective, productive, and discipline-reinforcing multidisciplinary care consists of the dual challenge of (a) strongly affirming disciplinary boundaries and (b) collaboratively establishing methods of interfacing, exchanging, and working together toward common clinical goals. In good multidisciplinary care unidisciplinary contributions do not cease to exist; on the contrary, they are fostered and supported by other disciplines. Likewise, disciplines also converge on a set of multidisciplinary care goals, to govern not only what they pursue together but also what they pursue within their own disciplines. This convergence requires that disciplines work to understand what they can expect from each other; what they need from each other in terms of assessment, planning, intervention, and evaluation information; and what they can offer other disciplines in terms of such information. At the risk of sounding pedantic, we would argue that good multidisciplinary care is like a good relationship with a significant other: the identity and integrity of each is preserved, and the functioning of each is stimulated and enriched by mutual interchange, feedback, reinforcement, and correction.

NURSING INTERVENTIONS

Communication

As cognitive impairment worsens, a patient's ability to communicate changes as well. It is commonly believed that patients rapidly lose communication ability and that communication is quasi-impossible with severely impaired patients. This is certainly the case for verbal communication, yet cognitively impaired elderly retain for quite a long time a sensitivity for nonverbal modes of communication. Communication is an inherent part of any nursing intervention in addition to being an intervention in itself. Throughout the process of decline, nurses must change their verbal and nonverbal communication strategies to stay in touch with their patients—including a gradual shift from predominantly verbal communication that is supported by congruent nonverbal communication to mostly nonverbal modes.

Beck and Heacock (1988) offer several verbal and nonverbal communication strategies, which we summarize and paraphrase here (see Beck & Heacock, 1988, for specific examples):

Verbal:
◆ Use congruent nonverbal communication to accompany verbal communication.
◆ Use matter-of-fact speech and yes/no questions.
◆ Provide positive direction; eliminate unnecessary choices.
◆ Be concrete.
◆ Speak slowly, using single words; keep voice low but resonant.
◆ Use a calm, reassuring tone of voice, projecting a sense of control.
◆ Eliminate competing or distracting background stimuli.
◆ Look directly at the person; identify yourself; obtain the individual's undivided attention.
◆ Give the person sufficient time to respond; if there is no response in 1 to 2 minutes, repeat yourself verbally and nonverbally in the same way.
◆ Consistently use the word for an item or a task that is most familiar to the person.
◆ Provide affectionate encouragement; use humor and diversion.
◆ If the elder is able to use only single words, construct verbal communication to match his or her ability.
◆ If the person's verbalizations do not make sense, search for clue words and repeat them to evoke the feeling of being connected.
◆ Break down tasks into individual steps.
◆ Do not agree with communication that you do not understand; do not pretend to understand.
◆ Do not attempt to force a patient to do anything; if you cannot gain cooperation, leave and come back later.
◆ Elicit listening behaviors and maintain attention by touching.

Nonverbal:
◆ Match your own verbal and nonverbal communication and cues.
◆ Be sensitive to the person's nonverbal behavior; use your nonverbal behavior in a therapeutic and planned manner.
◆ Remember that your emotions, positive and negative, will be communicated and that the patient will react to them.
◆ Adapt facial expressions; eyes especially can promote a feeling of understanding and empathy.
◆ Touch is important because often cognitively impaired individuals' affective and touch needs are unmet.
◆ Use all sensory channels.
◆ If the individual displays nonreceptive behaviors, convey your understanding that she or he does not want to talk now, and approach her or him later.
◆ Use positive, pleasant, nonverbal behaviors that are reassuring and

encouraging; observe which nonverbal modes the patient finds pleasurable and which ones make him or her uncomfortable.
♦   Use behaviors that show that you want to communicate with the individual.

Physical Care

Perhaps one of the reasons that caring for older adults, particularly those with cognitive impairment, is viewed as professionally less appealing to nurses is that much of the care provided has to do with basic functions of life—not heroically restoring vital functions (as in intensive care) but assuring that so-called ADLs, from the simple hygienic to the more complex instrumental, are maintained or that their loss is temporarily delayed.

Nutrition and Feeding

Importance

It is beyond question that good and appropriate nutrition is essential. Two reasons add to the significance of good nutrition for older adults with cognitive impairment. First, apart from aging and therefore having altered nutritional metabolic requirements, dementia patients often exhibit agitated behaviors that increase their caloric use. Second, irreversible cognitive impairment can be compromised further by reversible cognitive loss due to nutritional/metabolic dysfunction (Abraham, Holroyd et al., 1994; National Institutes of Health, 1987), specifically hypo- and hyperglycemia, hypercalcemia, and vitamin B_{12}, folate, or thiamine deficiency.

Nutrition is more than the quality of nutritional intake. Nutrition also includes the praxic ability to eat: from planning what, when, and how to eat to the ability to chew and swallow. It has social and environmental dimensions. Within this context, Norberg and Athlin (1989) argue that interventions to promote eating in cognitively impaired patients should target the appropriate problem:

1.   Problems associated with the task aspect; this refers to the ability to eat and drink.
2.   Problems associated with the relationship aspect; this refers to the social dimension of eating.

   3. Problems associated with the environmental aspect; this refers to the impact of the physical and social environment.

Hall (1994b) focuses attention on the importance of feeding problems in the ambulatory stage of dementia, the phase in which feeding problems begin to manifest themselves most acutely and in which nursing staff often revert to passive interventions. Patients may exhibit a loss of interest in eating, or they may be eating constantly. They lose the ability to select and prepare food or even to recognize food as food. The meal environment may be sensorily overwhelming. Food intake may also be compromised by fatigue, decreased attention span, slowness, or motor apraxia. All of this may occur when, at the same time, pacing, increased activity levels, or agitation increase caloric use, thus requiring higher caloric intake.

Interventions

The design of nutritious and appropriate meals is a dietary responsibility. However, there are some recommendations relevant to nursing in terms of general principles, facilitating food intake, providing snacks between meals, and the interface between certain nutrients/agents and behavior. These principles include a well-balanced diet with a caloric value appropriate to the needs of the person and considerate of the person's activity and mobility level. Diets must include sufficient complex carbohydrates (Beck & Heacock, 1988). If the food intake by the patient does not provide sufficient caloric intake, high-calorie liquids should be offered during or between meals (Harvis, 1990). There is some evidence that dementia patients may prefer sweet food, especially if its color stands out (De Maesschalck & Abraham, 1994). This preference may lead to a carbohydrate-high meal, which may be calorically high but nutritionally unbalanced. Caffeinated beverages should be avoided (Beck & Heacock, 1988), replaced by non- or decaffeinated alternatives. For many of the current generation of elderly people, coffee has a social dimension ("having a cup of coffee together"). Switching to decaffeinated coffee preserves the relationship aspect of drinking coffee (see Norberg & Athlin's [1989] advice mentioned earlier).

   Meals should be presented as much as possible in a pleasant and calm environment (Beck & Heacock, 1988; Hall, 1994b). Meals should be taken as long as possible in the company of others, whether family members at home or other residents in a residential environment. On the other hand, Hall (1994b) defends taking meals in one's room if this assures the needed quiet environment. The environment can also be enhanced by the use of food aromas (Hall, 1994b).

Food intake can be stimulated by offering food that is easy to chew (Beck & Heacock, 1988). In more advanced cases of cognitive impairment and/or for patients with impaired praxic ability, finger foods and drinkable foods (e.g., soup) might be indicated (Harvis, 1990). Patients who ambulate continuously and cannot sit still for prolonged periods of time may be given frequent high-calorie snacks, finger foods, or "brown bag" meals that they can carry along (Hall, 1994b). It might also help to provide nutritious snacks on a table where they are highly visible, leaving the decision of what to eat at what time of day to the patient (Harvis, 1990). Given that people with cognitive impairment have difficulty making decisions and may become agitated when confronted with situations in which they have to make a choice, single-dish offerings should be considered (Beck & Heacock, 1988). Another method may be to use small plates and frequent feedings to assure sufficient caloric intake and to counter feelings of being overwhelmed.

Considering patients' difficulty in making choices, De Maesschalck and Abraham (1994) investigated whether the mode of presentation of the components of a meal had an impact on food and caloric intake. Over a 5-week period, nursing home residents with significant cognitive impairment received the main meal of the day either unstructured—"all at once" on a tray—(Weeks 1, 3, and 5) or structured in separate sequential steps (Weeks 2 and 4). During the weeks that the meal was presented structured in the logical sequence of its components, food intake increased significantly, and residual food and caloric values of food left on the trays decreased significantly. Caloric intake showed a similar pattern of increase and decrease during respective structured and unstructured weeks as well but did not attain statistical significance.

This study suggests that demented nursing home residents eat more and leave less food untouched if their food is presented sequentially rather than all at once. The fact that the 5-week pattern of variation in caloric intake did not attain statistical significance can be attributed to the fact that almost all residents ate their carbohydrate-rich desserts (typically, pastry- or custard-type). This study also suggests the importance of nursing care focused on substitution of the cognitive tasks involved in an ADL such as eating. Structured presentation of food thus becomes a nursing intervention, in which the nurse assumes the role of cognition as mediator and regulator of cognitive and executive processes.

Dining rooms in residential settings can be noisy due to food handling, movement by staff and residents, resident behavior, furniture moving, and so on. Van Ort and Phillips (1992) observed that "meal times consistently [make] an already chaotic environment even noisier and more active" (p. 250). Goddaer and Abraham (1994) registered average decibel levels well above 60db(A). Consequently, agitation during meals in response to noise stress is not uncommon among severely demented residents, as can be predicted from the PLST model. In turn, agitated behaviors disrupt the meals of other residents and often lead to the disruptive patient's being served in the social isolation of his or her room. Goddaer and Abraham (1994) studied the effects of relaxing music on agitation among nursing home residents with severe cognitive impairment. Over a 4-week period, relaxing music was (Weeks 2 and 4) or was not (Weeks 1 and 3) played at a few decibels above the mean environmental noise level during the main meal of the day. Agitated behaviors decreased significantly during the weeks with relaxing music, compared with the weeks during which no such music was played during mealtimes. This study underscores the environmental impact on meals and the relevance of nursing interventions that manipulate the environment (as opposed to the patient). It also adds support to Gerdner and Swanson's (1993) interesting case studies on how individualized music reduced agitated behaviors in five Alzheimer's disease patients.

Van Ort and Phillips (1992) studied functional behaviors on the part of staff and residents that may inhibit or promote food intake. The behaviors on the part of the feeder are particularly relevant to this chapter. The authors distinguish between extinguishing behaviors, sustaining behaviors, and eliciting functional feeding behaviors. An extinguishing behavior was defined as a behavior by the feeder in which a feeding episode was begun but aborted before food reached the mouth. Extinguishing behaviors observed by Van Ort and Phillips included feeders failing to respond to resident cues, repeatedly interrupting the feeding, aborting feeding attempts, leaving to feed other residents, and removing the food tray. Eliciting behaviors by the feeder included putting food on the spoon, leaning toward the resident when presenting the food, calling the resident by name, and touching the resident. Sustaining behaviors assure continuous contact between feeder and resident: the feeder talks to the resident, reorients the resident to the meal, offers drink between food offerings, kisses or hugs the resident, holds the spoon ready for a bite, and touches the resident continually. In this regard note also that for severely demented patients, assigning the same care provider to assist with eating or feeding might be indicated. Athlin and Norberg (1987) found that care providers felt more certain about how to interpret the eating behavior of patients when their feeding responsibilities were changed from a task-assignment system to a patient-assignment system.

On the basis of their initial study, Van Ort and Phillips (1994) developed and tested both contextual and behavioral interventions to promote functional feeding. The *contextual intervention* consisted of structuring the feeding environment by minimizing noise and distractions, placing all subjects at the dining table, placing the food on a placemat directly in front of the subject, using a name card, placing finger food in subjects' hands at the beginning of the meal, positioning functionally impaired subjects next to self-feeding subjects, and avoiding staff feeder interruptions during the meal. The contextual intervention was found to lead to more food and drink intake, less food refusal, and more self-feeding. It did not extend the mealtime. The *behavioral intervention* focused on verbal and tactile prompts, role modeling, cue synchronization, and reinforcement. This intervention increased food and drink intake as well as self-feeding; however, there was a higher food refusal rate, and the mealtime was extended. Notwithstanding these differences between the contextual and behavioral interventions, it is clear that both interventions assured food and drink intake and promoted self-feeding, thus decreasing relative dependence in this ADL dimension.

Bathing

Importance

Many agitated behaviors, including physical and verbal aggression, occur during bathing. As Buckwalter (1994) points out, an older adult with cognitive impairment may experience bathing as a physical or sexual assault and react with an assaultive response in turn.

Interventions

Some strategies have been identified that may reduce patients' agitation: changing the time of day or frequency of bathing, using a comfortable shower chair, offering the choice of shower or tub bath (Rader, 1994), and using alternatives such as a towel bed bath (Rader, 1994; Sloane et al.,

1994; Wright, 1990) or sponge baths at the sink (Rader, 1994). It might also be helpful to move away from standard bath days (Rader, 1994; Sloane et al., 1994), as long as health, hygiene, and infection control are not compromised and social and personal factors are met (Sloane et al., 1994). Yet one must also realize that, at least in long-term care, regulations may allow only partial implementation of these suggested measures. Sloane et al. (1994) present consensus recommendations regarding staff–patient interactions and staff approaches related to bathing:

◆ Bathing must be an individualized process, which requires flexibility on the part of the caregiver.
◆ The caregiver should focus on the resident rather than on the task of bathing.
◆ The home environment and bathing experiences at home should be the point of reference from which to plan and implement bathing care.
◆ The resident's perceptions are always valid, thus recognizing the validity of resident experiences associated with the bathing process (including, for instance, the experience of physical or sexual assault).
◆ Persuasion should be used instead of coercion.
◆ Perfect solutions rarely exist for severe bathing problems, thus placing the onus for creativity and responsibility even more on the caregiver.

These recommendations for staff behavior and intervention must be complemented with environmental manipulations and appropriate communication. Thus, Sloane et al. (1994) stress the importance of a pleasant bathing environment: private and personal, warm and relaxing, with adjusted lighting, reduced noise, homelike furnishings, use of aromas, and comfortable and functional equipment. They also offer numerous communication techniques to motivate and engage older adults with cognitive impairment in the bathing process: communicating in a calm, personal, and gentle manner; using distraction and persuasion; offering a reason to participate; addressing the person in familiar terms; providing information; using past memories to convince or reassure; and offering choice, positive feedback, and rewards.

Dressing

Importance

Getting dressed is a complex process that encompasses selecting clothes, organizing them in the appropriate order and for the function they serve, and putting them on, using gross and fine motor skills. Beck (1988) developed the Beck Dressing Performance Scale, which identifies 43 separate dressing components with which older adults may need assistance. The types of assistance and, by extension, the degree of dependence are rated at the levels of no assistance, stimulus control, initial verbal prompt, repeated verbal prompt, gestures/modeling, complete physical guidance, and complete assistance.

Dressing has a personal/emotional dimension. It is a personal expression of oneself, regardless of age and cognitive status. It influences how people feel; for example, being forced to wear pajamas during the day leads people more readily to assume the sick role or feel embarrassed or inferior. Dressing also has a social dimension. It reflects our well-being, our capacity to take care of ourselves. Appropriate dress allows us to be around other people and/or stimulates us to want to be around other people.

As in bathing, dressing has a privacy component. Dressing a person may lead to the desirable end result of having the person dressed, but it is often experienced as an intrusion into privacy. Coupled with the poor impulse control that characterizes people with cognitive impairment, it often results in the understandable reactions of agitation and violence.

Interventions

Nursing interventions related to dressing must focus on the praxic skill of dressing, with cognitive substitution as necessary, as well as on the management of patients' responses to the dressing situation. Beck and associates (Beck, Heacock, Mercer, Walton, & Shook, 1991) distinguish between general and specific strategies, both of which include interactional (see also verbal and nonverbal communication above) and environmental strategies:

1. General strategies: Interactional
   - Restrict conversation to dressing.
   - Speak clearly in a calm voice with low pitch, using simple sentences (even one or two words when possible).
   - Call the elder by name.
   - Consistently use the same word for the same dressing item or action.
2. General strategies: Environmental
   - Make up the bed.
   - Eliminate improper clothing options to reduce number of choices and decisions.

- ◆ Minimize clutter of nonclothing items in the area.
- ◆ Put other clothing out of the elder's sight to avoid distraction.
- ◆ Increase lighting.

3. Specific strategies: Interactional-verbal
    - ◆ Give the patient concrete, one-step verbal commands.
    - ◆ Offer praise after each step of the dressing process is completed.
    - ◆ Give praise regarding appearance after completion of dressing.

4. Specific strategies: Interactional-nonverbal
    - ◆ Dress bottom half, then top half of the body.
    - ◆ Hand clothing items to the elder in the correct position; with less-impaired patients, lay out clothing in correct position. In other words, provide the cognitive substitution to compensate for the patient's loss of cognitive ability to plan and execute complex tasks.
    - ◆ Place shoes beside the foot on which the elder will put them, another example of cognitive substitution.
    - ◆ Use gestures to indicate what you want the elder to do.
    - ◆ Gestures can be complemented by modeling activities.
    - ◆ Use physical touch to indicate to the elder which body part you want moved or used.
    - ◆ Use graduated physical guidance to start the elder's movement, and then allow the elder to complete the action without help.
    - ◆ Use touch by giving the elder a pat on the back or a hug after completing each dressing step.

5. Specific strategies: Environmental
    - ◆ Prepare a consistent environment.
    - ◆ Use a dark bedspread to contrast with clothing.
    - ◆ Lay clothes face down in the order in which they will be used.
    - ◆ Cluster matching outfits on hangers.
    - ◆ Introduce one item of clothing at a time.
    - ◆ Reduce the number of clothing options.
    - ◆ Provide an incentive for completing dressing.
    - ◆ Reduce external stimuli (turn off radio/television, reduce number of people in the room).
    - ◆ Provide privacy.

The importance of staff interaction during dressing has been underscored by a study of 239 staff–resident interactions during dressing on a unit for Alzheimer's disease patients (Burgener & Barton, 1991). Relaxed behavior by staff was associated with flexible, relaxed, calm, and cooperative behaviors in the residents. Personal approaches were better received than authoritarian or task-oriented approaches. Interruptions in interactions were disruptive to both residents and staff. Distraction, redirection, praise, and a lighthearted approach were helpful when residents became upset or paranoid.

Sleep

Importance

Disturbances in the sleep-wake cycle are highly prevalent among older adults with irreversible cognitive impairment. Furthermore, contrary to common belief, older adults in general may require less sleep than younger adults do. Irregular sleep-wake cycles, nighttime awakening with or without agitation, and excessive daytime napping are significant nursing problems.

Interventions

Stewart (1991) offers some basic principles that should be kept in mind. Obviously, caffeine use should be avoided. Activity or age- and condition-appropriate exercise during the day should be increased. The bedroom should be kept cool and quiet. If possible, hypnotic medications should be avoided; if necessary, use a short-acting benzodiazepine. Note that these agents may help patients fall asleep, but they are also known to cause vivid, if not disturbing, dreams in some people and thus affect overall sleep quality. Drowsiness is a common side effect as well and may increase the likelihood of falls. Other helpful strategies include flexibility in institutional routines related to sleep (Beck & Heacock, 1988) and, on the nutrition side, offering warm milk at bedtime (Alessi, 1991).

There is quite a bit of clinical controversy about the appropriateness of daytime napping (see e.g., Stewart, 1991). Our position is that some naps may be helpful if they are in tune with circadian rhythms and sleep processes. Typical human circadian rhythms show a dip in the early afternoon, and for young adults a brief nap at this time is not inappropriate. However, the elderly tend to take either longer naps or frequent short naps during the day. This pattern of napping disrupts the circadian sleep-wake cycle and the quality of night rest. What is most often disrupted among the cognitively impaired elderly is rapid eye movement (REM) sleep, the phase of sleep that gives one the feeling of being rested (subjective sleep quality). For the cognitively impaired elderly, a morning nap of moderate length (e.g., 30 to 60 minutes) might be helpful, as it can be hypothesized that it will emulate the disturbed REM sleep. The patient will feel more rested, and the likelihood of agitated behavior later in the day is likely to decrease. Thus, morning naps not only contribute to the restoration of the disturbed sleep process but also reenergize a person to be better able to manage stressful stimuli during the remainder of the day (cf. PLST hypothesis).

Conclusion

This section on promoting ADLs illustrates various ways in which nursing care can maintain or improve function. More hidden, but not less important, are the policy implications. From a policy perspective, ADLs are seen as "static" indicators that can be used to determine eligibility for various levels of care. Within this perspective, ADLs are seen as skills people lose, not skills that people may regain, maintain, or lose less rapidly. Policy related to long-term care should adopt a dynamic perspective on ADLs, abandoning ADLs as a means or needs test and adopting a clinical perspective that substitutes for the passive "lost is lost" assumption an active "not all is lost that seems lost" assumption.

COGNITIVE INTERVENTIONS

Recent years have seen a growth in the application of cognitive interventions to either enhance or slow down the decline of cognitive functions. Much of this work is still in a developmental stage, even though some approaches have received considerable clinical attention. For instance, reality orientation methods continue to be advocated (e.g., Gropper-Katz, 1987; McMahon, 1988) and used in clinical settings, even though the empirical evidence for this long-used intervention is ambivalent at best. One of the few randomized nursing studies (Hogstel, 1979) did not find a significant effect. Validation therapy is rapidly gaining acceptance, perhaps because of its clinically intuitive appeal, namely, focusing on the emotional content of a demented elderly person's statements and expressions. In the absence of stronger empirical evidence than that available today (e.g., Bleathman & Morton, 1988), this intervention may have more strength as a method of empowering care providers than as de facto help for patients. Likewise, remotivation therapy (Janssen & Giberson, 1988) must be validated empirically through well-designed studies. Again, this intervention is a clinically appealing one; however, the seriousness of cognitive impairment does not permit experimentation with interventions that do not withstand the test of systematic investigation.

Perhaps one of the reasons some cognitive interventions have failed to yield empirically verifiable results is that these interventions are developed as solutions to problems but often have little theoretical foundation in cognitive theories. They pay little attention to the role, purposes, and processes of cognition; neither do they differentiate between different types of cognitive processes. The future may lie in the development of interventions that are grounded in a view of cognition as a set of dynamic processes; in the recognition that cognition, as a dynamic entity, may respond to interventions that specifically attempt to stimulate selected cognitive functions; and the abandonment of the idea that superficial cognitive functions (e.g., orientation) are important to older adults with cognitive impairment, thus leading to the adoption of a perspective of stimulating "life-relevant" cognitive functions that play a role in people's ability to function (the so-called higher cortical cognitive processes).

Individual Cognitive Nursing Interventions

A study of 20 cognitively impaired older adults showed that cognitive skills remediation through systematic cognitive exercises (Carter, Caruso, Languirand, & Berard, 1980) significantly improved memory function as measured by recalling numbers in a list (Beck, Heacock, Mercer, Thatcher, & Sparkman, 1988). A study with traumatic brain injury patients, even though the pathology is different from dementing illness, showed that comprehensive and intensive cognitive retraining led to improvements in such cognitive tasks as sequencing objects in logical order, recognition and reproduction of geometric designs, and task completion (Grinspun, 1987).

Group Cognitive Nursing Interventions

A qualitative study of four cognitively impaired elders showed that participation in a psychotherapeutic group increased verbal activity and some higher functioning processes more than expected (Akerlund &

Norberg, 1986). Abraham, Neundorfer, and Currie (1992) reported a study in which 76 older adults with mild to moderate cognitive impairment participated in one of three 24-week group intervention protocols: cognitive-behavioral therapy, focused visual imagery, and educational discussion groups, the latter being a control condition (for protocols, see Abraham, Niles, Thiel, Siarkowski, & Cowling, 1991).

Cognitive-behavioral therapy and focused visual imagery are both cognitive interventions but require the activation of different cognitive resources. Cognitive-behavioral therapy engages people in rigorous examination of their thinking and behavior and encourages them to change faulty ways of thinking about themselves and their interactions with their physical and social environment. Visual imagery therapy is an intensely cognitive effort, requiring unique cognitive skills such as imagination, memory storage and retrieval in both verbal and visual codes (Hill, Evankovich, Sheikh, & Yesavage, 1987; Stern & Stern, 1989), recognition and recall, and naming to achieve the goal of "thinking in pictures." At the clinical level, cognitive-behavioral therapy influences people's cognitive abilities and processes, whereas in visual imagery, cognitive abilities and processes are the means to achieve therapeutic outcomes. Thus, the former aims at changes in cognitive abilities and processes (cognition as dynamic outcome), and the latter utilizes cognitive processes and abilities (cognition as dynamic process).

Significant improvement in overall cognitive functioning, as measured by the Modified Mini-Mental State Exam (Teng & Chui, 1987), was observed from baseline after 8 and 12 weeks of treatment and 4 weeks following completion of the 24-week protocol in subjects participating in cognitive-behavioral and focused visual imagery groups. The latter groups showed slightly more, but statistically nonsignificant, improvement over the former (Abraham, Neundorfer, & Currie, 1992). To further elucidate the cognitive gains made by subjects, Abraham and Reel (1992) reanalyzed the data, focusing on the 15 neurocognitive parameters tested by the Modified Mini-Mental State Exam. Main effects for intervention were observed on neurocognitive operations involving abstraction and conceptual thinking, concentration and linguistic manipulation, and execution of auditorily presented language skills. Main effects for time were noted on short- and medium-term recall, fluency of category retrieval, abstraction and conceptual thinking, concentration and linguistic manipulation, and execution of visually presented commands. Interaction effects for intervention and time were found on subjects' ability to visually and linguistically identify objects and on their praxic ability to recognize and redraw simple intersection geometric figures. There were no effects on the various orientation items or on the task of immediately repeating three words upon their verbal presentation.

It can be inferred that the cognitive improvement among cognitive-behavioral and visual imagery subjects was due predominantly to the activation of cognitive resources. Why this improvement occurs is not well understood but may be related to the amount, type, and intensity of cognitive resources that are activated in the course of the three group interventions. Educational discussion groups rely on basic and primary cognitive skills used routinely by elderly people in their daily life, even in the constrained environment of a long-term-care facility. Cognitive-behavioral group therapy requires some of these same skills but at a more intensive level. Furthermore, it requires the higher cognitive skills of reflecting on one's own and others' cognitive errors, verbalizing these reflections and one's reactions to them, and learning other modes of thinking and behaving. Visual imagery requires still different cognitive skills: imagination, construction of mental images, storage and retrieval from short- and long-term memory in both verbal and visual codes, recognition and recall, naming and other linguistic skills, and reproduction. The cognitive skills activated in this mode are perhaps the most unusual and least used in the daily life of older adults.

Even though the evidence is only beginning to accumulate in nursing, there are clear indications that cognition can be improved (or at least its decline slowed) by means of specific nursing interventions. Reanalysis (Abraham & Reel, 1992) of the original cognitive effects reported by Abraham, Neundorfer, and Currie (1992) showed that the cognitive gains made by subjects involved brain functions at higher cortical and subcortical/limbic levels. In contrast, cognitive interventions had no effect on lower and more basic cortical functions: orientation to self, time, and space and repeating words immediately after their presentation. This differential effect raises questions, not only about the extent to which interventions can affect these lower-level cognitive functions but also as to whether nursing should even be involved in trying to improve or maintain lower-level functions. In the case of the nursing home residents in this study who were old and frail in addition to mildly to moderately cognitively impaired, knowing when and where they were born, what the date is, and the exact address or location of where they are may just not be important. See in this regard our concern above about the relevance (regardless of effectiveness) of reality orientation therapies.

The findings also underscore the importance of higher cognitive functions within the perspective of cognition as dynamic processes of mediation, regulation, and modulation. Thus, nursing should aim to develop interventions that focus on higher cortical and subcortical/limbic functions. These functions have the closest link to and are of the greatest relevance to maintaining, improving, sustaining, or substituting functional performance. This is an area with significant future opportunities for research. However, it will be important to conduct these studies in collaboration with other disciplines, which can strengthen the focus on differential cognitive processes (e.g., neuropsychology, geriatric neurology, geriatric psychiatry).

IMPLICATIONS AND DIRECTIONS FOR FUTURE RESEARCH

The selective issues addressed in this chapter signal that the care of cognitively impaired older adults is not as discouraging as is often believed. Clinical achievements are possible, even though it requires a fundamental rethinking as to what are successful clinical outcomes with and quality care for this population. The challenge continues to be to design, implement, and test nursing interventions that directly or indirectly affect the daily functioning and health care needs of individuals.

Further research is needed to improve the quality of care for older adults with cognitive impairment. Beck et al. (Beck, Heacock, Rapp, & Shue, 1993) argue that instruments must be developed and tested that can accurately identify competencies and deficits and detect subtle changes in cognitive and functional status. They also point to the need to design and evaluate interventions that use remaining cognitive abilities. For this, it will be necessary to better understand the association between the level of functional disability and cognitive dysfunction. Finally, these authors point out the need for interface between the biological sciences and nursing.

The case needs to be made (again and again) for a stronger commitment to research on the effectiveness and outcomes of nursing interventions for the cognitively impaired elderly. Research on interventions should increase in amount and broaden in scope. In general, nursing research on interventions constitutes only about one tenth of all the research done in nursing (Abraham, Chalifoux, & Evers, 1992). Intervention research on the elderly, cognitively intact or impaired, constitutes a small fraction of these studies; moreover, there are proportionately more intervention studies involving elderly subjects conducted in Europe than in North America (Abraham, Chalifoux, Evers, & De Geest, 1995). To stimulate nursing intervention research with the elderly and the cognitively impaired in particular, this area should be identified as a priority for funding—realizing full well that intervention research is more expensive on a per subject basis than nonintervention research. In addition, there is not just a need for more intervention research but equally a need for conceptual frameworks in which to embed this research (e.g., the PLST model discussed earlier).

The conclusion is self-evident: without more, better, and larger-scale research using specific and sensitive research methodologies attuned to the realities of aging and older adults, nurses will continue to be forced to base much of their practice on clinical experience. Although it is not necessary (nor practical) to achieve an empirically sustained knowledge base about nursing care of cognitively impaired elderly, it is critical that a broadly based repertoire of empirically tested interventions be made available to support and improve care.

REFERENCES

Abraham, I. L. (1994). Beyond continuity and towards fluidity of care: Rethinking long-term care for an aging society. *Acta Hospitalia, 33*(4), 71–75.

Abraham, I. L. (1995). Differentiated neural cognitive screening assessment of nursing home residents: Algorithms from Factor-Analytic Studies of variants on the Mini-Mental State Examination. In B. Vellas (Ed.), *Facts and research in gerontology* (pp. 81–93). New York: Springer Publishing Co.

Abraham, I. L., Chalifoux, Z. L., & Evers, G. C. M. (1992). Conditions, interventions, and outcomes: A quantitative analysis of nursing research (1981–1990). In P. Moritz (Ed.), *Patient outcomes research: Examining the effectiveness of nursing practice* (NIH Publication No. 93-3411, pp. 70–87). Bethesda, MD: National Institutes of Health.

Abraham, I. L., Chalifoux, Z. L., Evers, G. C. M., & De Geest, S. (1995). Conditions, interventions, and outcomes in nursing research: A comparative analysis of North American and European/international journals (1981–1990). *International Journal of Nursing Studies, 32,* 173–187.

Abraham, I. L., Chalifoux, Z. L., Snustad, D. G. Buckwalter, K. C., Fulmer, T., Beck, C. K., & Evers, G. C. (1993). Beyond the role of extender: Independent and interdependent contributions of nursing to geriatric rehabilitation. *Neurorehabilitation, 3,* 12–25.

Abraham, I. L., Fox, J. M., Harrington, D. P., Snustad, D. G., Steiner, D. A.,

Abraham, L. H., & Brashear, H. R. (1990). A psychogeriatric nursing assessment protocol for use in multidisciplinary practice. *Archives of Psychiatric Nursing, 4,* 242–259.

Abraham, I. L., Holroyd, S., Brashear, H. R., Snustad, D. G., Diamond, P., Manning, C. A., & Thompson-Heisterman, A. A. (1994). Multidisciplinary assessment of patients with Alzheimer's disease. *Nursing Clinics of North America, 29,* 113–128.

Abraham, I. L., Manning, C. A., Boyd, M., Neese, J. B., Newman, M., Plowfield, L., & Reel, S. (1993). Cognitive screening of nursing home residents: Factor structure of the Modified Mini-Mental State (3MS) Examination. *International Journal of Geriatric Psychiatry, 8,* 133–138.

Abraham, I. L., Manning, C. A., Newman, M. C., Brashear, H. A., Snustad, D. G., & Wofford, A. B. (1994). Cognitive screening of nursing home residents: Factor structures of the Mini-Mental State Examination (MMSE). *Journal of the American Geriatrics Society, 42,* 750–756.

Abraham, I. L., Neundorfer, M. M., & Currie, L. J. (1992). Effects of group interventions on cognition and depression in nursing home residents. *Nursing Research, 41,* 196–202.

Abraham, I. L., Niles, S. A., Thiel, B. P., Siarkowski, K. I., & Cowling, W. R. (1991). Therapeutic group work with depressed elderly. *Nursing Clinics of North America, 26,* 635–650.

Abraham, I. L., Onega, L., Chalifoux, Z. L., & Maes, M.-J. (1994). Care environments for patients with Alzheimer's disease. *Nursing Clinics of North America, 29,* 157–172.

Abraham, I. L., & Reel, S. J. (1992). Cognitive nursing interventions with long-term care residents: Effects on neurocognitive dimensions. *Archives of Psychiatric Nursing, 6,* 356–365.

Abraham, I. L., Smullen, D. E., & Thompson-Heisterman, A. A. (1992). Geriatric mental health: Assessing geropsychiatric patients. *Journal of Psychosocial Nursing and Mental Health Services, 30*(9), 13–19.

Akerlund, B., & Norberg, A. (1986). Group psychotherapy with demented patients. *Geriatric Nursing, 6,* 83–84.

Alessi, C. A. (1991). Managing the behavioral problems of dementia in the home. *Clinics in Geriatric Medicine, 7,* 787–801.

Athlin, E., & Norberg, A. (1987). Caregivers' attitudes to and interpretations of the behavior of severely demented patients during feeding in a patient assignment care system. *International Journal of Nursing Studies, 24,* 145–153.

Beck, C. (1988). Measurement of dressing performance in persons with dementia. *American Journal of Alzheimer's Care and Related Disorders and Research, 3*(3), 21–25.

Beck, C., & Heacock, P. (1988). Nursing interventions for patients with Alzheimer's disease. *Nursing Clinics of North America, 23,* 95–124.

Beck, C., Heacock, P., Mercer, S., Thatcher, R., & Sparkman, C. (1988). The impact of cognitive skills remediation training on persons with Alzheimer's disease or mixed dementia. *Journal of Geriatric Psychiatry, 11,* 73–88.

Beck, C., Heacock, P., Mercer, S., Walton, C. G., & Shook, J. (1991). Dressing for success: Promoting independence among cognitively impaired elderly. *Journal of Psychosocial Nursing and Mental Health Services, 29*(7), 30–35.

Beck, C. K., Heacock, P., Rapp, C. G., & Shue, V. (1993). Cognitive impairment in the elderly. *Nursing Clinics of North America, 28,* 335–347.

Bleathman, C., & Morton, I. (1988). Validation therapy with the demented elderly. *Journal of Advanced Nursing, 13,* 511–514.

Buckwalter, K. C. (1994). To bathe or not to bathe: That is the question [Introduction]. *Journal of Gerontological Nursing, 20*(9), 53.

Burgener, S. C., & Barton, D. (1991). Nursing care of cognitively impaired institutionalized elderly. *Journal of Gerontological Nursing, 17*(4), 37–43.

Carter, L. T., Caruso, J. L., Languirand, M. A., & Berard, M. A. (1980). *The thinking skills workbook: A cognitive skills remediation manual for adults.* Springfield, IL: Charles C Thomas.

De Maesschalck, L., & Abraham, I. L. (1994). *The effects of structured versus unstructured presentation of meals on food and caloric intake among elderly with dementia.* Manuscript submitted for publication.

Frances, A., Dysken, M. W., Christensen, R., Maletta, G., Schut, L., & Wilson, B. (1988). A multidisciplinary approach to primary degenerative dementia. *Hospital and Community Psychiatry, 39,* 1145–1148.

Gerdner, L. A., & Swanson, E. A. (1993). Effects of individualized music on confused and agitated elderly patients. *Archives of Psychiatric Nursing, 7,* 284–291.

Goddaer, J., & Abraham, I. L. (1994). Effects of relaxing music on agitation during meals among cognitively impaired nursing home residents. *Archives of Psychiatric Nursing, 8,* 150–158.

Grinspun, D. R. (1987). Nursing intervention in cognitive retraining of the traumatic brain injury client. *Rehabilitation Nursing, 12,* 323, 324, 329, 330.

Gropper-Katz, E. (1987). Reality orientation research. *Journal of Gerontological Nursing, 13*(8), 13–18.

Hall, G. R. (1988). Care of the patient with Alzheimer's disease living at home. *Nursing Clinics of North America, 23,* 31–46.

Hall, G. R. (1994a). Caring for people with Alzheimer's disease using the conceptual model of progressively lowered stress threshold in the clinical setting. *Nursing Clinics of North America, 29,* 129–141.

Hall, G. R. (1994b). Chronic dementia: Challenges in feeding a patient. *Journal of Gerontological Nursing, 20*(4), 21–30.

Hall, G. R., & Buckwalter, K. C. (1987). Progressively lowered stress threshold: A conceptual model for care of adults with Alzheimer's disease. *Archives of Psychiatric Nursing, 1,* 399–406.

Hall, G. R., & Buckwalter, K. C. (1991). Whole disease care planning: Fitting the program to the client with Alzheimer's disease. *Journal of Gerontological Nursing, 17*(3), 38–41.

Harvis, K. A. (1990). Care plan approach to dementia. *Geriatric Nursing, 11,* 76–80.

Hill, R. D., Evankovich, K. D., Sheikh, J. I., & Yesavage, J. A. (1987). Imagery mnemonic training in a patient with primary degenerative dementia. *Psychology of Aging, 2,* 204–205.

Hirst, S. P. (1989). Gerontic nurse specialists: An examination of their roles with dementia sufferers and their caregivers. *Clinical Nurse Specialist, 3,* 105–108.

Hogstel, M. O. (1979). Use of reality orientation with aging confused patients. *Nursing Research, 28,* 161–165.

Janssen, J. A., & Giberson, D. L. (1988). Remotivation therapy. *Journal of Gerontological Nursing, 14*(6), 31–34.

Maas, M. L., Swanson, E., Specht, J., & Buckwalter, K. C. (1994). Alzheimer's special care units. *Nursing Clinics of North America, 29,* 173–194.

McMahon, R. (1988). The "24-hour reality orientation" type of approach to the confused elderly: A minimum standard for care. *Journal of Advanced Nursing, 13,* 693–700.

National Institutes of Health, Consensus Conference on Differential Diagnosis of Dementing Diseases. (1987). *Journal of the American Medical Association, 258,* 3411–3416.

Norberg, A., & Athlin, E. (1989). Eating problems in severely demented patients: Issues and ethical dilemmas. *Nursing Clinics of North America, 24,* 781–789.

Rader, J. (1994). To bathe or not to bathe: That is the question. *Journal of Gerontological Nursing, 20*(9), 53–54.

Ryden, M. B., & Feldt, K. S. (1992). Goal-directed care: Caring for aggressive nursing home residents with dementia. *Journal of Gerontological Nursing, 18*(11), 35–42.

Sloane, P. D., Rader, J., Barrick, A.-L., Hoeffer, B., Dwyer, S., McKenzie, D., Lavelle, M., Buckwalter, K., Ourington, L., & Pruitt, T. (1994). *Bathing persons with dementia.* Manuscript submitted for publication.

Stern, J. M., & Stern, B. (1989). Visual imagery as a cognitive means of compensation for brain injury. *Brain Injury, 3,* 413–419.

Stewart, J. T. (1991). Managing the care of patients with dementia. *Postgraduate Medicine, 90*(4), 45–49.

Teng, E. L., & Chui, H. C. (1987). The Modified Mini-Mental State (3MS) Examination. *Journal of Clinical Psychiatry, 48,* 314–317.

Thompson-Heisterman, A. A., Smullen, D. E., & Abraham, I. L. (1992). Psychogeriatric nursing assessment. In K. C. Buckwalter (Ed.), *Geriatric mental health nursing: Current and future challenges* (pp. 17–26). Thorofare, NJ: Slack.

Van Ort, S., & Phillips, L. (1992). Feeding nursing home residents with Alzheimer's disease. *Geriatric Nursing, 13,* 249–253.

Van Ort, S., & Phillips, L. (1994). *Nursing interventions to promote functional feeding.* Manuscript submitted for publication.

Wright, L. (1990). Bathing by towel. *Nursing Times, 86*(4), 36–39.

CHAPTER 6

The Nature of the Family Caregiving Role and Nursing Interventions for Caregiving Families

Patricia G. Archbold and
Barbara J. Stewart

The role of nursing in providing care to impaired older people and their families is extremely important in today's health care system. As part of their care for impaired older people, nurses are often the health care professionals who interact with families about caregiving issues and concerns. In this chapter we review research on interventions for family caregivers, with an emphasis on the utility of these findings for nursing practice. In the review we also highlight studies elucidating caregiving processes related to the nature of the family caregiving role that point the way to new nursing interventions with caregiving families. We

Author notes: Patricia Archbold, RN, DNSc, FAAN, and Barbara Stewart, PhD, are professors at the School of Nursing, Oregon Health Sciences University, and Adjunct Investigators at the Center for Health Research at Kaiser Permanente. The authors wish to thank Jane Kirschling, Lotus Shyu, and Tara Shaw for their help with this chapter.

believe that the nature of the family caregiving role is a critical but under-studied concept that forms the foundation for the unique role of nursing in current and future interventions for caregiving families.

BACKGROUND

The family is the major provider of long-term and medically related services to older people in the community (Shanas, 1979; Stone, Cafferata, & Sangl, 1987). About half of the family caregivers for older people in this country have been providing unpaid assistance for 1 to 4 years, and another quarter have been providing assistance for 5 years or more. Eighty percent of family caregivers provide unpaid assistance 7 days a week and spend an average of 4 extra hours per day—more than a half-time job—on caregiving tasks (Stone et al., 1987). Recent estimates indicate that the average care costs incurred by families of dementia patients were $4,564 for a 3-month period, with 71% of the costs for unpaid labor (Stommel, Collins, & Given, 1994).

Of particular interest to policymakers in the United States is the relationship of family caregiving to health care costs. Although people aged 65 and over represent only 12% of the population, they account for 31% of all hospital discharges and 42% of all short-stay hospital days of care (U.S. Senate Committee on Aging, 1991). The cost of health care for older people accounts for more than one third of the country's total health care expenditures, and it is attributable mainly to acute and highly technical care often required for exacerbations of chronic conditions. Of every 1,000 persons aged 75 and over, 440 were discharged from a hospital in 1991 (U.S. Bureau of Census, 1993).

Typically, families take on caregiving responsibilities with little or no preparation from nurses or other health care professionals. Moreover, Medicare reimbursement guidelines have severely limited the opportunity for home health nurses to provide families with more than minimal assistance (Polich et al., 1990). These restrictive policies may, in the long run, be costly, in that provision of care by family members who are unprepared for and unsupported in their caregiving has been linked to higher acute care utilization and costs for the care receiver (Anderson, 1990; Berry & Evans, 1985/86).

Multiple studies of the effects of caregiving on families indicate that, for some family caregivers, caregiving is very difficult (Horowitz, 1985).

Yet in our previous studies we found that families wanted to provide care in the home: 80% of caregivers reported that they were willing to sacrifice "quite a bit" or "practically anything" to continue taking care of the care receiver (Archbold & Stewart, 1988). In addition, older people want to remain in their homes for as long as possible (McAuley & Blieszner, 1985). We think, therefore, that nursing and the health care system should support families in their caregiving activities.

Development of Caregiving Research

Research on caregiving for frail older people has developed rapidly over the past two decades. Initially, the focus of this research was on identifying caregiving as a phenomenon and describing its negative consequences. The next phase of work focused on clarifying the variables in caregiving and developing measures for them. The conceptual approaches to the study of caregiving during the two decades have included stress and coping (adaptation) theory (e.g., Pearlin, Mullan, Semple, & Skaff, 1990), role theory (e.g., Archbold, Stewart, Greenlick, & Harvath, 1990), social exchange theory (e.g., Walker, Martin, & Jones, 1992), and feminist theory (e.g., Abel & Nelson, 1990). Current research efforts focus on understanding caregiving processes, caregiving in specific disease conditions, and the evaluation of interventions with caregivers. The interested reader can find excellent reviews covering the two decades of research on caregiving (Biegel, Sales, & Schulz, 1991; Given & Given, 1991; Horowitz, 1985; Kahana, Biegel, & Wykle, 1994), with several focused on analyzing interventions with family caregivers (Collins, Given, & Given, 1994; Gallagher, 1985; Knight, Lutzky, & Macofsky-Urban, 1993; Toseland & Rossiter, 1989).

Nurse researchers have contributed substantially to the development of knowledge about caregiving. Their contributions include exploratory work to identify salient variables in caregiving (Bowers, 1987; Bull, 1992; Harvath, 1994; Hirschfeld, 1983), instrument development (Archbold, Stewart, Greenlick, & Harvath, 1992; Given et al., 1992; Oberst, Thomas, Gass, & Ward, 1989; Phillips, Morrison, & Chae, 1990a, 1990b; Phillips, Rempusheski, & Morrison, 1989; Stommel, Wang, Given, & Given, 1992), longitudinal and correlational work to explore caregiving processes (Archbold et al., 1990; Given et al., 1993; Oberst et al., 1989), and the evaluation of interventions with caregivers (Archbold et al., 1995; Farran

& Keane-Hagarty, 1994; Mohide et al., 1990; Naylor et al., 1994; Quayhagen, Quayhagen, Corbeil, Roth, & Rodgers, 1995).

INTERVENTIONS

In this chapter we have chosen to describe in detail those intervention studies that we think are particularly relevant for nursing. We have grouped the selected interventions into seven types: psychoeducational, respite, health services, in-home nursing, transitional care, telephone, and support groups.

Psychoeducational Interventions

Most of the research on psychoeducational interventions with caregivers has been done by disciplines other than nursing; however, the interventions used can, for the most part, be done by nurses with advanced preparation. Some psychoeducational interventions are directed toward increasing the caregiver's problem-solving skills (Zarit, Anthony, & Boutselis, 1987), feelings of competence (Chiverton & Caine, 1989), and social skills (Robinson, 1988), and others are aimed at reducing caregiver stress (Haley, Brown, & Levine, 1987). Still others focus on helping caregivers moderate their negative response to caregiving problems, such as depression and anger (Gallagher-Thompson, 1993; Lovett & Gallagher, 1988). These interventions may be delivered in group counseling (Haley et al., 1987; Lovett & Gallagher, 1988; Robinson, 1988) or individual counseling (Zarit et al., 1987).

Studies of psychoeducational interventions have shared some common features. The target of the psychoeducational interventions in these studies was mainly the caregiver, not the care receiver or the family as a unit. These studies used volunteer samples, and thus the results may not be generalizable to the population of caregivers. To target the intervention to caregivers who needed it, many of the studies selected their samples on the basis of high baseline scores on such variables as strain, depression, and anger. Many of these interventions were not comprehensive but instead were focused on a specific aspect of caregiving (e.g., caregiver anger, stress). The psychoeducational interventions studied were usually short term and were not set up to respond to transitions in the caregiving situation. Finally, psychoeducational interventions required caregivers to leave their homes to come to the intervention site.

Example of a Psychoeducational Intervention Study

Recently, nurse researchers Farran and Keane-Hagarty (1994) examined the effectiveness of a brief (eight 2-hour sessions) educational and support group for caregivers of people with dementia. Group sessions focused on understanding the impact of dementia on functional abilities, developing an environment to compensate for functional losses, managing problematic behaviors, meeting physical care needs, enhancing self-care for caregivers, using formal and informal resources, and understanding legal and financial options. The structure of the sessions was based on caregiver input and the group leader's evaluation of the caregivers' response to the content. Pre- to posttest change revealed an unexpected increase in caregiver distress with cognitive incapacities, life impact, and total burden. Findings such as these are not uncommon among caregiving intervention studies; however, they often occur in concert with high levels of satisfaction with the intervention. Because such interventions focus in part on the caregivers' expression of feelings about caregiving, the intervention may have enhanced caregivers' willingness to express negative affect.

Effectiveness of Psychoeducational Interventions

Despite the limitations of psychoeducational interventions, they appear to be effective in reducing strain and depression in some caregivers. Knight et al. (1993) conducted a meta-analysis of interventions for caregivers, including 10 controlled studies of psychoeducational interventions that attempted to change emotional distress in caregivers; emotional distress included subjective caregiver burden and emotional dysphoria (i.e., depression, anxiety, hostility). They reported average effect sizes for group interventions as follows: .15 for burden (5 studies, 95% confidence interval [CI] = $-.43$ to .73) and .31 for emotional dysphoria (7 studies, 95% CI = $-.38$ to 1.00). The average effect sizes for individual interventions were .41 for burden (5 studies, 95% CI = $-.04$ to .86) and .58 for emotional dysphoria (3 studies, 95% CI = $-.17$ to 1.33). Thus, on the average, the group interventions had small effect sizes, and the individual interventions had moderate effect sizes, with a greater effect on emotional dysphoria than on subjective caregiver burden in both group and individual interventions. The wide confidence intervals also reflect the degree to which intervention effectiveness varied across studies, ranging from large positive effect sizes to small negative effect sizes. When effect sizes reported by Knight and colleagues are summarized by the randomization status of the studies, the results on effectiveness are less definitive; the median effect size in studies not fully randomized was .73 (range = .03 to 1.03), whereas the median effect size in studies where caregivers were randomly assigned to conditions was only .16 (range = −.22 to .66).

Relevance for Nursing

Despite mixed results, we believe that psychoeducational interventions should be considered by nurses when the caregiver has identified high strain or negative affect as a problem. The following example illustrates how and when a nurse might use psychoeducational interventions. In a recent presentation, Gallagher-Thompson (1993) gave the example of a caregiver who responded with anger to an incontinence episode in the morning and generalized her anger response to the entire day. Gallagher-Thompson's anger intervention helped the caregiver to give herself self-supportive statements (e.g., "Incontinence is something that happens in my family member; I have gone through this before; I can make it through"). A nurse might use this strategy with a family after determining that the care receiver's incontinence was not treatable. The first strategies proposed to the family would be focused on modifying the incontinence itself, then on the management of the incontinence so that it was less difficult for the caregiver, and finally on the caregiver's anger response.

Respite Studies

Respite care is a method of providing relief to the caregiver from the burden and strain of caregiving activities. It includes such interventions as day care, adult day health, and in-home respite. In some cases, respite involves the temporary admission of the care receiver to a hospital or long-term-care facility overnight or for a longer period. With the exception of two studies (Lawton, Brody, & Saperstein, 1989; Montgomery & Borgatta, 1989), studies of respite care have not used true experimental designs. In Montgomery and Borgatta's (1989) study, 94 caregivers received respite only; 89 caregivers received respite plus education, a family consultant, and a support group; 85 caregivers formed the control group. Although the findings of Montgomery and Borgatta are encouraging regarding the beneficial effects of respite in reducing subjective burden (effect sizes = .74 and .75), the results by Lawton and colleagues (1989) are not as promising with regard to burden (effect size = .08), perhaps because the comparison group received high levels of respite from other community sources. However, families with respite care ($n = 317$) in Lawton's study maintained the patient with Alzheimer's disease in the community an average of 22 days longer than did families in the control group ($n = 315$). Because previous research suggests that respite can be beneficial to families, it is one strategy that nurses should use with family caregivers who need relief from caregiving activities.

Health Services

Interdisciplinary Home Care Team

In a randomized controlled study ($n = 82$ experimental and $n = 76$ control), Zimmer, Groth-Juncker, and McCusker (1985) evaluated the effects of 6 months of in-home services and 24-hour-per-day emergency telephone support provided by an interdisciplinary health care team (physician, nurse practitioner, and social worker) to homebound chronically and terminally ill older people. The outcome variables examined were health care utilization, functional status and satisfaction of the ill older people, and the satisfaction of their family caregiver.

The in-home services included the provision of primary health care, including physician house calls. Initial assessments of patients in the home were done by each team member, after which an interdisciplinary care plan was developed, with one team member designated as the primary care provider. The nurse practitioner prepared at the master's level conducted other routine and emergency assessments in the home and was responsible for the nursing plan. Social, emotional, and financial problems were handled by the social worker. The team provided physical and psychological support to families and friends of the patient, encouraging them to begin or continue their informal care. Experimental patients had significantly fewer hospitalizations, nursing home admissions, and outpatient visits than did controls. Both patients and family caregivers in the experimental group expressed significantly higher levels of satisfaction than did patients and caregivers in the control condition. Although the overall costs for the experimental group were lower, as hypothesized, no significant differences were found in patient health care costs. Because health care in the United States is shifting out of institutions and into the home and community, this model of interdisciplinary collaboration may prove very useful to nurses engaged in planning such health care delivery changes.

Posthospital Support Program

Oktay and Volland (1990) used a quasi-experimental design (control condition administered in Year 1, experimental condition in Year 2 to sequential discharges of older people from a hospital) to evaluate the effects of a 1-year posthospital support program on family caregiver stress, patient functioning, and patient health care utilization and costs (n = 93 comparison, n = 98 treatment group). The intervention included assessment, case management, skilled nursing, counseling, referrals, respite care, education, a support group, medical backup, and on-call help. The intervention had no effect on patient functioning in activities of daily living (ADLs), instrumental activities of daily living (IADLs), or mental status. Because only 2 of the 15 comparisons between treatment and control groups on caregiver stress yielded significant differences, the evidence for an effect of the intervention on this variable is extremely limited. The intervention group experienced fewer hospitalizations than did the control group; however, the second year of the project coincided with the initiation of diagnostic related groupings, and thus the reduction in hospital utilization and cost in the experimental group is difficult to interpret. Nevertheless, providing focused interdisciplinary care after hospital discharge has the potential to benefit older people and families, but it needs to be evaluated with a true experimental design.

In-Home Nursing

Cognitive Stimulation of Patients with Alzheimer's Disease

Quayhagen, Quayhagen, Corbeil, Roth, and Rodgers (1995) assessed a home-based intervention focused on cognitive stimulation of patients with Alzheimer's disease. The goal of the cognitive stimulation program was to provide a structured plan of activities, including targeted conversation exercises, memory techniques, and interpersonal problem-solving skills. Family members were instructed to work 6 hours per week (1 hour per day) with the patient on the program. Experimental family dyads ($n = 25$) and comparison dyads ($n = 28$ placebo and $n = 25$ wait list controls) participated in the study for a period of 9 months. Statistically significant differences were found between the experimental and comparison patients. As predicted, care recipients in the wait list control group declined on the cognitive and behavioral outcomes, and the experimental group maintained baseline by the 9-month testing. Contrary to predictions that care recipients in the experimental group would maintain cognitive status, they actually exhibited cognitive improvements at the 3-month posttreatment testing. The other unanticipated findings were that care recipients in the placebo group maintained their mean scores on the memory factors, but as expected did decline below baseline in cognitive ability and fluency. This intervention seems to hold promise for nurses working with demented elders and their caregivers.

Caregiver Support Program

Mohide and colleagues (1990) used an experimental design to evaluate the effects of a 6-month caregiver support program, an intervention designed to enhance the competence and sense of control of caregivers to people with dementia. Caregivers were assigned to the experimental ($n = 30$) and control ($n = 30$) conditions using random block assignment. Three caregiver support nurses (CSNs) initially made weekly home visits to caregivers; the number of visits was increased or decreased depending on the needs of the caregiver. The caregiver's health was assessed, and where appropriate, caregivers were encouraged to seek medical attention. Nurses provided individualized caregiver education that focused on dementia. The CSNs assisted the caregiver in examining solutions to behavior problems. All caregivers were given a copy of the book, *The 36 Hour Day*. Four hours per week of respite care were provided to each caregiver, and support groups were made available to them. Members of the control group received community nursing care focused on the demented patient. The intervention had no significant effects on the study's outcome measures: caregiver depression, anxiety, and quality of life; however, the effect sizes were .26, .21, and .35, respectively, indicating a small effect. It is likely that the absence of significant differences between the control and experimental groups is attributable to an inadequate sample size; we believe that interventions such as this one may prove to be very valuable for older people with dementia and their families.

PREP System of Nursing Interventions

Archbold, Stewart, and colleagues (1995) conducted a pilot study of an expanded home health nursing intervention referred to as PREP, which was designed to increase *PRe*paredness, *E*nrichment, and *P*redictability in caregiving situations. PREP's first goal was for families to be competent in, and thereby feel more prepared for, their caregiving activities. PREP's second goal was to strengthen mutuality (the caregiver–care receiver bond) and increase rewards of caregiving by increasing the enrichment in caregiving situations. Enrichment is the process of endowing caregiving with positive meaning or pleasure for both the caregiver and care receiver (Cartwright, Archbold, Stewart, & Limandri, 1994) and involves enhancing caregiving through the pleasurable, the aesthetic, and the ceremonial (Archbold, 1991). PREP's third goal was to increase the predictability of caregiving activities, thereby increasing a sense of control, especially in unstable caregiving situations. On the basis of our previous research, we thought that caregiver role strain might be reduced by increasing preparedness, mutuality, rewards, and a sense of control and predictability (Archbold et al., 1990).

The practice of PREP nurses was not restricted by Medicare definitions of skilled care, and PREP nurses had control of the number and purpose of the home visits they made. PREP was distinguished by its family focus and had four components: (1) care planning and management; (2) the PREP Advice Line; (3) follow-up contact by the nurse, using the Keep-in-Touch system; and (4) completion, in which PREP nurses brought families' participation to closure.

The four main findings from the PREP pilot study, which compared 11 interventions (PREP) with 11 control families (standard home health), were as follows. First, the mean level of reported preparedness, enrichment, and predictability by PREP caregivers was significantly higher ($p < .05$) than that of controls, with an effect size of approximately 1 SD (Archbold et al., 1995). However, the intervention had no beneficial effect in reducing role strain or depression by the 12-week interview.

Second, PREP reduced the mean health care costs per family by $3,700 over the 3-month period immediately after referral for home health care (Miller, Hornbrook, Archbold, & Stewart, 1995). Third, PREP was acceptable to families as reported in exit interviews. Fourth, PREP was feasible for home health nurses as indicated in PREP charts and interviews with the PREP nurses. We are planning to evaluate PREP in a larger, randomized intervention trial.

Transitional Care

Transitional care by master's-level clinical nurse specialists was successful in producing beneficial outcomes in older people who were discharged from the hospital (Naylor et al., 1994). The total sample included 276 older patients ($n = 142$ with medical diagnoses, and $n = 134$ with surgical diagnoses) and 125 caregivers. The transitional care administered to those people randomized to the intervention group ($n = 140$ patients and 74 caregivers) involved a comprehensive assessment by the nurse of the functional status of the older person as well as the primary caregiver's postdischarge needs. Most care was provided in the hospital and involved at least two visits by the gerontological nurse specialist during the hospitalization. In addition, the intervention included the availability of a gerontological nurse specialist by phone during and after the hospitalization. Further, the nurse initiated at least two telephone contacts to the patient within the first 2 weeks after discharge. For patients having medical diagnoses, the intervention group exhibited significantly fewer rehospitalizations, shorter duration of rehospitalizations, and smaller charges for rehospitalizations than the control group. Differences were not found between the intervention and control patients with surgical diagnoses. Studies such as this one indicate the value in placing nurses with advanced practice skills in a position to provide transitional care.

Telephone Advice and Monitoring

Two types of telephone interventions—telephone advice lines and telephone monitoring—have been used with success in a variety of health care arenas. Telephone advice lines, through which families can receive timely responses to their health and caregiving questions from a professional familiar with their situation, have been used in hospice care since its inception and with frail older people and their families (Schler, Granadillo, & Vargas, 1985).

Telephone monitoring, in which a nurse or other health professional makes systematic assessments and, when needed, recommends interventions, has been used successfully in a broad range of health care situations (e.g., Gortner et al., 1988). In some of the interventions described earlier (e.g., Archbold et al., 1995; Naylor et al., 1994; Zimmer et al., 1985), the availability of advice lines and/or telephone monitoring was included in the system of care. At this point, we believe that evidence supports the institution of telephone monitoring and support systems for frail older people and their caregivers, and we would encourage health care delivery systems to build this service into their plans.

Support Groups

We chose to include a section on support groups because they are by far the most accessible intervention for caregivers, especially caregivers for persons with Alzheimer's disease. These groups vary considerably in purpose and nature, and rigorous evaluation of their effects is difficult because people self-select into them when they are ready, thus creating difficulties for randomizing to experimental and control conditions. The distinction between psychoeducational interventions and support group interventions is blurred, because most psychoeducational groups provide support and most support groups provide some education; however, we distinguish psychoeducational groups from support groups by their more systematic educational focus.

Most evaluations of support groups have been based on anecdotal comments from participants. Gonyea (1991), however, examined systematically the relationship between participation in a support group and the caregiver's sense of well-being. She concluded that although there were statistically significant ($p < .05$) Pearson correlations between support group participation and the three dependent variables of objective burden, subjective burden, and morale, the significant rs were small, with absolute values ranging from .10 to .19. Further, in multiple regression analyses, the strongest predictors of caregiver well-being were caregiver and elder characteristics. Because of the availability of support groups, nurses may want to recommend them to family caregivers who express a need to interact with people who share a common caregiving experience.

This recommendation should be made with the recognition, however, that the beneficial effects of support groups for elder caregivers have yet to be demonstrated empirically.

Distinguishing Features of the Seven Types of Interventions

We would like to highlight some of the main strengths and limitations of different types of interventions in terms of their relevance for nursing. Two strengths of the psychoeducational interventions are that they are the most fully evaluated of the caregiving interventions, and they are often targeted to specific caregiving problems. The health services and in-home nursing interventions have their long-term contact with the family as one important advantage; such sustained contact allows for monitoring of transitions and for the development of a therapeutic relationship with families. The health services interventions also have the advantage of an interdisciplinary approach to care and care planning that is tailored to the impaired older individuals and their families, but exactly how those interventions differed from usual care, except for there being more care, was not well described. In contrast, the nursing care provided as part of the interventions conducted by the Quayhagen, Mohide, and Archbold research teams was described in much more detail than the health services interventions.

In comparing these seven types of interventions, one sees that the underlying goals of the interventions vary widely. For example, the goals of psychoeducational interventions are mainly to provide information, teach problem-solving skills, and help caregivers deal with their negative responses to caregiving (e.g., burden, depression). The goal of respite is to provide relief from everyday caregiving activities. The goals of support groups are to provide opportunities to obtain support from and give support to other caregivers, who share the common experience of caregiving. The goals of most health services, in-home nursing, transitional care, and telephone interventions are to improve the well-being of the impaired older person by augmenting care, often around times of health transitions, and they include the goal of improving the way in which caregivers perform their caregiving role.

The main conclusion that we would like to highlight about distinguishing features of the seven types of interventions is this: When nurses are involved in caregiving interventions, they usually focus attention on the way in which care is delivered by the family—one aspect of the caregiving role. Because a priority for most caregivers is to do a good job in caregiving, they may be especially open to receiving assistance regarding the caregiving role. Therefore, we think that the current focus of nursing interventions on the caregiving role is appropriate and should be expanded.

RESEARCH ON THE NATURE OF THE CAREGIVING ROLE

In this section we summarize results of descriptive, correlational, and longitudinal research on the nature of the caregiving role that we think hold particular promise for nursing interventions. Similar to professionals in other disciplines, nurses intervene to help caregivers reduce burden, strain, or depression; in contrast to most other disciplines, however, nurses are in a unique position to work with family caregivers on how to carry out the caregiving role. The nature of the caregiving role includes (a) the type and amount of caregiving activities that are done, (b) the way the care is provided, (c) the quality of the care, and (d) transitions in the care provided.

In our opinion, the nature of the caregiving role is one of the most salient variables for nursing interventions. First, nurses are skilled caregivers themselves and possess knowledge that is useful for family caregivers. Second, nursing is one of the few professions that is privileged to care for a person's body, and thus nurses are able to assist families with physical and intimate care. Third, nurses in many settings have contact with older people and their family caregivers during times of health transitions, times when caregivers may feel unprepared for a new aspect of the caregiving role.

Type and Amount of Caregiving Activities

Researchers have focused on caregiving activities since the early 1980s. Prior to that time, a person either was a caregiver (i.e., did caregiving) or was not a caregiver. Later, caregiving activities were conceptualized and measured in terms of which caregiving tasks were performed (usually categorized as help with ADLs and IADLs) (Stone et al., 1987).

The amount of care pertains to the number of caregiving activities done, how frequently caregiving activities are done, and how much time it takes to do them. Amount of care has been measured in a number of ways. For example, Oberst et al. (1989) used a Caregiving Load Scale to quantify the time and energy that caregivers expend in caregiving tasks. The scale includes 10 tasks, which are rated on a 5-point scale ranging from "little or no" time and energy to "a great deal" of time and energy.

In the past decade, findings from research have helped us understand the underlying purposes and meanings of the caregiving role to caregivers (e.g., Albert, 1991; Bowers, 1987). Bowers (1987) identified five categories of caregiving activities reported by 31 offspring caregivers of impaired older people, including anticipatory caregiving (behaviors or decisions based on possible needs of the parent), preventive caregiving (activities engaged in to prevent illness, injury, complications, or deterioration in the parent), supervisory caregiving (activities such as arranging for, checking on, setting up), instrumental care (hands-on caregiving), and protective caregiving (protecting the parent from threats to his or her self-esteem). These findings could serve as the basis for new nursing interventions; for example, nurses within organized health systems could offer courses for potential caregivers (middle-aged and older people), providing information about the range of activities that might be involved in future caregiving and sources of support and help for these activities.

Albert (1991) reported on how family caregivers think about the tasks they perform. In his study, he treated caregiving tasks as a cognitive domain, asking caregivers to specify "what sorts of things they do regularly for their parent," then eliciting judgments from them of similarities in tasks, using a card sort. Using multidimensional scaling, Albert found that

> Caregivers think about the tasks they perform using three cross-cutting sets of distinctions: the type of impairment giving rise to the task (physical vs. cognitive-emotional limitation); where the task is performed (within the household vs. outside, involving others); and whether the task enhances parental autonomy or responds to a parent's incompetence. (p. 72)

Caregivers did not categorize tasks according to the extent they were burdensome. Albert concluded that caregivers have an organized lay or folk understanding of their caregiving activities that sometimes differs and sometimes coincides with the view of the clinician or researcher. It is important, therefore, to try to understand the caregiving role from the caregiver's view.

Although evidence suggests that there are many commonalities in caregiving activities across illness categories (Kirschling, Stewart, & Archbold, 1994), it is also important to understand how caregiving differs across these categories. In all disease categories, caregivers provide help with personal care, transportation, housekeeping, and emotional support. On the other hand, researchers have identified important and clinically relevant differences in the nature of the family caregiving role, such as pain management in cancer (Given & Given, 1994), managing behavior problems in dementia (Pearlin et al., 1990), and assistance because of slowness in moving in Parkinson's disease (Stewart, Archbold, Carter, & Inoue, 1993).

The Way Care Is Provided and the Quality of Care

Currently, we have a great deal of information about *what* activities caregivers do but not a lot of information about *the way* caregivers do these activities (Biegel et al., 1991). Intervention planning by nurses has been hampered because of the lack of systematic information describing what caregivers try, what works, and what does not work. Much of the research that does exist on the way in which family members provide care has been conducted by nurses. Cartwright and colleagues (1994) described ways in which caregivers report using enrichment processes to enhance caregiving; the two main types of enrichment processes identified were customary routines (e.g., bedtime rituals) and innovative routine breakers (e.g., enjoying a special dessert). Gilliss and Belza (1992) described ways in which caregivers provide comfort to people who have had open heart surgery. Comfort measures included helping the patients get up and out of chairs, beds, and couches and providing and positioning pillows while the patient is sitting up or lying down. Harvath (1994) described strategies used by caregivers to manage dementia-related behavior problems, including such strategies as going along, putting off, and guiding.

In contrast to looking at task-specific caregiving, nurses may also benefit from understanding how caregivers organize the totality of the role they need to perform. Nkongho and Archbold (in press) found that

African-American caregivers engaged in a process of "working out systems" of care. These systems facilitated caregiving by creating routines of care that attended to the needs of the older person and other family members and to the work roles of the caregiver. Caregivers reported that it took time to work out a system, and systems had to be modified on the basis of changes in the health status of the care receiver or other family members.

We think that the contribution of nursing to interventions with caregivers may be greatest with respect to *how* caregiving activities are done. Nurses are skilled in many of the processes of care that family members must learn and perform. However, many caregivers have also become experts in the caregiving role, and nurses could improve their interventions with caregiving families by systematically studying these expert caregivers and the way in which they provide care.

At this point, there is no standard measure of the quality of family care. Work in the area to date has produced tools to detect poor-quality care (e.g., neglect and abuse) (Phillips et al., 1990a, 1990b) but not to measure the positive extreme of quality. Clinical determination of skill in care is confounded by legal issues (e.g., assignment of blame). Because a main goal of nursing interventions may be to improve the quality of care provided by families, we think it is very important to develop measures of the quality of family care that are sensitive to the effects of nursing interventions (Stewart & Archbold, 1992, 1993). Further, although there is some research linking amount of care provided to burden and strain (Oberst et al., 1989), little research exists about the association between the caregiving role variables of how care is provided and the quality of care and such responses to caregiving as burden, strain, rewards, and depression.

Transitions in the Care Provided

In a longitudinal study of caregiving to 103 posthospitalized older people, one quarter of caregivers interviewed at 6 weeks after discharge reported that as time went on caregiving had become somewhat or much more difficult for them, indicating difficulty in ongoing caregiving transitions (Archbold & Stewart, 1988). Between 6 weeks and 9 months after hospital discharge, 3% of the caregivers had died and 16% of the care receivers had died. In the year after entry to the study, more than 60% of the care receivers were rehospitalized: 28% were hospitalized once, 22% were hospitalized two or three times, and 11% were hospitalized four times or more. These findings illustrate the magnitude and frequency of transitions that occur in caregiving. Bull (1992) found that in the transition from hospital to home care, caregivers worried about (a) learning new skills needed to manage the medical condition, (b) modifying the environment, and (c) changing roles or functions within the family unit.

Specific disease categories and trajectories have been linked to transitions within caregiving. Given and Given (1994), for example, describe the process of shifting caregiver role responsibilities as the person undergoing cancer treatment is more or less able to perform her/his normal and illness-related roles. The model presented by these authors suggests that the following transitions to and within caregiving may occur: (a) transition to the acute, diagnosis period; (b) transitions to and across adjutant therapies (chemotherapy, radiation, hormone); and (c) transition to palliative care. Even within one of the treatment categories (radiation) there may be multiple shifts required in the caregiving role because of the patient's experience of physical (e.g., fatigue) and psychological effects of the treatment (Oberst et al., 1989).

In acute conditions the caregiving role changes with the progression of the disease, the effects of treatment, and the rate of recovery. For example, Gilliss and Belza (1992) delineate changes in the priority goal of care and predominant caregiver work types for each week following cardiac surgery. Initially, the caregiver's goal is managing the illness, and the predominant work types are comfort and monitoring. In the second week, the goal shifts to managing everyday life, and predominant work types are functional and monitoring. Similar shifts in priority goals and work types continue through the fifth postoperative week. Preliminary evidence from the Parkinson's Spouses Study indicates that as this chronic disease progresses, caregivers do more of almost every type of caregiving activity, even those that one might assume are part of a regular spousal role, such as sitting and spending time with one's spouse (Stewart, Archbold, Carter, & Inoue, 1993).

Such findings suggest that when caregivers experience transitions, they are sometimes faced with issues for which they are unprepared. We think that transition points may be times when caregivers are especially open to nursing interventions. Interventions such as Naylor and colleagues' (1994) may be particularly useful at such times.

Creating Partnerships with Family Caregivers

Recent expansion of managed care options in this country, as well as proposed revisions in the health care system (White House Domestic Policy Council, 1993), create incentives for providing care in the least expensive setting: outside hospitals and long-term care institutions. In light of these proposed changes, it will be important for nurses and other health care providers to consider families as partners in the provision of health care to frail older people and to develop innovative ways in which to collaborate with families in this endeavor.

Descriptive research has provided a basis for understanding how family members create partnerships to manage chronic illness (Corbin & Strauss, 1988) and how family caregivers view their relationships with nursing home staff (Duncan & Morgan, 1994). Recently, nurses and other professionals have experimented with innovative strategies for developing partnerships with family caregivers (Harvath et al., 1994; Maas et al., 1993; Wilken, Farran, Hellen, & Boggess, 1992). For example, Wilken and colleagues (1992) developed a program called Partners in Care for family caregivers and nursing home staff. This 8-week program provided a forum in which caregivers and staff shared their knowledge about caregiving and clarified caregiving roles in the nursing home. Preliminary findings suggest that the program was very successful in enhancing collaboration and communication among family and nursing home staff in the planning of care for older residents with Alzheimer's disease. For example, the dietitian indicated that "she found the group most helpful because family caregivers gave her specialized (idiosyncratic) information about food choices of care receivers, information that does not appear on standard dietary request forms" (p. 14).

CONCLUSIONS

The contributions of standard nursing practice and health care delivery to the health and well-being of caregiving families has not been studied systematically. However, caregivers of older persons recently discharged from the hospital reported that they used multiple sources of information in learning to provide care, including talking with professionals such as doctors, nurses, and social workers (69%); using a trial-and-error approach (59%); talking with friends or relatives (53%); reading books and articles

(37%); and calling on the experience gained from a previous job taking care of a sick or disabled person (15%) (Stewart, Archbold, Harvath, & Nkongho, 1993). Of these information sources, caregivers reported learning the most about how to take care of the care receiver's physical needs and how to find out about and set up services for the care receiver from health professionals. In sharp contrast, however, health professionals were among the two poorest sources of information about taking care of the care receiver's emotional needs and handling the stress of caregiving. These findings suggest that health professionals, including nurses, may not be addressing caregivers' needs to learn how to handle the care receivers' emotional problems or the stress of caregiving—two important components of the caregiving role.

In this chapter we have argued that nurses have an important role in providing services to family caregivers in the area of the nature of the caregiving role. Nursing intervention strategies in this area, such as transitional care and expanded in-home care, are in their infancy but show promise. Finally, recent research about the nature of the caregiving role provides directions for the creation of new interventions that may be helpful in preparing families for caregiving.

REFERENCES

Abel, E. K., & Nelson, M. K. (1990). *Circles of care.* New York: State University of New York.

Albert, S. M. (1991). Cognition of caregiving tasks: Multidimensional scaling of the caregiver task domain. *The Gerontologist, 31,* 726–734.

Anderson, J. M. (1990). Home care management in chronic illness and the self-care movement: An analysis of ideologies and economic processes influencing policy decisions. *Advances in Nursing Science, 12*(2), 71–83.

Archbold, P. G. (1991). An interdisciplinary approach to family caregiving research. *Communicating Nursing Research, 24,* 27–42.

Archbold, P. G., & Stewart, B. J. (1988). *The effects of organized caregiver relief: Final report to NCNR* (R01 NU/AG 01140). Portland: Oregon Health Sciences University.

Archbold, P. G., Stewart, B. J., Greenlick, M. R., & Harvath, T. (1990). Mutuality and preparedness as predictors of caregiver role strain. *Research in Nursing and Health, 13,* 375–384.

Archbold, P. G., Stewart, B. J., Greenlick, M. R., & Harvath, T. A. (1992). The clinical assessment of mutuality and preparedness in family caregivers to frail older people. In S. G. Funk, E. M. Tornquist, M. T. Champagne, & R.

A. Wiese (Eds.), *Key aspects of elder care: Managing falls, incontinence, and cognitive impairment* (pp. 328–339). New York: Springer Publishing Co.

Archbold, P. G., Stewart, B. J., Miller, L. L., Harvath, T. A., Greenlick, M. R., VanBuren, L., Kirschling, J. M., Valanis, B. G., Brody, K K., Schook, J. E., & Hagan, J. M. (1995). The PREP system of nursing interventions: A pilot test with families caring for older members. *Research in Nursing and Health, 18*(1), 3–16.

Berry, N. J., & Evans, J. M. (1985/86). Cost effectiveness of home health care as an alternative to inpatient care. *Home Health Care Services Quarterly, 6*(4), 11–25.

Biegel, D. E., Sales, E., & Schulz, R. (1991). *Family caregiving in chronic illness.* Newbury Park, CA: Sage.

Bowers, B. J. (1987). Intergenerational caregiving: Adult caregivers and their aging parents. *Advances in Nursing Science, 9*(2), 20–31.

Bull, M. J. (1992). Managing the transition from hospital to home. *Qualitative Health Research, 2*(1), 27–41.

Cartwright, J. C., Archbold, P. G., Stewart, B. J., & Limandri, B. J. (1994). Enrichment processes in family caregiving to frail elders. *Advances in Nursing Science, 17*(1), 31–43.

Chiverton, P., & Caine, E. D. (1989). Education to assist spouses in coping with Alzheimer's disease: A controlled trial. *Journal of the American Geriatrics Society, 37,* 593–598.

Collins, C. E., Given, B. A., & Given, C. W. (1994). Interventions with family caregivers of persons with Alzheimer's disease. *Nursing Clinics of North America, 29*(1), 195–207.

Corbin, J. M., & Strauss, A. (1988). *Unending work and care: Managing chronic illness at home.* San Francisco: Jossey-Bass.

Duncan, M. T., & Morgan, D. L. (1994). Sharing the caring: Family caregivers' views of their relationships with nursing home staff. *The Gerontologist, 34,* 235–244.

Farran, C. J., & Keane-Hagarty, E. (1994). Multi-modal intervention strategies for caregivers of persons with dementia. In E. Light, G. Niederehe, & B. D. Lebowitz (Eds.), *Stress effects on family caregivers of Alzheimer's patients* (pp. 237–254). New York: Springer Publishing Co.

Gallagher, D. E. (1985). Intervention strategies to assist caregivers of frail elders: Current research status and future research directions. *Annual Review of Gerontology and Geriatrics, 5,* 249–282.

Gallagher-Thompson, D. (1993, September). *Development of psycho-educational programs for family caregivers.* Paper presented at Families at Risk: State-of-the-Art Caregiving for the Elderly in the 21st Century, Burlingame, CA.

Gilliss, C. L., & Belza, B. L. (1992). A framework for understanding family caregivers' recovery work after cardiac surgery. *Family and Community Health, 15*(3), 41–48.

Given, B. A., & Given, W. C. (1991). Family caregiving for the elderly. In J. J. Fitzpatrick & J. S. Stevenson (Eds.), *Annual review of nursing research, Vol. 9,* (pp. 77–92). New York: Springer Publishing Co.

Given, C. W., & Given, B. A. (1994). The home care of a patient with cancer: The midlife crisis. In E. Kahana, D. Biegel, & M. Wykle (Eds.), *Family caregiving across the lifespan* (pp. 241–261). Thousand Oaks, CA: Sage.

Given, C. W., Given, B., Stommel, M., Collins, C., King, S., & Franklin, S. (1992). The caregiver reaction assessment (CRA) for caregivers to persons with chronic physical and mental impairments. *Research in Nursing and Health, 15,* 271–283.

Given, C. W., Stommel, M., Given, B., Osuch, J., Kurtz, M. E., & Kurtz, J. C. (1993). The influence of cancer patients' symptoms and functional states on patients' depression and family caregivers' reaction and depression. *Health Psychology, 12,* 277–285.

Gonyea, J. G. (1991). Alzheimer's disease support group participation and caregiver well-being. *Clinical Gerontologist, 10*(2), 17–34.

Gortner, S. R., Gilliss, C. L., Shinn, J. A., Sparacino, P. A., Rankin, S., Leavitt, M., Price, M., & Hudes, M. (1988). Improving recovery following cardiac surgery: A randomized clinical trial. *Journal of Advanced Nursing, 13,* 649–661.

Haley, W. E., Brown, S. L., & Levine, E. G. (1987). Experimental evaluation of the effectiveness of group interventions for dementia caregivers. *The Gerontologist, 27,* 376–382.

Harvath, T. A. (1994). Interpretation and management of dementia-related behavior problems. *Clinical Nursing Research, 3,* 7–26.

Harvath, T. A., Archbold, P. G., Stewart, B. J., Gadow, S., Kirschling, J. M., Miller, L., Hagan, J., Brody, K., & Schook, J. (1994). Establishing partnerships with family caregivers: Local and cosmopolitan knowledge. *Journal of Gerontological Nursing, 20*(2), 29–35.

Hirschfeld, M. J. (1983). Homecare versus institutionalization: Family caregiving and senile brain disease. *International Journal of Nursing Studies, 20,* 23–32.

Horowitz, A. (1985). Family caregiving to the frail elderly. *Annual Review of Gerontology and Geriatrics, 5,* 194–246.

Kahana, E., Biegel, D. E., & Wykle, M. L. (Eds.). (1994). *Family caregiving across the lifespan.* Thousand Oaks, CA: Sage.

Kirschling, J. M., Stewart, B. J., & Archbold, P. G. (1994). Family caregivers of post-hospitalized older persons and persons receiving hospice: Similarities and differences. *Home Health Care Services Quarterly, 14*(4), 117–140.

Knight, B. G., Lutzky, S. M., & Macofsky-Urban, F. (1993). A meta-analytic review of interventions for caregiver distress: Recommendations for future research. *The Gerontologist, 33,* 240–248.

Lawton, M. P., Brody, E., & Saperstein, A. R. (1989). A controlled study of respite service for caregivers of Alzheimer's patients. *The Gerontologist, 29,* 8–16.

Lovett, S., & Gallagher, D. (1988). Psychoeducational interventions for family caregivers: Preliminary efficacy data. *Behavior Therapy, 19,* 321–330.

Maas, M., Swanson, E., Buckwalter, K. C., Tripp-Reimer, T., Weiler, K., & Specht, J. (1993). Nursing intervention for family members of patients with Alzheimer's disease: Family involvement in care (FIC). In B. Vaughn-Cole,

M. A. Johnson, L. Walker, & J. Malone (Eds.), *Family nursing interventions.* Rockville, MD: Aspen.

McAuley, W. J., & Blieszner, R. (1985). Selection of long-term care arrangements by older community residents. *The Gerontologist, 25,* 188–193.

Miller, L. L., Hornbrook, M., Archbold, P. G., & Stewart, B. J. (1995). *Home health care services for frail, elderly patients and family caregivers: Measuring use, costs and outcomes of an innovative program.* Manuscript submitted for publication.

Mohide, E. A., Pringle, D. M., Streiner, D. L., Gilbert, J. R., Muir, G., & Tew, M. (1990). A randomized trial of family caregiver support in the home management of dementia. *Journal of the American Geriatric Society, 38,* 446–454.

Montgomery, R. J. V., & Borgatta, E. F. (1989). The effects of alternative support strategies on family caregiving. *The Gerontologist, 29,* 457–464.

Naylor, M., Brooten, D., Jones, R., Lavizzo-Mourey, R., Mezey, M., & Pauly, M. (1994). Comprehensive discharge planning for the hospitalized elderly: A randomized clinical trial. *Annals of Internal Medicine, 120,* 999–1006.

Nkongho, N., & Archbold, P. (in press). Working out caregiving systems in African American families. *Applied Nursing Research.*

Oberst, M. T., Thomas, S. E., Gass, K. A., & Ward, S. E. (1989). Caregiving demands and appraisal of stress among family caregivers. *Cancer Nursing, 12,* 209–215.

Oktay, J. S., & Volland, P. J. (1990). Post-hospital support program for the frail elderly and their caregivers: A quasi-experimental evaluation. *American Journal of Public Health, 80,* 39–46.

Pearlin, L. I., Mullan, J. T., Semple, S. J., & Skaff, M. M. (1990). Caregiving and the stress process: An overview of concepts and their measures. *The Gerontologist, 30,* 583–594.

Phillips, L. R., Morrison, E. F., & Chae, Y. M. (1990a). The QUALCARE scale: Developing an instrument to measure quality of home care. *International Journal of Nursing Studies, 27,* 61–75.

Phillips, L. R., Morrison, E. F., & Chae, Y. M. (1990b). The QUALCARE scale: Testing of a measurement instrument for clinical practice. *International Journal of Nursing Studies, 27,* 77–91.

Phillips, L. R., Rempusheski, V. F., & Morrison, E. (1989). Developing and testing the beliefs about caregiving scale. *Research in Nursing and Health, 12,* 207–220.

Polich, C., Parker, M., Bernstein, L. H., Krulewitch, H., Fischer, L. R., Pastor, W., & Pitt, L. (1990). The provision of home health services through health maintenance organizations: The role of the physician. *Quality Review Bulletin, 16*(5), 170–181.

Quayhagen, M. P., Quayhagen, M., Corbeil, R. R., Roth, P. A., & Rodgers, J. A. (1995). A dyadic remediation program for care recipients with dementia. *Nursing Research, 44,* 153–159.

Robinson, K. M. (1988). A social skills training program for adult caregivers. *Advances in Nursing Science, 10*(2), 59–72.

Schler, S. H., Granadillo, O. R., & Vargas, L. (1985). Extended health team availability improves utilization of health resources [Summary]. *The Gerontologist, 25,* 222.

Shanas, E. (1979). The family as a social support system in old age. *The Gerontologist, 19,* 169–174.

Stewart, B. J., & Archbold, P. G. (1992). Nursing intervention studies require outcome measures that are sensitive to change: Part 1. *Research in Nursing and Health, 15,* 477–481.

Stewart, B. J., & Archbold, P. G. (1993). Nursing intervention studies require outcome measures that are sensitive to change: Part 2. *Research in Nursing and Health, 16,* 77–81.

Stewart, B. J., Archbold, P. G., Carter, J. H., & Inoue, I. (1993, September). *Spousal caregiving to people with Parkinson's disease.* Paper presented at Families at Risk: State-of-the-Art Caregiving for the Elderly in the 21st Century, Burlingame, CA.

Stewart, B. J., Archbold, P. G., Harvath, T. A., & Nkongho, N. O. (1993). Role acquisition in family caregivers for older people who have been discharged from the hospital. In S. G. Funk, E. M. Tornquist, M. T. Champagne, & R. A. Wiese (Eds.), *Key aspects of caring for the chronically ill: Hospital and home* (pp. 219–231). New York: Springer Publishing Co.

Stommel, M., Collins, C. E., & Given, B. A. (1994). The costs of family contributions to the care of persons with dementia. *The Gerontologist, 34,* 199–205.

Stommel, M., Wang, S., Given, C. W., & Given, B. (1992). Confirmatory factor analysis (CFA) as a method to assess measurement equivalence. *Research in Nursing and Health, 15,* 399–405.

Stone, R., Cafferata, G. L., & Sangl, J. (1987). Caregivers of the frail elderly: A national profile. *The Gerontologist, 27,* 616–626.

Toseland, R. W., & Rossiter, C. M. (1989). Group interventions to support family caregivers: A review and analysis. *The Gerontologist, 29,* 438–448.

U.S. Bureau of the Census. (1993). *Statistical abstract of the United States: 1993* (113th ed.). Washington, DC: U.S. Government Printing Office.

U.S. Senate Committee on Aging, the American Association of Retired Persons, the Federal Council on the Aging, & the U.S. Administration of Aging. (1991). *Aging America trends and projections* (DHHS Publication No. [FCoA] 91-28001). Washington DC: U.S. Department of Health and Human Services.

Walker, A. J., Martin, S. S. K., & Jones, L. L. (1992). The benefits and costs of caregiving and care receiving for daughters and mothers. *Journals of Gerontology, 47,* S130–S139.

White House Domestic Policy Council. (1993). *The president's health security plan.* New York: Random House.

Wilken, C. S., Farran, C. J., Hellen, C. R., & Boggess, J. E. (1992). Partners in care: A program for family caregivers and nursing home staff. *American Journal of Alzheimer's Care and Related Disorders and Research, 7*(4), 8–14, 22.

Zarit, S. H., Anthony, C. R., & Boutselis, M. (1987). Interventions with care givers of dementia patients: Comparison of two approaches. *Psychology and Aging, 2,* 225–232.

Zimmer, J. G., Groth-Juncker, A., & McCusker, J. (1985). A randomized controlled study of a home health care team. *American Journal of Public Health, 75*(2), 134–141.

CHAPTER 7

Ethnic Elderly: Care Issues

Veronica F. Rempusheski

Beliefs, values, and patterns of care emerge from an individual's heritage and are grounded in ethnic identity. Ethnic identity, which is the statement of one's ethnicity or membership in an ethnic group, is an issue in elder care because of its integrating nature. An elder's meaning of the care process is symbolized in ritual practice, moral commitment, and behaviors specific to an ethnic group. Rules for actions and exchanges, unique to an ethnic elder's interpretation of the care process, determine the kind of caregiving/care receiving relationship developed between an elder and a care provider (Rempusheski, 1988). Outside anthropology, race has dominated the research literature as a variable in comparative studies of elders. Edwards (1992), however, argues that "ethnicity appears to be replacing terms which traditionally have been used to designate race" (p. 31). Yet each discipline concerned with ethnicity seems to use its own conceptualization and measurement, with little consistency in the approach used to identify ethnicity of subjects. Some authors assign subjects to ethnic categories without defining the ethnicity variable used in their study. Other approaches used by researchers to assign subjects to ethnic categories include self-declared ethnicity, surnames, country of birth, and language spoken at home as proxy measures; assignment by health professionals who have contact with subjects in a study; a child's race and maternal country of origin; and complex algorithms that incorporate a number of criteria (Edwards,

1992). Few have attempted to quantify ethnicity. One example is the Identificational Ethnicity Scale, which has been used with Italian American (Martinelli, 1984) and Polish American elderly (Rempusheski, 1986). (Note: The omission of a hyphen in these two ethnic titles is intentional, based on the defined ethnic sample in these studies.)

This chapter presents the state of knowledge and selected care issues of ethnic elderly. Terms used interchangeably with ethnicity or used to portray the notion of ethnicity in the literature are defined, described, and differentiated so as to delineate the domain of meaning of ethnic elderly. This domain of meaning provides the framework for evaluating the state of knowledge about ethnic elderly, for thinking about the care issues of ethnic elderly, and for interpreting the variations, similarities, differences, and potential universals of care expected and care received by ethnic elderly.

CLARIFICATION OF TERMS

Basic to an evaluation of the state of knowledge about ethnic elderly is the identification of terms used as variables to elicit the notion of elders' perceptions of belonging to a sociocultural unit with origins, rules, and contrasts. Once the term has been identified, its meaning as used or implied in a study must be evaluated for its ability to capture the notion intended. Use of a term—race, minority, or ethnicity—is based not only on its common usage in society but also on its conceptual and operational definitions, its appropriateness of use, and its relevance to the question and study purpose. Analysis, interpretation, and applicability of a study of ethnic elderly must be consistent with the definitions and measurement of ethnic variables.

Race

Much has been written about race as a concept and a theory. Race is a biological term referring to hereditary traits. A race is a group of people with a large number of inherited traits in common or, owing to their common ancestry, sharing a general tendency to produce certain physical types identifiable by having the same kind of skin color, hair, eyes, head shape, body build, stature, face, and nose. The science of race has been the domain of geneticists and anthropologists. The myth of race arises from confusing hereditary traits with traits that are socially acquired, wherein there is an erroneous integration of biological and behavioral classification systems used interchangeably (Hertz, 1928; McLemore, 1994; Mead, Dobzhansky, Tobach, & Light, 1968; Montagu, 1964; Ringer & Lawless, 1989).

"Geneticists believe that anthropologists have decided what a race is. Ethnologists assume that their classifications embody principles which genetic science has proved to be correct. Politicians believe that their prejudices have the sanction of genetic laws and the findings of physical anthropology to sustain them" (Hogben, 1932, p. 122). Those comments were published pre–World War II, when some people still viewed race in its somewhat pure state of Caucasoid, Negroid, and Mongoloid. Precipitated by the atrocities of World War II, which were the result of linking religious beliefs, language, and superior abilities to race, an international panel of social scientists was convened, and on July 18, 1950, a statement on race was issued by the United Nations Educational, Scientific, and Cultural Organization (UNESCO). This statement was subsequently critiqued by a group of anthropologists and geneticists, and a new statement was released by UNESCO in September 1952. Whereas the 1950 statement recommended the use of the term *ethnic groups* instead of *race,* the 1952 statement recognized the tendency of society to identify perceptions of peoples by physical appearance. It noted the appropriate use of *race*—the major classifications that combine elements of geographic location and heredity—and the need to recognize that no race is pure, each being the result of evolution of the highly complex processes of gene mutation, selection, adaptation, and isolation (UNESCO, 1952).

Race identity and descriptors for race have since changed. Earlier beliefs about race have evolved beyond an all-or-none phenomenon of presence and distribution of genes in a population and the frequency with which certain physical traits are revealed over time. To this end, investigators may specify the presence and/or frequency of particular traits when studying a population (Tripp-Reimer & Lauer, 1987). The resulting descriptors for race classification today include a combination of the original terms and geographic origin, such as Caucasian (or white), black, Native American Indian, Asian, and Hispanic. Often the concepts of race and ethnicity are aggregated, the terms used interchangeably, and both are revealed in a classification of groups that combines the racial categories listed above with a hyphenated or nonhyphenated subclassification, such as black South African and white South African. A racial classification framework is implied when racial groups of Native Americans, Asians, and Hispanics are compared to whites. An ethnicity framework is presumed when the racial groups are subclassified by country of origin, region, and language and compared to each other.

Minority

Minority is a relative term referring to a group of people outside the majority group that occupies a geographic area. There are ethnic minorities and racial minorities, within which exist elders who wish to maintain their ethnic identities. At issue is the maintenance of ethnic identity of elders living as members of minority groups within a pluralistic society. Pluralistic societies like the United States, within which there exist racially visible minorities, pose unique problems for elders who wish to maintain their ethnic identities. In some areas of the United States, ethnic minorities are buffeted between shifting political, social, religious, and geographic boundaries. Maintaining an ethnic identity within ethnic minorities poses unique problems that vary by region, locale, and composition of the majority group and other minorities.

Minorities in the United States have become defined partially in relation to the three major periods of immigration in U.S. history: (a) 1820–1860, (b) 1880–1920, and (c) 1965–present. Between 1820 and 1860, approximately 5 million immigrants entered the United States, mostly Irish and German. During the 1880–1920 period, there were 23 million immigrants, mostly from southern, central, and eastern Europe. Since 1965, more than 10 million immigrants have entered the United States, mostly from Asian and Latin American countries (Parrillo, 1991). The evolving definition of minority in the United States today is characteristic of the more than 30% of annual immigrants from Latin America, nearly 50% from Asian countries, 10% from Europe, and 3% from Africa (U.S. Immigration and Naturalization Service, 1990). The sociological and anthropological literature abounds with accounts of "ethnic neighborhoods" created in cities throughout the United States by immigrants primarily of low socioeconomic status. A similar pattern is seen today as new classifications of minority groups are perceived and defined (Parrillo, 1991).

Minority has been defined as "members of ethnic and racial groups who share in common a relative lack of power and suffer the effects of discrimination based upon real or perceived racial or cultural differences" (Padgett, 1989, p. 214). This definition is interpreted by Padgett (1989) to refer mainly to blacks, Hispanics, and Native Americans, though Pacific Islanders and some Asian ethnic groups may be included. She admits that "members of some white ethnic groups may also suffer from discrimination or some Hispanic and Asian groups appear to be exempt from minority status, which makes the concept difficult to operationalize" (p. 215). To further clarify the concept, Padgett noted the need to be explicit about each minority or ethnic group: black Americans may be native-born or come from West Indian (e.g., Jamaican, Bahamian) backgrounds; Hispanic groups include Mexican, Puerto Rican, and Cuban Americans and others from Central and South American countries; white ethnic groups may be Polish, Italian, Greek, or Hungarian or originate from other European countries. Minority elders, as Padgett defines them, have experienced the profound lifelong effects of inequality and racial/ethnic discrimination; however, European immigrants have had to make similar adjustments to inequality further complicated by barriers of language and culture. The relative nature of the term *minority* allows individual interpretation of its definition, depending on the geographic location of the group and the historical, political, and social environment within which it exists.

Ethnicity

Ethnicity has been defined as a "condition of belonging to a social group within a cultural and social system that claims or is accorded special status on the basis of complex, often variable traits including religious, linguistic, ancestral or physical characteristics" (Edwards, 1992, p. 31). A number of factors are used to determine ethnicity, including past origins, symbolic identification, subcultural social relations, territoriality, and kinship. Presumed in these factors is the idea of boundary, in which exchange within or across an ethnic boundary is dictated by the rules of an ethnic group.

Ethnicity is grounded in an individual's beliefs and values, which are associated with origins (heritage), rules (for actions and behaviors), and contrasts (differentiation) (DeVos & Romanucci-Ross, 1975). From these origins, rules, and contrasts emerge rituals, moral commitments, and behaviors unique to each ethnic group. This uniqueness may be measured on nine dimensions in the Identificational Ethnicity Scale (IES), with a single ethnic group specified. The IES yields a degree of ethnic identity by individual and group scores. IES items are scored 1 or 2 for association with an ethnic group (e.g., degree to which one thinks of self within an ethnic group, feels close to others in the same ethnic group, and feels pride in others with similar ethnic background) (see Table 7.1). Ethnic name is the determining factor for the ethnic association in the IES. The underlying assumption is that if an individual has not changed his or her ethnic name, then there are shared beliefs and values specific to an ethnic group. The potential exists, however, that the IES may be measuring what Gans (1979) calls symbolic ethnicity, wherein an external characteristic, such as a name, serves as a social, political, or economic symbol perceived to create a particular desired image. Psychometric properties of the IES have not been published.

In summary, terms used as variables to elicit the notion of elders' perceptions of belonging to a sociocultural unit with origins, rules, and contrasts incorporate specifications of (a) an ethnic identity by country of origin, religion, and language and (b) racial or minority categories that refine or further define the heterogeneity of the ethnic identity. Definitions and rationale for subject classifications should be clearly communicated by the author. The terms, their definitions, and rationale should be logical and consistent with the hypothesis or research question and study purpose. Comparing the literature on ethnic elderly entails not only searches using all of the above terms but also careful examination of how the terms are defined, used, and discussed in each research study.

STATE OF KNOWLEDGE
ABOUT ETHNIC ELDERLY

Ethnic elderly classifications that appear in the literature include (a) racial terms alone (e.g., black, white, Anglo, Hispanic, Latino, Asian), (b) country of origin or language alone (e.g., Polish American, Italian American, Greek), (c) combined racial terms with country of origin (e.g., Cuban-American Hispanic), and (d) religion or religious sect (e.g., Jewish, Amish). This diverse classification precludes comparison of like studies for the presentation of substantive topics. Therefore, the state of knowledge about ethnic elderly will be discussed as it pertains to theoretical and methodological issues and the confounding aspects of comparing studies of ethnic elderly. It is hoped that this perspective will sensitize

TABLE 7.1   Ethnic Identity Interview Questions for Polish Americans

1. How do you think of yourself?	a. Polish [2]
	b. Polish American [2]
	c. American Polish [1]
	d. American of Polish descent [1]
	e. American [0]
2. If you thought it would help you socially or professionally, would you change your Polish name?	a. Yes [0] b. No. [1]
3. Do you feel any special sense of closeness to Polish Americans?	a. Yes [1]. Go to question #4
	b. No [0]. Go to question #5
4. How close would you say you feel to Polish Americans?	a. Slight sense of closeness [1]
	b. Moderate sense of closeness [1]
	c. Strong sense of closeness [2]
	d. Very strong sense of closeness [2]
5. When you meet a Polish American for the first time, how do you feel?	a. I assume we have something in common [1]
	b. It is just like meeting anyone else [0]
6. Do you ever feel proud when you see someone with a Polish name do well or succeed, for example, in sports, business, academics, or entertainment?	a. Yes [1] b. No. [0]
	c. I never notice Polish names [0]
7. Does it bother you when Polish names appear in connection with criminal activities or other negative events?	a. Yes [1] b. No [0]
	c. I never notice Polish names [0]
8. If during an election you had to choose between two people you thought had equal ability, with no real political differences, and one was Polish American and the other was not, would you vote for the Polish American?	a. Yes [1] b. No. [0]
9. Some people think that Polish Americans face prejudice and discrimination. Would you agree with them?	a. Yes [1] b. No [0]

Rempusheski, 1986, pp. 171–172. Adapted from the Identificational Ethnicity Scale for Italian Americans (Martinelli, 1984). *Key:* [ ] = number of points allotted for answer. Points are summed for total score. Maximum score is 11; a total score of 1–11 is evidence of ethnic identity in that person. The quality of the ethnic identity is not presumed, just that a "degree" of ethnic identity exists.

readers to the issues that must be considered in the development, dissemination, and use of knowledge specific to care of ethnic elderly.

Theoretical and Methodological Issues

Key to approaching teaching about, study of, and care of ethnic elderly is a sensitivity to understanding one's own perceptions and how they influence the choice of an orientation, theoretical approach, framework, or model, whether in the direct or indirect care of ethnic elders, teaching about their care, or conducting research. Dressler (1993) contends that the problem of care of ethnic persons stems from the failure of scientists to formulate empirically useful theories of ethnicity, theories that can be used to evaluate the observations of ethnic group differences in health in ways that reflect the biocultural complexity of the phenomenon. Because the purpose of this chapter is to focus on the domain of ethnic elderly, no attempt has been made to do an inclusive review of all the existing frameworks, theories, and conceptual models and how they may articulate with the care or study of ethnic elderly. Rather, the overall orientation of ethnic elderly serves as a kind of framework or way of directing one's attention. Several kinds of frameworks that sensitize the researcher to ethnic or cultural diversity can be found, not only in the transcultural nursing literature but also in the disciplines of anthropology, psychology, and sociology. The Triandis model is a psychosocial model that has demonstrated utility for enhancing cultural sensitivity in nursing science (Facione, 1993).

A "conceptual model of race," developed by LaVeist (1994), is intended to address the definitional, conceptual, and measurement problems of race and to predict observed health outcomes. His model specifies race as a latent factor for which skin color is the manifest indicator, and thus he stipulates physiognomy as the force that drives a categorization of individuals into risk/behavior groups. LaVeist hypothesized that the interaction between societal factors (e.g., socioeconomic status) and cultural/ethnic factors (e.g., cultural norms and practices) produces observed morbidity and mortality differentials across racial groups.

Age as a societal factor could be incorporated into the LaVeist model; however, none of the previous models specifically incorporates the variable of age nor accounts for the theoretical and methodological issues of age and its confounding effects in research (Phillips, 1989). Models specific to care of ethnic elders are rare, including other models that have been tested on ethnic elderly. Phillips and Rempusheski's (1985) decision-making model for elder abuse and neglect was empirically generated; it includes a variable labeled "cultural stereotypes" as evidenced by "judgments about the ethnic backgrounds of the elder and caregiver" (p. 136) being assessed by the nurse and social worker. This model has not been tested. As this variable is only one piece of the total model, it may be more relevant as a theme that emerged from the literature.

Confounding Aspects of Comparing Studies

It is not uncommon to search the literature for "ethnic" studies and find upon reading them that although the term *ethnic, ethnicity,* or *ethnic identity* was used in the title, subtitle, or content of the article, the actual orientation being used is one of race (e.g., black elders compared to white elders, as in Clark, Maddox, & Steinhauser, 1993; Crimmins & Saito, 1993; Fillenbaum et al., 1993; Ulbrich & Bradsher, 1993), or the sample consists of a single race (e.g., black, white, or Hispanic [Latino] elders, as in Bazargan, Barbre, & Hamm, 1993; Zsembik, 1993). When black/white comparisons are used, the genetically determined variable of skin color or tone appears to be the component of race being measured, whereas when a single racial group is studied, socially or culturally influenced variables are incorporated or used to support findings. Conclusions are, for the most part, drawn from a sample defined by race (all of one race aggregated together without differentiation by ethnic identity) and interpreted as an ethnic difference with regard to various kinds of health behaviors. This approach is the most common form of confusing the terms previously described.

Another kind of racial aggregation is seen when Anglos (presumed to represent whites) are compared to non-Anglos, with the latter term further classified into blacks, Asians, and Hispanics (Graveley & Oseasohn, 1991). One study used "Anglo-born" to mean a person born in the United Kingdom, in contrast to those in the sample who were Canadian-born (Jones & van Amelsvoort-Jones, 1986). "Anglo" in this latter example is an ethnic orientation.

Less common yet no less evident in the literature is use of the term *race* or *minority* in the title, subtitle, or content of the article, when the actual orientation is one of ethnicity. For example, confusion precipitated by the use of both racial terms (i.e., Hispanic, non-Hispanic) and ethnicity in the title of one study (Mintzer et al., 1992) was made clear in the sample description, in which non-Hispanic was defined as white and further differentiated by country of origin, region, and religion (i.e., Eastern European Jewish, Western European Protestant, and Irish Catholic). Hispanics in the Mintzer study were further defined as Cuban-American Hispanics. Additionally, minority group classification may refer to either racial or ethnic minority, or a combination of both, within one study (Angel, Angel, & Himes, 1992).

Additional confusion of terms and their meaning may occur. Race may be presumed with the use of such terms as African American and Euro-American; black is the presumed race in the former term and white in the latter term (Dressler, 1993; Wallace, Snyder, Walker, & Ingman, 1992). Here again, what appears to be an ethnic orientation to the classification of subjects may be a racial orientation. The racial or ethnic orientation of a study is revealed in the author's use of more than one term to mean the same thing (when terms are not defined), either in the results or in the discussion when the results are compared to the existing literature.

Eisenberg (1979) used the term *ethnic background* in one of his sub-headings, but in subsequent paragraphs he used the term *race*. The last sentence of this section of the article makes reference to the "ethnic origin of the patient" (p. 959) as it may influence diagnoses. Although Eisenberg does not define these terms, he is using race synonymously with ethnic background. It becomes evident that this author is using a racial framework rather than an ethnic framework because he extrapolates from the literature those study data that compare blacks and whites; skin color is the variable compared.

Throughout the literature on race, skin color, particularly black, emerges as a variable that appears to influence the care of ethnic elderly. Skin color is a continuous variable; however, it is typically dichotomized. There are no specific guidelines for determining the point in the continuum at which the line of demarcation is drawn. This decision is left to societal interpretation or researcher observation (LaVeist, 1994). Keith and Herring (1991) suggest that the continuing disadvantage that darker blacks experience is due to persisting discrimination against them in the United States. Race as a dummy or binary variable has been used to measure ethnicity, skin color (predominately dichotomous skin color), and nationality. Measurement error, erroneous interpretations of research findings, and ineffective health care decisions and policies have resulted from not knowing what is being measured. Skin tone and stratification in ethnic elder communities may be the more important variables to be measured, not as proxy variables for race but to differentiate various skin tones with their association with care issues of ethnic elderly.

CARE ISSUES OF ETHNIC ELDERLY

This section will address four issues viewed as important to the care of ethnic elderly: (a) poverty, (b) access, (c) decision making, and (d) family and community.

Poverty

Poverty among ethnic elderly emerges as a dominant theme in the literature across those studies that examine race, minority groups, and ethnic groups. Variations of this theme were included in discussions of inadequate income to meet basic needs (such as nutrition, environment, transportation) and health care needs (such as diagnosis and treatment of pathologies, prescription drugs, and care services for themselves or primary caregivers). A cycle of illness or disability is evident among the poor ethnic elderly in that they are more likely to have a greater number and more severe states of illnesses and disabilities. Poverty is revealed as the underlying issue in noncompliance for drug treatment, in which an inability to have a prescription filled (first-stage compliance), because of its cost, and the subsequent use of over-the-counter (OTC) drugs as an adaptive strategy are attempts by ethnic elders to compensate for their poverty (Bazargan et al., 1993). The way in which care is provided can offset the influence of poverty on the health of ethnic elderly. Attention to elders' health beliefs and behaviors that are relative to the specific problem created by the poverty need to be incorporated into the following:

- ◆ Potential programs to decrease the financial burden of the cost of care.
- ◆ Evaluation of the care regimen.
- ◆ Perception or understanding by elderly about their treatment and care and about expected outcomes.
- ◆ Evaluation of perceived severity and scope of illness by ethnic elders.
- ◆ Elderly persons' perception of their control relative to their care.

Access to Care

Where and to whom is care offered? Is the care delivery aimed at being convenient to ethnic elders as recipients of care or to the care providers? Access to care is related to an elder's resources: economic resources to pay for care, cognitive resources to investigate what services are available and how to obtain them, and mobility and transportation resources to get to the place where services are offered. In addition, access to care is related to the complex process of gaining entrée into a system for care and the actual services received. Specifically, these aspects of access focus on (a) *placement of services* relative to where the elderly are located and to their abilities and needs (e.g., available home-care, office, clinic, hospital, hospice, and rehabilitation services within boundaries that are conveniently reached by the elderly person or his or her care provider); (b) *delivery of care* that is appropriate to the elder, comprehensive, and consistent, in order to maintain that person in the best health and function possible; and (c) the *nature of the elder–care provider relationship,* including the degrees of responsibility and investment in care by recipients and providers. This last focus is revealed in a shared understanding of the beliefs and values underlying the care process and outcomes. Beliefs and values guide an elder's interpretation and understanding of a health care problem and its treatment.

Are health care beliefs and values of ethnic elders assessed and understood by providers? Palmer's (1992) study of the beliefs and practices of an Amish group was precipitated by her observations of nurses who did not seek to understand them. Their lack of understanding affected the kind of care they gave. If health beliefs and practices are not elicited or understood, the lack of knowledge and misperception may lead to potential prejudice or bias in giving care to ethnic elders. The inequality of high mortality and morbidity rates linked to racial groups (e.g., blacks have the highest death rate in 13 of the 15 leading causes of death in the United States; 25% of blacks are diagnosed with hypertension, compared to 10% of whites) is not an ethnic or race issue. Rather, this inequality is an access-to-care issue, with the economic aspects of access (e.g., poverty, lack of or insufficient insurance) exerting a major influence on disparities in health care (Dressler, 1993; Funkhouser & Moser, 1990).

Studies claiming race, minority status, or ethnicity of elders as a significant factor in prescription and nonprescription drug use (Bazargan et al., 1993; Fillenbaum et al., 1993) and participation in cervical screening

(White, Begg, Fishman, Guthrie, & Fagan, 1993) are actually measuring access to care. It is unclear how the term *race* (comparing black to white elders) is defined or determined, other than the color of skin. For example, even when Fillenbaum et al. (1993) state that "blacks are less likely than their white counterparts to be married and to have supplemental health insurance, are less educated, and have more strained economic circumstances" (p. 1579), they remain convinced that "with other factors controlled, race made a statistically significant, if substantively small, contribution to explaining prescription drug use" (p. 1581). What is actually being captured in the race variable? The authors assume that the similar poor health status of both black and white elders in their sample would lead elders to use the available health care services, to be treated with prescribed drugs, and that this treatment would be consistent among all elders and all providers. These assumptions suggest that the authors believe the care process is purely objective; it is not.

Decision Making

Recognizing subjectivity in clinical assessment and decisions is the first step in identifying individual biases and the effect of those biases on ethnic elders to whom care is delivered. Most important is not to assume that one's own perspective of a care activity, such as personal hygiene, and the rituals associated with that activity are the norm for all ethnic elderly. Rempusheski (1989) suggested a list of assessment categories and questions to elicit the rituals, beliefs, and symbols that elders associate with sleep, personal hygiene, and eating. Eliciting rules for sleep, including bedtime and awakening rituals, avoids bias about the kinds of activities a professional may believe should take place at bedtime or upon awakening.

Ethnic bias is acknowledged as a factor in clinical decision making by health care providers (Eisenberg, 1979; Phillips & Rempusheski, 1985). Eisenberg (1979) summarized the medical decision-making literature. He said that most of the literature is based on normative concepts, or on how decisions *should* be made, rather than on how they *are* made. He noted that there has been a tendency by clinicians to deny the effect of non-biomedical variables on their diagnostic and therapeutic decisions. Treatment decisions are presumed not to differ across patient populations. There is, however, considerable evidence to support the effect of sociocultural variables on the diagnosis and treatment of individuals.

Although some questions were raised as to the adequacy of the methods employed (particularly control by case mix and severity of disease), diagnosis and treatment differed by social class in several studies. Rating of normalcy versus pathology for a diagnosis, kind and length of treatment, and referral to surgeons and other specialists differed for lower-, middle-, and upper-class patients. According to Eisenberg, income and race are variables subsumed within the definition of class. Such hidden variables contribute to misinterpretation of data, lack of knowledge about the care needs of ethnic elderly, and denial that ethnicity plays a role in clinical decision making. Subjectivity was hypothesized as having more influence than objective assessment in diagnostic and treatment decisions. This situation was detected as a discrepancy between a physician's actual diagnosis and the views he or she expressed during an interview.

Nursing decision-making literature has revealed similar problems with subjectivity in diagnostic and intervention decisions for elders. The presumed path of an "objective" diagnosis and obstacle-free intervention is analogous to the way decisions *should* be made. However, in a study that interviewed nurses and social workers about their assessment of elder–family caregiver abusive relationships, the most common decision paths incorporated a value decision composed of interpretation of social roles and interactions of elders and caregivers, cultural stereotypes, personal values, and professional values. The least common path used by these care providers was one that assessed only the nature of the situation and the caregiver's role performance, resulting in a diagnosis and intervention (Phillips & Rempusheski, 1985). Among the cultural reasons for decisions given by these subjects were ones denoting the *origin* of the elder or caregiver (e.g., "He is a man from Greece"), the *rules* for actions and behaviors (e.g., "He expects certain things and maybe this doesn't go over so well with the children"), and *contrasts* (e.g., "I can see why maybe somebody would get upset with him, because he's from a different culture and his reactions are different") (Phillips & Rempusheski, 1985, p. 137).

Family and Community

Values, beliefs, structure, process, composition, boundaries, and roles of ethnic families and ethnic communities comprise some of the variables to be considered for elder ethnic care. Family and community issues may be examined together when family members, including elders, are within close proximity to each other and/or comprise a large network of persons who share similar values and beliefs within a circumscribed geographic boundary. Ethnic communities in urban, suburban, and rural settings provide the backdrop for support for ethnic elderly. The history of migration of ethnic groups into the United States is evidence of the re-creation of ethnic communities, some originating from agricultural communities and transformed into urban areas while maintaining their basic values.

Family, health, and home ownership were among the values held by Poles and Polish Americans in Rempusheski's (1988) review of the literature. She found that family life, family support, and loyalty were held to the highest standard, that family relationships were valued over professional or occupational satisfaction, that the need for care and confidence was invested in one's own children and family, and that children were regarded as a sign of status, particularly in Catholic families. Dispersal of families away from prescribed geographic boundaries challenges these values. A conflict arises, therefore, when values are not shared among the generations of an ethnic family and is compounded by dispersal of families geographically. Expectations not met by family members may be met, at least partially, by a community. Rempusheski's sample was of Polish-American elders who had moved to the Southwest from ethnic communities in northeastern states, leaving family members behind. These elders re-created an ethnic community in which language, values, beliefs, and rituals were shared. Care and support for unmarried and widowed elders were partially met by this community.

Solitary living arrangements among the elderly increased after World War II with the growth in retirement plans and the expansion of Social Security. Although this trend affected all groups, Angel et al. (1992) noted a significant variation between racial and ethnic groups as a result of family size and ethnic values related to care of aging parents. They noted that the larger family size among Latinos, combined with obligations felt by children to care for their parents, increased the probability that elderly who were ill would be cared for at home. However, the probability of living with others, such as children, was influenced by health and proximity of children. They concluded that, "although institutionalization is a clear option in the case of serious declines in health, it is an option that is rarely exercised by blacks or Latinos" (p. 513). In a large-scale survey of ethnic elderly in New York City, Cantor (1985) found that higher levels of family assistance and family solidarity differentiated Hispanics from blacks and whites.

Family roles, proximity, values, and community geography emerge as key variables for elder care among Old Order Amish (Palmer, 1992; Tripp-Reimer, Sorofman, Lauer, Martin, & Afifi, 1988). Both Palmer's (1992) case study of Amish in Pennsylvania and Tripp-Reimer and colleagues' (1988) interviews with Amish in Iowa revealed values and examples of elders cared for by family or members of the community, all within a circumscribed geographic area. Interestingly, however, neither respite nor support existed for the caregiver, particularly when the primary caregiver was an unmarried daughter (Tripp-Reimer et al., 1988). Although it is rare for Amish elders to be institutionalized, these authors noted evidence that some elders were placed in an Amish nursing home.

Questions remain about the gaps in care that exist for ethnic elders who are unmarried or widowed, are geographically distanced or without family, and choose to live alone. With the onset of serious illness, declining health, or declining function, these elders have three options: (a) to continue to live alone despite safety concerns and diminishing health; (b) to move in with others who can provide assistance, supervision, or direct care; or (c) to enter a long-term care institution and receive formal care. Among the factors influencing the option chosen by an elderly person are the availability of other relatives who are willing or able to serve as caregivers; the elder's financial resources; ethnic values of expected care (by the elder) or responsibility and duty for care by family members; and community factors, such as support from nonfamily members or informal and formal caregivers, available housing or long-term-care facilities, and the rapidity of health/function decline of the elder.

Families desiring to keep their elders at home are challenged to provide care in balance with other family responsibilities, which often include full-time employment, child care, and relationship with a spouse and children. Adult day care (ADC) centers provide family caregivers with a supervised daytime location for elders. The goals of the ADC centers sampled in one study (Wallace et al., 1992) included respite to caregivers, socialization, rehabilitation, therapeutic diets, nursing services, and physical therapy for elders. Wallace et al. (1992) found, even after controlling for geographic distribution of ADC centers that favor African Americans, that African Americans used ADC centers at over twice the rate of use by older whites. Interestingly, after controlling for either Medicaid or family characteristics, the authors found that race did not appear as a significant variable. They suggested that their findings reveal that the immediate cause of racial differences in ADC-center use is primarily a function of economics and family status. More important, however, they concluded that African-American elderly are much more likely than white elderly to depend on children as primary caregivers and to rely on Medicaid. Providing ADC centers as respite for family caregivers crosses ethnic, racial, and minority boundaries. The more important concern here is to assist family support systems when family members may be struggling to maintain a balance financially and psychologically as caregivers to their elders.

CONCLUSIONS

The selected care issues presented in this chapter pose dilemmas that challenge some basic values of nursing: shared responsibility for care and individualizing care versus generalizing care based on universal concepts of caring for elders. Nurses, for the most part, subscribe to a common belief that the care provider and the care recipient have a shared responsibility for care. It is important for nurses, in uncovering the health beliefs and behaviors of ethnic elderly, to address both the elder's and the provider's perspectives on the care expected and the care received. Input from family members or from persons aware of the ethnic elder's health beliefs and previous life behaviors is incorporated into the plan of care, taking into account those ethnic beliefs and behaviors thought to be most significant to the elder when he or she is unable to participate in the care.

Maintaining a care plan that focuses on the ethnic elder's individuality, in contrast to universal concepts of care, is another challenge to nurses' basic values of care. What are the universal care needs of ethnic elders, the particulars of giving and receiving care that cut across sociocultural boundaries? What is it about those universal care needs that make them unique or individualize them to a population of ethnic elderly? For example, touch has been proposed as a universal care need of elders. However, the rules for ways to touch, how to touch, appropriate places to touch, and who may touch vary by ethnic group. Perhaps it is the way in which the care need is met, including the use of symbols and rituals, that is unique for each ethnic elder population. Finally, there may be care needs that vary by individuals within an ethnic elderly population, and care providers need to be sensitive to investigating the unique care needs of the ethnic elderly for whom they give care.

REFERENCES

Angel, R. J., Angel, J. L., & Himes, C. L. (1992). Minority group status, health transitions, and community living arrangements among the elderly. *Research on Aging, 14,* 496–521.

Bazargan, M., Barbre, A. R., & Hamm, V. (1993). Failure to have prescriptions filled among black elderly. *Journal of Aging and Health, 5,* 264–282.

Cantor, M. H. (1985). The informal support system of New York's inner city elderly: Is ethnicity a factor? In D. E. Gelfand & A. J. Kutzik (Eds.), *Ethnicity and aging: Theory, research and policy* (pp. 153–174). New York: Springer Publishing Co.

Clark, D. O., Maddox, G. L., & Steinhauser, K. (1993). Race, aging, and functional health. *Journal of Aging and Health, 5,* 536–553.

Crimmins, E. M., & Saito, Y. (1993). Getting better and getting worse: Transitions in functional status among older Americans. *Journal of Aging and Health, 5,* 3–36.

DeVos, G., & Romanucci-Ross, L. (1975). Ethnicity: Vessel of meaning and emblem of contrast. In G. DeVos & L. Romanucci-Ross (Eds.), *Ethnic identity: Cultural continuities and change* (pp. 363–390). Palo Alto, CA: Mayfield.

Dressler, W. W. (1993). Health in the African American community: Accounting for health inequalities. *Medical Anthropology Quarterly, 7*(4), 325–345.

Edwards, N. C. (1992). Important considerations in the use of ethnicity as a study variable. *Canadian Journal of Public Health, 83*(1), 31–33.

Eisenberg, J. M. (1979). Sociologic influences on decision-making by clinicians. *Annals of Internal Medicine, 90,* 957–964.

Facione, N. C. (1993). The Triandis model for the study of health and illness behavior: A social behavior theory with sensitivity to diversity. *Advances in Nursing Science, 15*(3), 49–58.

Fillenbaum, G. G., Hanlon, J. T., Corder, E. H., Ziqubu-Page, T., Wall, W. E., & Brock, D. (1993). Prescription and nonprescription drug use among black and white community-residing elderly. *American Journal of Public Health, 83,* 1577–1582.

Funkhouser, S. W., & Moser, D. K. (1990). Is health care racist? *Advances in Nursing Science, 12*(2), 47–55.

Gans, H. J. (1979). Symbolic ethnicity: The future of ethnic groups in America. *Ethnic and Racial Studies, 2,* 1–20.

Graveley, E. A., & Oseasohn, C. S. (1991). Multiple drug regimens: Medication compliance among veterans 65 years and older. *Research in Nursing and Health, 14*(1), 51–58.

Hertz, F. (1928). *Race and civilization.* New York: Macmillan.

Hogben, L. (1932). *Genetic principles in medicine and social science.* New York: Knopf.

Jones, D. C., & van Amelsvoort-Jones, G. M. M. (1986). Communication patterns between nursing staff and the ethnic elderly in a long-term care facility. *Journal of Advanced Nursing, 11*(3), 265–272.

Keith, V. M., & Herring, C. (1991). Skin tone and stratification in the black community. *American Journal of Sociology, 97,* 760–778.

LaVeist, T. A. (1994). Beyond dummy variables and sample selection: What health services researchers ought to know about race as a variable. *HSR: Health Services Research, 29*(1), 1–16.

Martinelli, P. C. (1984). Ethnicity in the sunbelt: Italian American migrants in Scottsdale, Arizona (Doctoral dissertation, Arizona State University, 1984). *Dissertation Abstracts International, 45,* 2664A.

McLemore, S. D. (1994). *Racial and ethnic relations in America* (4th ed.). Boston: Allyn and Bacon.

Mead, M., Dobzhansky, T., Tobach, E., & Light, R. E. (Eds.). (1968). *Science and the concept of race.* New York: Columbia University Press.

Mintzer, J. E., Rubert, M. P., Loewenstein, D., Gamez, E., Millor, A., Quinteros, R., Flores, L., Miller, M., Rainerman, A., & Eisdorfer, C. (1992). Daughters caregiving for Hispanic and non-Hispanic Alzheimer patients: Does ethnicity make a difference? *Community Mental Health Journal, 28*(4), 293–303.

Montagu, A. (1964). *Man's most dangerous myth: The fallacy of race* (4th ed.). New York: World.

Padgett, D. (1989). Aging minority women: Issues in research and health policy. *Women and Health, 14*(3/4), 213–225.

Palmer, C. V. (1992). The health beliefs and practices of an Old Order Amish family. *Journal of the American Academy of Nurse Practitioners, 4,* 117–122.

Parrillo, V. N. (1991). Rethinking today's minorities. In V. N. Parrillo (Ed.), *Rethinking today's minorities* (pp. 3–14). New York: Greenwood Press.

Phillips, L. R. (1989). Age: A truly confounding variable. *Western Journal of Nursing Research, 11,* 181–195.

Phillips, L. R., & Rempusheski, V. F. (1985). A decision-making model for diagnosing and intervening in elder abuse and neglect. *Nursing Research, 34,* 134–139.

Rempusheski, V. F. (1986). Exploration and description of caring for self and others with second generation Polish American elders (Doctoral dissertation, University of Arizona, 1985). *Dissertation Abstracts International, 46,* 3785B.

Rempusheski, V. F. (1988). Caring for self and others: Second generation Polish American elders in an ethnic club. *Journal of Cross-Cultural Gerontology, 3,* 223–271.

Rempusheski, V. F. (1989). The role of ethnicity in elder care. *Nursing Clinics of North America, 24*(3), 717–724.

Ringer, B. B., & Lawless, E. R. (1989). *Race-ethnicity and society.* New York: Routledge.

Tripp-Reimer, T., & Lauer, G. M. (1987) Ethnicity and families with chronic illness. In L. M. Wright & M. Leahey (Eds.), *Families and chronic illness* (pp. 77–100). Springhouse, PA: Springhouse Corp.

Tripp-Reimer, T., Sorofman, B., Lauer, G., Martin, M., & Afifi, L. (1988). To be different from the world: Patterns of elder care among Iowa Old Order Amish. *Journal of Cross-Cultural Gerontology, 3,* 185–195.

Ulbrich, P. M., & Bradsher, J. E. (1993). Perceived support, help seeking, and adaptation to stress among older black and white women living alone. *Journal of Aging and Health, 5,* 365–386.

UNESCO. (1952). *What is race?* Paris: United Nations Educational, Scientific, and Cultural Organization.

U.S. Immigration and Naturalization Service (INS). (1990). *Statistical yearbook: 1989.* Washington, DC: U.S. Government Printing Office.

Wallace, S. P., Snyder, J. L., Walker, G. K., & Ingman, S. R. (1992). Racial differences among users of long-term care: The case of adult day care. *Research on Aging, 14,* 471–495.

White, J. E., Begg, L., Fishman, N. W., Guthrie, B., & Fagan, J. K. (1993). Increasing cervical cancer screening among minority elderly. *Journal of Gerontological Nursing, 19*(5), 28–34.

Zsembik, B. A. (1993). Determinants of living alone among older Hispanics. *Research on Aging, 15,* 449–464.

CHAPTER 8

Health and Experiences of Older Homeless Adults

Sharon M. Wallsten and A. T. Panter

In *Healthy People 2000* (U.S. Department of Health and Human Services [DHHS], 1990), three broad national goals are stated: (a) increase the span of healthy life for Americans, (b) reduce health disparities among Americans, and (c) achieve access to preventive services for all Americans. Homeless individuals in this country constitute the group of people who have benefited least from any of these stated goals. They are often silent, unnoticed, and they have few advocates, so their plight is poorly understood. Although homeless people have some of the most complex and extreme social and health problems, organized community efforts on their behalf are provided primarily by volunteers and a relatively few paid professionals, who work with minimal resources to provide shelter, meals, guidance, and health care.

Author notes. The authors thank Joan Scovill for her assistance with data collection in the study reported in this chapter. Address correspondence to Sharon M. Wallsten, Duke University, School of Nursing, Box 3322 Medical Center, Durham, NC 27710 (email: walls001@mc.duke.edu)

This chapter begins with a brief review of the history of homelessness in the United States, provides an operational definition of homelessness, and describes the people affected by homelessness and their social and health problems. The chapter also discusses two groups of homeless individuals who have been particularly difficult for researchers to identify and target: homeless people in rural areas and homeless older adults. We conclude by reviewing findings from a study we conducted to investigate the overall health and social support of homeless older adults in five North Carolina counties and by discussing implications for practice and interventions.

HISTORY OF HOMELESSNESS IN THE UNITED STATES

Early History (1700s–1800s)

Contemporary discussion and debate regarding homelessness occur "in an historical vacuum," as if there were no prior evidence on this topic (Kusmer, 1987, p. 21). Yet a 1987 exhibition organized by the Museum of the City of New York chronicles the existence of homeless individuals in New Amsterdam as early as 1653 (MacDonald, 1987). In the 17th and 18th centuries the majority of colonial towns had no institutions to house dependent individuals. Only Philadelphia, Boston, and New York had institutions, usually referred to as almshouses (also known as poorhouses or county farms), that housed the poor and destitute. Rather, policies of colonial communities made provisions for dependent members of the community while simultaneously protecting the community from potentially dependent newcomers or transients. Whereas "outsiders" (including single dependent women) were evicted from the community, the town provided small amounts of money to help the family or family surrogate of the "insider" (Martin, 1987; Rothman, 1987).

Rothman (1987) suggested that the notion of "neighbor" and "stranger" (p. 12) was replaced in the early 19th century by "worthy" and "unworthy" poor. The worthy were eligible for town help, and the unworthy were eligible for shelter and food in the town almshouse. Thus, the destitute were no longer banished from the town but sent to the almshouse, in the belief that "the poor were the victims of their own inadequacy and guilty of poverty" (p. 12). Almshouses were run with a great deal of regimentation, with the purpose of reforming the occupants. For example, residents could not leave without permission, and any infraction of the rules resulted in punishment such as solitary confinement or reduced food rations. Not only healthy homeless men were relegated to these institutions; individuals with mental illness, children, and widows lived in almshouses (Quigley, 1992).

Kusmer (1987) described an increase in the homeless population in cities in the 1840s and 1850s, which was followed by a temporary decline during the Civil War years. However, another large increase in homelessness occurred after the Civil War and lasted through the depressions of the 1870s and 1930s. Even before vast numbers of people were made destitute by the Great Depression, homeless people included veterans of the Civil War and people who held transient jobs, such as building railroads or picking crops (Quigley, 1992). The depression of the 1870s gave rise to vagrants and tramps who sometimes traveled by railroad as unpaying "hobos." During the 1930s, women as well as men traveled the rails, and both groups were convicted of vagrancy (Kusmer, 1987; Martin, 1987).

Kusmer (1987) hypothesized that the increase in the underclass during this time resulted from the country's rapid change from an agricultural, small-town society to an industrial economy centered in large cities. Many people left agricultural areas and migrated to industrial centers. However, the new economy was not able to handle the influx of workers. Because few provisions were made to ensure employee safety, many workers were left jobless because of industrial accidents or diseases related to their jobs. Moreover, the absence of child labor laws encouraged employers to hire children rather than adults. The migration from rural to urban areas resulted in increasing numbers of unemployed and homeless men and women searching for places to stay in urban areas. Kusmer also referred to a writer who interviewed "derelict women" (p. 24) of the New York Bowery (later referred to as "skid row") in 1927; they talked about former homes, lost husbands, and lost children.

"Skid row" is a term coined from a road in Seattle that was used to skid logs to the mill. Thousands of men went to the Northwest in the late 19th century to work in the logging industry. Saloons and brothels frequented by loggers grew up along roads that were later called "skid row" (Jackson, 1987). This term was subsequently used to denote a rundown, undesirable area. Outside skid row areas, homeless women, children, men, mentally ill, and mentally retarded stayed in almshouses.

Introduction of Social Services (Early to Mid-1900s)

In response to these conditions, in the early 1900s a number of public services were instituted: adoption and foster care services were founded, shelters were built for mentally ill and retarded individuals, and government stipends were provided to widows and injured workers. The economic depression of the 1930s caused massive social upheaval that resulted in large, incalculable numbers of homeless people. The New Deal reforms of the 1940s, such as the provision of Social Security and the recruitment for World War II, reduced the numbers of homeless people considerably by the 1950s. Those remaining homeless were primarily older white alcoholic males (Quigley, 1992).

Thus, homelessness in the United States in the 1930s through the 1950s primarily was a problem of unmarried white males, with an average age of 50, who were chronic alcoholics living in skid row areas of large cities. These men were employed intermittently, and approximately 25% were on Social Security. When they had sufficient income, they paid to sleep in flophouses, in cheap hotels, or in beds at missions (Foscarinis, 1991; Kiesler, 1991; Rossi, 1990). Single room occupancy (SRO) hotels served as minimal housing for the poor in urban areas. According to Ovrebo, Minkler, and Liljestrand (1991), the elderly poor are the largest single group of SRO users. Since the 1970s, however, this SRO option has been rapidly disappearing. For example, between 1970 and 1983, 89% of SRO units and other low-cost and substandard housing were demolished; San Francisco lost 40% of its SRO units between 1975 and 1982 (Hooyman & Kiyak, 1993). The tragedy is not the elimination of unsafe, substandard housing but the replacement of affordable units by expensive condominiums or other units that are out of financial reach of the poor. Despite far from ideal living conditions in SROs, few individuals had to sleep on the streets in the past, and society generally was shielded from seeing such problems of homelessness in daily life. As a result, public policymakers could easily neglect problems related to homelessness. In recent years the poorest of the poor have been forced out of housing due to demolition or conversion to more expensive property. Growing numbers of poor families have been forced to double and triple up, a condition that makes them more and more vulnerable to becoming homeless (Foscarinis, 1991; Kiesler, 1991; Rossi, 1989, 1990).

New Visibility and Federal Programs (Early 1980s on)

In the early 1980s the picture of homelessness in America began to change. The "new homeless" became more visible as they searched for shelter and food in public areas—and their presence made other people feel uncomfortable. In 1983, Congress established the Federal Emergency Management Agency's (FEMA) Emergency Food and Shelter Program, which was the first federal program established in response to the growing problem of homelessness in the United States. Contrary to the belief that homelessness would be a temporary problem, the continuous increase of homeless people proved otherwise (Wassem, 1993). Therefore, after considerable grass-roots lobbying on the part of activists, President Reagan signed the Stewart B. McKinney Homeless Assistance Act into law on July 22, 1987. This act was the federal government's first comprehensive approach to addressing the homelessness issue, encompassing both emergency and chronic needs.

According to Foscarinis (1991), just 5 years earlier Reagan had been publicly quoted in the *Boston Globe* on June 17, 1982, as saying "no one is living on the streets," and in 1983 his advisor, Edwin Meese, had stated that soup kitchens were a "free lunch" for persons not really in need. Kondratas (1991) reported that the Bush administration funded the McKinney Act more fully; when Jack Kemp became the Department of Housing and Urban Development (HUD) secretary in 1989, he established priorities for the department and consolidated the McKinney Act programs. The McKinney programs now include emergency services, nonemergency housing, mental health services, primary health services, comprehensive social services, and prevention. In the 1980s, emergency services comprised the largest funding category under the McKinney programs, with a shift toward housing services in recent years (Wassem & Robinson, 1993). Although the service delivery programs financed under the McKinney Act meet important needs, they do not address underlying problems and are inadequate to meet the demands (Foscarinis, 1991).

On May 19, 1993, President Clinton signed Executive Order 12848, which mandated 17 agencies comprising the Interagency Council of the Homeless (established under the Stewart B. McKinney Homeless Assistance

Act) to develop, within 9 months, "a single coordinated Federal plan for breaking the cycle of existing homelessness and for preventing future homelessness" (President, 1993). Onlookers anticipated that the Clinton administration would end a 12-year period of conflicting views between advocates for the homeless and government officials (Deparle, 1994). The recently distributed federal plan titled *Priority: Home! The Federal Plan to Break the Cycle of Homelessness* (U.S. Department of Housing and Urban Development [HUD],1994) extends the prior administration's scope of homelessness. The report recognizes homelessness as a large-scale problem and does not attempt to downplay its scope (DeParle, 1994). The report refers to a study indicating that 7 million people were homeless at some point during the 1980s and that they were not just those suffering from drug, alcohol, or mental illness problems. Rather, these individuals suffered from poverty, racism, and past federal budget cuts. The prior administration repeatedly cited studies showing that 600,000 individuals, the majority of whom were drug and alcohol abusers and/or suffering from mental illness, were homeless on any given night. This new report differentiates between a visible group of homeless people (including individuals with mental illness or those suffering from drug and alcohol problems) and a more hidden group (including individuals suffering from chronic poverty). The federal plan also blames economic and structural changes in society for the loss of shelter for 37 million poor Americans ("Invisible Parade," 1994). The report calls for increased appropriations to HUD to compensate for past budget cuts, to reorganize massively the McKinney services programs, to improve delivery of services by non-profit groups, and to expand programs for the mentally ill to include aggressive outreach efforts. Currently the federal McKinney programs provide a complicated array of 20 categorical programs administered by six agencies. The 1995 fiscal year budget proposes that the Emergency Food and Shelter Program, now under FEMA, be transferred to HUD and that linkages be developed between McKinney programs and existing programs in local areas. A comprehensive approach is described, beginning with aggressive outreach and assessment, the provision of emergency shelter with movement to transitional housing, and finally, permanent or supportive housing. Simultaneously, individuals with chronic problems or problems needing special attention should be given additional help, such as counseling and job training. The overall goal is to help the individual or family move from homelessness to independent living.

In the past there has been considerable disagreement as to whether money is best targeted to emergency or supportive services (Wassem & Robinson, 1993), and unfortunately, as with so many social welfare programs, little longitudinal research has evaluated the kinds of programs that have helped people leave and stay out of homeless circumstances. As it stands, we know more about the scope of the problem than about the kinds of programs that have helped or hindered efforts to solve the problem.

Although at present an estimated 700,000 people are homeless on any one night in the United States (with an estimated yearly growth rate of about 25%), little action has been taken to examine and respond to the underlying causes of and pathways to homelessness (Foscarinis, 1991; Waxman & Reyes, 1990). Foscarinis (1991) argued that "the legitimization of homelessness has removed some of the political riskiness that previously impeded remedial action" (p. 1234), thus allowing society to feel more comfortable with the presence of homeless individuals, more complacent about the problem at large, and more willing to establish crisis infrastructure to deal with homeless people. Although establishing crisis infrastructure has provided temporary solutions (e.g., establishing schools for homeless children), it can be argued that the legitimization process moves attention away from creating the permanent infrastructure necessary to enable homeless individuals to make the transition to more stable living situations.

HOMELESSNESS TODAY

Operational Definition

Researchers in this field struggle to define operationally the concept of homelessness. One operational definition of homeless individuals is provided in *Outcasts on Main Street: The Report of the Federal Task Force on Homelessness and Severe Mental Illness* (DHHS, 1992). The report defines a homeless person as one "who lacks a fixed, regular, and adequate nighttime residence" and whose main nighttime residence is a "supervised public or private shelter designed to provide temporary living accommodations; an institution that provides a temporary residence for individuals intended to be institutionalized; or a public or private place not designed for, or ordinarily used as, a regular sleeping accommodation for human beings" (p. 7). This definition, then, excludes individuals living on the brink of homelessness with dangerously low incomes, in substandard or condemned housing, or those who are temporarily living with others. These excluded conditions clearly warrant attention.

Current Demographics

Who Are the Homeless?

It is estimated that more than one third of the homeless population are members of homeless families, one fourth are children, and one fourth are employed full- or part-time (Jordan, 1988; Waxman & Reyes, 1990). In 1990 the U.S. Conference of Mayors surveyed 30 cities and found that the homeless population was 51% single men, 34% families with young children, 12% single women, and 3% unaccompanied youth. Overall, 23% of the homeless population was children. The survey also found the population to be composed of 46% black, 34% white, 15% Hispanic, 3% Native American, and 1% Asian individuals. The survey identified 28% as mentally ill, 38% as substance abusers, and 6% as having AIDS or HIV-related illness. In addition, 24% were employed full- or part-time, and 26% were veterans (Waxman & Reyes, 1990).

A 1988 study focusing on the homeless in northern Virginia reported that almost 83% of the 7,100 people staying in northern Virginia's homeless shelters held jobs and that many held full-time jobs (Jordan, 1988). Despite full-time employment, however, their salaries were insufficient to afford available housing. Data also showed that 67% of those in the shelters arrived with a family member, and 36% were children.

Vulnerability to Homelessness

The Conference of Mayors survey also indicated that 29 of the 30 cities reported that a lack of affordable housing was the main cause of homelessness. Other frequently cited causes were mental illness coupled with a lack of mental health services, substance abuse coupled with a lack of treatment programs, unemployment, employment problems, poverty or lack of income, and inadequate levels of public assistance (Waxman & Reyes, 1990). According to Kiesler (1991), homeless individuals are disproportionately from minority groups and are much poorer than their "homeless predecessors" (p. 1245). The homeless also include the elderly (Keigher,

1991). The new homeless are less the result of deinstitutionalization and more the result of economic policies that led to significant decreases in available affordable housing, increases in health care costs for large numbers of uninsured people, regressive tax policies, and reduced financing for welfare programs such as Aid to Families with Dependent Children (Kiesler, 1991).

Douglass et al. (1988) suggest several precursors to homelessness, including being deinstitutionalized at 50 years of age from a mental institution; being released from prison at midlife or later; being an alcoholic or drug addict with no success at treatment; being exploited, abused and abandoned by family members; losing a home and assets; not being able to afford housing; being without a supportive family; and having poor education and job skills. In addition, poverty, combined with any of the above, is cited as influential in the transformation to homelessness.

Impoverished families who rent or own their homes pay over 70% of their income to housing (Shapiro, 1989). Thus, for many poor Americans, any unexpected expense, such as one arising from a serious medical problem or a change in employment status, can propel them toward homelessness. The new homeless are often shelterless as well as homeless. Some homeless people are turned away when shelters have reached maximum occupancy, and some prefer to stay in outside areas because they fear for their safety in public shelters. Some people even prefer staying in their own unconventional public place, such as an abandoned car, rather than spend time in group shelters.

Extent of Homelessness

Estimates of the extent of homelessness in this country vary greatly. A frequently cited estimate of 600,000 homeless individuals in the United States (Burt & Cohen, 1989), as provided in the *Report of the Federal Task Force on Homelessness and Severe Mental Illness* (DHHS, 1992), is nearly double a 1984 HUD (1984) estimate of 250,000 to 350,000. Shelter and Street Night (S-Night) operation for the 1990 U.S. census counted a total of 178,828 people in shelters and 49,793 on the streets throughout the United States (National Coalition for the Homeless, 1991). These data were collected on one particular night, and no attempt was made to randomize identification days. At the state level, census takers in North Carolina counted 2,637 persons in shelters and 259 in the streets. And yet a separate survey conducted by the North Carolina Division of Community Assistance (1988) identified 8,045 homeless people.

Through telephone interviews with shelter managers in five North Carolina counties, Wallsten and Panter (1994) found an average census of 549 people staying in the shelters on any given night. The five counties included a mixture of rural and urban areas, excluding several major cities in the state and excluding those individuals staying outside or in unconventional places. Given that the state includes 100 counties, we can extrapolate and estimate a total homeless population of between 10,000 and 11,000 in North Carolina shelters alone. The disparate conclusions reached in any of the estimates above reflect the substantial methodological difficulties involved in tracking down and defining the sample.

Extent of Mental Illness Among the Homeless

It has taken considerable research to dispel the belief that the majority of homeless people are mentally ill (Dennis, Buckner, Lipton, & Levine, 1991). Ten studies supported by the National Institute of Mental Health (NIMH) from 1982 to 1986 have found mental illness prevalence rates among the homeless ranging from 28% to 37% (Tessler & Dennis, 1989). The *Report of the Federal Task Force on Homelessness and Severe Mental Illness* (DHHS, 1992) estimated that 4 million people in the United States are severely mentally ill and that approximately 1 of 20 of them is homeless. Moreover, of the estimated 600,000 homeless people, approximately one third of the single adults have a severe mental illness (DHHS, 1992). Although about one third to one half of homeless people have a diagnosable mental disorder, the percentage with serious or chronic mental illness is estimated to range from 10% to 15%. The diagnosable illnesses and conditions are diverse and include alcohol and drug abuse or dependency, anxiety disorders, mild depression, and schizophrenia. Douglass et al. (1988) found that 33% of elderly homeless respondents in Detroit reported having been patients in mental hospitals, and 31% reported having been in alcohol or drug detoxification hospitals. In Detroit, hospitalization was more likely among women than men and among whites rather than African Americans. Although whites were more likely to have been in mental institutions, African Americans were more likely to have been imprisoned.

Goodman, Saxe, and Harvey (1991) and Kiesler (1991) maintained that homelessness itself is a risk factor for emotional disorder. Depression was found to be prevalent among the Detroit sample, and as Douglass et al. (1988) suggested, one cannot resolve issues of causality in determining whether the homelessness or the depression came first. Examining homeless elderly men and those living in flophouses and apartments in the Bowery in Manhattan, Cohen, Teresi, and Holmes (1988a) found that physical health and depression were highly correlated. They also reported high interrelations among stress, unfulfilled needs, and depression. Although the rate of mental hospitalizations among the homeless group was 23% and rates of gross organic mental symptoms were relatively low, the depression rate was 1½ times greater than that of the control group.

Methodological Issues in Studying Homelessness

Several methodological issues confront those doing research on the homeless. The first major issue concerns the definition of homelessness itself, because many newly homeless people live temporarily with other family units before presenting themselves in shelters. Second, some homeless individuals prefer not to stay in shelters, choosing more covert, unconventional places, such as in cars or trucks, outside areas, or condemned and dilapidated buildings. Conventional issues in conducting cross-sectional research are compounded by specific problems in regulations pertaining to length of shelter stay. Cross-sectional studies of homelessness often confuse precursors and consequences and oversample the long-time homeless relative to the new homeless who may have left the sampling frame. People who leave homeless circumstances more rapidly may differ substantially from the long-term homeless with respect to certain health indicators such as social ties, mental and physical health status, and support services obtained (Shinn, Knickerman, & Weitzman, 1991).

Defining the rural population is laden with problems, and defining the characteristics of the homeless population is even more problematic (Toomey, First, Greenlee, & Cummins, 1990). For example, the definition of rural and urban geographic areas employed is critical in data interpretation. Yet the Housing Assistance Council, Inc. (HAC, 1991) reported a half dozen definitions of *rural* used by federal agencies. These varied criteria make it difficult for researchers to decide on the best operational definition to adopt. An even more basic issue is the definition of homelessness, which can include people found in shelters, on the street, in shacks, and in temporary residence with friends or relatives, as well as those who come to community kitchens for meals but not shelter. Also, cross-sectional studies that involve interviews conducted at different time points might easily include the same respondents, who may travel from shelter to shelter. Another possible problem stems from the question of whether respondents' rural or urban living circumstances are based on the shelter or other outside location or on the place where the individual last had a residence he or she considered stable. In a pilot study conducted by Wallsten and Panter in 1994 (described later), there was evidence that respondents interviewed in urban shelters had come directly from rural counties. Other problems include obtaining a random sample of homeless people in rural and urban communities so that they can be compared.

OLDER HOMELESS ADULTS AND RURAL HOMELESS

Estimating Numbers of Older Homeless Adults

The numerous methodological issues described above help explain why estimating the numbers of homeless who are elderly is such a great challenge. The 1984 HUD survey mentioned earlier reported that about 6% of the 250,000 to 350,000 homeless were elderly. More recent surveys, conducted by the Aging Health Policy Center, estimated that the percentage of persons aged 50 and over living in shelters in eight cities was between 14.5% and 28% (Cohen et al., 1988a). Street outreach programs, such as the one conducted by the Coalition for the Homeless (1984) in New York City, reported proportions of older persons ranging as high as 50%. In a review of several studies, Kutza and Keigher (1991) described a Nashville study, with 22% who were 60 and older, and an eight-city study mentioned above, with 27% aged 60 and over. An unknown number of elderly individuals live in deplorable conditions in isolated areas such as abandoned buildings; these people stay hidden and thus may not be counted as homeless (Keigher, Berman, & Greenblatt, 1991).

   Cohen, Teresi, Holmes, and Roth (1988) suggest that these figures are underestimates. Many elderly people stay away from public shelters because of fear of being mugged or of being treated with insensitivity. In addition, the elderly tend to avoid formal assistance because of the fear of being institutionalized. Thus, studies that base their samples on Department of Social Service records or on a city's users of emergency services are likely to be excluding a sizable number of older adults who are trying to stay concealed from public notice.

Profile of Older Homeless Adults

Deinstitutionalization in the 1950s through the 1970s was accompanied by very little effort in discharge planning and too few community mental health centers to meet the demands of outpatient treatment and follow-up. With the passage of the 1963 Community Mental Health Center Act, 768 centers were developed, but this number was only half that initially proposed. Also, the establishment of Medicaid in 1963 and the federal Supplemental Security Income (SSI) and Supplemental Security Disability Insurance (SSDI) programs provided direct entitlements to mentally disabled persons living in community-based facilities, thereby providing incentives to discharge patients from state hospitals. Consequently, many former patients with chronic mental illness returned to communities and ultimately became part of the homeless scene. Nationally, 50 state hospitals closed, and many others were consolidated. As a result of changing laws and policies, the state hospital census dropped nationally from 560,000 in 1955 to 216,00 in 1974; by 1989 the census had fallen to 100,000 (Dorwart, 1988; DHHS, 1992; National Institute of Mental Health, 1991).

Economic policies and housing policies contributed even more to the growing numbers and different profiles of the homeless (Kiesler, 1991). Urban redevelopment projects eliminated a considerable number of low-cost housing options for poor people (Foscarinis, 1991), and growing numbers of impoverished families doubled or tripled up in single housing units as affordable housing became scarce (Rossi, 1989). A sizable proportion of residents in these renewal areas were the elderly poor renting rooms in houses, residential hotels, and missions (Boondas, 1985). Many older homes and apartments were renovated and priced out of reach for the poor and near-poor, the former residents of the renewed districts.

Keigher (1991) noted that despite paying relatively large percentages of their incomes for housing, the elderly poor experience housing problems such as overpricing, substandard units, and crowded conditions, and they seldom have the resources to deal with these problems. As increasing numbers of the elderly live longer, more individuals will be searching for affordable housing. Thus, there is a threat that increasing numbers of the elderly poor may become homeless. As the numbers of elderly persons increase and as low-rent housing in small communities becomes increasingly unavailable, many of the elderly, already on the fringes of poverty, may face homeless conditions. As noted by the National Resource Center for Rural Elderly (1992), many low-income rental units in rural vacation areas have been converted to condominiums and rentals for upper-income retirees. This shift may become a significant problem in locations such as North Carolina's coastal and mountain communities, which are known areas for retirees. In a study by the Housing Risks of the Elderly Project, conducted in Chicago in 1988, Keigher (1991) reported that precipitating forces of homelessness are diminished mental capacity, loss of income, loss of financially supportive persons, and evictions. She further suggested that even without these "trigger" events, elderly remain in subminimal and deplorable living conditions.

Although poverty rates among the elderly declined considerably during the past 20 years, certain groups remain particularly vulnerable to the effects of poverty. Elderly African Americans are three times as likely as whites to have incomes below the poverty level, and elderly Hispanics are more than twice as likely. In addition, women are twice as likely as men to live in poverty. Even more significantly, almost 50% of the elderly living alone are poor or near-poor. These vulnerable individuals have little income for anything other than basic necessities (Chen, 1991; Commonwealth Fund Commission, 1988; Keigher, 1991). Income reduction in old age, when compounded by a lack of government services and the occurrence of any unexpected strain, can catapult a vulnerable individual to the streets (Boondas, 1985).

In addition, many elderly homeless persons are eligible for benefits under the Social Security Act but do not receive them. It is estimated that 35% of all homeless individuals are eligible for these benefits, yet only 4% receive them (Congressional Budget Office, 1990; DeParle, 1990; Tessler & Dennis, 1989). Often mentally unstable, without family supports or close friends, homeless elderly persons tend not to be aware of available resources or to be unable to deal with the complexities of application without having an advocate present to help them.

Moreover, although some older adults are covered by Medicaid, only 25% of poor older North Carolinians and 31% of the poor older adults nationally avail themselves of the program (Division of Aging and CARES, 1991). Thus, any major medical or social event, such as the purchase of expensive medication or the death of a spouse, could conceivably stress older adults beyond a coping point. In a hearing before the House Subcommittee on Health and the Environment, Dr. James Wright (1990) pointed out that the conventional health care system is inadequate for the homeless because they are unlikely to have insurance and are often unwelcome in public clinics.

In the Detroit field study (Douglass et al., 1988), the homeless elderly population was composed largely of "young" old rather than "old" old. With an age range of 54 to 86 years, over half of the sample was younger than 65 years. Doolin (1986) also talks about the premature aging of homeless elderly, suggesting that these young-old often have physiological problems similar to a those of a 70-year-old, but they may be 20 years younger and therefore ineligible for certain health care entitlements. Williams, Sobol, Alker, and Lozier (1991) reported that the average age of death for homeless people is young; for example, in San Francisco the average age of death was 41 years, and in Atlanta it was 31 years.

Douglass et al. (1988) suggested that the numbers of elderly homeless decrease with advancing years because of high mortality rates and the development of medical problems that lead to Medicaid nursing home placement. In addition, they noted that elderly homeless who reach age 65 and receive Social Security or other economic entitlements may finally accrue sufficient money to pay for shelter. However, many individuals eligible for entitlements cannot receive them because they lack a permanent address.

Health Problems of Homeless Elders

Homelessness necessitates adapting to harsh living circumstances in which food and shelter are priority daily concerns. Cohen, Teresi, Holmes, and Roth (1988) referred to homeless elderly men as survivors; they provide for their daily needs despite deplorable circumstances, although this may be jeopardized by illness or disability. The life-style of the homeless essentially negates the pursuit of disease prevention and health promotion practices and interferes with organized attempts to treat acute or chronic problems. In a June 1989 hearing before the House Subcommittee on Health and the Environment, Janelle Goetcheus (1990), medical director of Health Care for the Homeless Project in Washington, DC, described regularly seeing numbers of individuals with untreated chronic health problems such as tuberculosis, diabetes, and high blood pressure, in addition to acute problems such as frozen appendages or burns from grates. She described treating people in their 50s who had health problems that mirrored those of the frail elderly with chronic illness. She even reported finding people dying in advanced stages of cancer.

It is often difficult, under the best life conditions, to modify one's normal environment to accommodate to disabilities or chronic conditions. In the general population, at least four of five persons aged 65 and older have a minimum of one chronic health condition. The most common problems are related to conditions such as arthritis, heart disease, hypertension, and stroke, often made worse by sensory impairments and mobility problems (Persily & Albury, 1991). Doolin (1986) suggested that being elderly and homeless constitute double jeopardy, in that problems commonly associated with aging are compounded by the problems inherently associated with being homeless (i.e., no residence, lack of food and clothing, no regular medical services, few reliable social supports). Moreover, as Doolin pointed out, physical disorders of the homeless elderly are generally similar to those of their nonhomeless peers but are magnified by disordered living conditions. The lack of a supportive environment to manage a personal program of preventive medicine, the overcrowding in shelters, and the hardships of having to live continually in stressful situations would compromise the heartiest individual, regardless of age. The paramount needs perceived by the elderly homeless are food and shelter; thus, immediate health care needs get little attention (Doolin, 1986). Being homeless is associated with greater incidence of morbidity and mortality and increased risk from communicable diseases, injuries, hypothermia, and malnutrition (Brickner et al., 1984; Lindsey, 1989). Clearly, to survive in homeless conditions, the elderly must adapt to a harsh life-style and must be particularly resourceful. This process may be jeopardized by illness or disability.

Brickner et al. (1984) identified certain unique problems that stem from homelessness, such as consequences of trauma or criminal assault, infestation with scabies or lice, peripheral vascular disease, cellulitis and leg ulcers, frostbite or burns from grates, and pulmonary tuberculosis. Given a questionnaire that included 11 medical disorders, elderly homeless Bowery men reported significantly more somatic and respiratory symptoms and more cases of hearing disorder, hypertension, and edema than did elderly in the nonhomeless population (Cohen, Teresi, & Holmes, 1988b). The 10 most frequently self-reported chronic health problems among the elderly homeless in Detroit were dental problems, arthritis, hypertension, circulatory problems, emphysema or bronchitis, heart trouble, ulcers or stomach ailments, glaucoma, asthma, anemia, and diabetes (Hodgkins, Douglass, & Lam, 1990).

Rural Homeless Older Adults

Another source of vulnerability for older homeless adults is their location, urban or rural. The head of the Ohio Coalition for the Homeless observed that "rural homelessness is growing faster than we can keep track of it. People are living in railroad cars and tarpaper shacks. Shelters in tiny towns we've never heard of are operating at or above capacity and are turning people away" (Wilkerson, 1989, p. A1). In a 1988 national survey of 2,200 rural and urban shelters conducted by the HAC, rural people accounted for 25% of all stays in homeless shelters (Wilkerson, 1989). Whereas 11.6% of housing is dilapidated in the worst areas in New York City, 49% of rental housing in some rural southern counties is dilapidated and lacks all plumbing facilities (National Coalition for the Homeless, 1987). The National Coalition for the Homeless (1987) suggests that rural homelessness is less visible than urban homelessness because the land area is less densely populated, and extreme conditions of impoverished living go unnoticed. Migration probably occurs from rural areas to urban areas, thereby transferring numbers of homeless people to urban centers. Also, overcrowding, as a result of multiple generations living together, is overlooked and accepted. The coalition also suggests that rural people respond to homelessness differently from their urban counterparts. With few or no formal supportive services available, they continue to live in extreme housing deficiencies. Statewide estimates of the nonmetropolitan homeless in Iowa, Colorado, and Pennsylvania are between 40% and 50% of the figures in metropolitan areas (HAC, 1991).

In 1983, HAC began to document growing signs of homelessness in the nation. Their literature review found that the bulk of documentation of rural homelessness could be obtained only through public hearing records, needs assessments, planning documents, and descriptive reports and that most data had not been collected with a specific focus on rural homelessness (HAC, 1991). An exception to this, noted by HAC, is a series of studies conducted in Ohio that were explicitly designed to look at rural homelessness. According to Roth, Toomey, and First (1992), the first Ohio Department of Mental Health study, which was conducted between 1983 and 1985, used a combination of purposive and random sampling, drawing on urban areas, small city areas, and rural counties. Roth and Bean (1986) reported that 20% of 979 interviews were carried out in rural settings. Rural respondents were younger, included a higher proportion of women, were mostly white (a reflection of the state's ethnic breakdown), and were more likely to be married than were urban homeless people. In subsequent analysis of this study, Burt and Cohen (1989) reported a rate of 2.4 homeless persons per 10,000, with 29% aged 50 and over.

In a second Ohio study, viewed as the first comprehensive study of rural homelessness in the country, interviews were held with 921 homeless adults in 21 randomly selected rural counties (First, Rife, & Toomey, 1994). Results showed that minorities were overrepresented, and 7.7% of the sample were age 50 and over. Five major groups of homeless persons were identified: young families, people employed full- or part-time but with too little income to support housing, women unable to work because of dependent children or limited skills, older men (who tend to be homeless longer and more likely to be disabled, with fewer social supports than women), and disabled persons without the social networks and social programs to help them live independently. Unfortunately, an urban comparison group was not included. HAC (1991) noted that although similar patterns have been found in other reported studies reviewed by their office, the rural homeless are diverse, and great caution must be taken in comparing studies that have little, if any, common methodology.

Variables Influencing Social Supports and the Elderly Homeless

Shinn et al. (1991) described several paths linking social relationships to homelessness. Members of social networks may provide help in finding or maintaining housing, or they may provide emotional support in coping with problems. They can also promote homelessness by making current living conditions impossible or simply by having their resources used up by the individual. The authors suggested that although lack of social ties and social isolation may contribute to homelessness, lack of stable living conditions may also influence the stability of one's social ties. According to Rossi, Wright, Fisher, and Willis (1987), families and friends provide help to the limits of their potential, and undue strain on the relationship or resources may move the individual to homeless circumstances. In their review of the literature, Shinn et al. (1991) also caution about interpreting findings from cross-sectional studies because the directionality of the observed effects cannot be easily disentangled.

In the Detroit study described earlier in this chapter (Douglass et al., 1988), the elderly homeless were generally alone, with few family supports. Even when kin were in the same city, 56% of the respondents were opposed to living with them, 31% were in favor of living with them, and 13% did not know whether or not they wanted to live with relatives. Less than 50% of the respondents had had recent contact with relatives. On the other hand, 61% of those surveyed indicated having at least one friend they could count on. As Douglass et al. (1988) suggested, it would be interesting to understand the kinds and extent of resources friends provide. Cohen et al. (1988) reported a paucity of social relationships among the homeless elderly, compared to a community sample. However, their Bowery dwelling group had some semblance of a social network among group members.

Shinn et al. (1991) compared social relationships of mothers requesting shelter with those of poor housed mothers and found that homeless families reported more network members than did housed families. Also, sheltered families had seen family and friends more recently. However, sheltered families were less likely than housed families to believe that network members would provide them with housing for more than a few days. Families had sought shelter after seeking help from their respective families and friends, who may themselves have had few extra financial or emotional resources. The authors suggested that homeless mothers are not socially isolated, but rather their social ties may have been strained by recent events.

Using data from the National Survey of Personal Health Practices and Consequences, Auslander (1988) found that the poor had significantly fewer close friends and relatives than the more affluent had. The poor who had more friends that they saw more often were healthier than those who had fewer friends. However, this result did not hold true for those who had more relatives, including a spouse. Auslander suggested that the reason family ties of the poor are not perceived as helpful is that the supporters frequently have limited resources themselves and make demands on the one who needs their support.

The combination of social stressors, physical and mental health status, and unemployability due to age and health problems make a compelling case to take steps to help the elderly homeless lead the remainder of their lives in more dignity. The nation's goals should include providing food, clothing, and comfortable shelter to all elderly.

STUDY OF HOMELESS OLDER ADULTS IN FIVE NORTH CAROLINA COUNTIES

Purpose of Study

The remaining part of this chapter describes the Wallsten and Panter (1995) study. This study occurred in two phases. Phase 1 examined census characteristics and shelter services of a subset of shelters in the Piedmont area of North Carolina, which we will be reporting elsewhere. Phase 2 involved personal interviews with older homeless adults from the shelters.

Wallsten and Panter conducted the study to

- ◆ estimate the numbers of homeless older adults in five North Carolina counties;
- ◆ determine whether homeless older adults stayed in rural areas;
- ◆ describe the fundamental health, economic, housing, and social problems confronting North Carolina's homeless older adults;
- ◆ obtain a general sense of the migration patterns of elderly persons living in rural areas needing shelter;
- ◆ examine specifically the numbers and kinds of social supports and their relationship to depression and extent of mental health problems.

In this chapter, we present some basic descriptive information about the older homeless adults we interviewed and provide a general profile of their experiences.

Method

Procedures

The study was conducted in two phases. Briefly, the first phase involved telephone interviews with shelter managers of all shelters within the five designated counties to determine the kinds of shelter services provided, the overall census, and the census of older adults. Residents at all shelter sites with older homeless adults participated in the second phase, which consisted of face-to-face interviews. These interviews were held in the most private areas available within the respective shelters, which ranged from private rooms to corners of hallways. Fewer than five interviews were held outdoors near the shelter, and one was held in a community kitchen. All respondents seemed interested and pleased to have attention directed at them. In many cases, tears fell from the respondents' eyes as they discussed personal matters. Interviewers were carefully trained to handle sensitive issues.

Sample

Participants were 63 individuals (56 males, 7 females). Approximately 80% of the respondents were interviewed in shelters in predominantly urban counties, and the remainder were interviewed in rural counties. Of those interviewed in urban counties, approximately 32% reported having come from rural counties (the U. S. Bureau of the Census defines rural areas as those with 2,500 or fewer residents). The sample included 43 whites, 18 African Americans, 1 Native American, and 1 Hispanic. They ranged in age from 50 to 81 years. The majority (66.7%) were separated or divorced; 17.5% were single and never married, 12.7% were widowed, and 1.6% were currently married. (In the Detroit sample, by comparison, 37.3% were divorced or separated, 19.3% were widowed, and 31.3% were single and never married.) In the North Carolina study, more than half of the respondents were between 50 and 60 years of age. Approximately half (51.6%) of the sample had an educational level of eleventh grade or less. However, 17.7% had achieved a high school education, 24.2% had achieved some post–high school or college training, 3.2% had graduated from college, and 3.2% had completed graduate school or professional school.

The majority of respondents (77.7%) indicated that they did not have a place they considered to be their home, and 69.8% reported that this was the first time that they had been without their own place to live. Eighty-six percent could recall the first night they made the decision to stay in an emergency shelter. Interestingly, 92% revealed never having experienced homelessness as a child. About half of the respondents indicated living with someone else prior to becoming homeless; 26.9% said that the person was a friend or unrelated adult, 11.1% said the person was a spouse, 12.7% said the person was a relative, and 6.3% said the person was a child.

Instrument

The questionnaire involved an interview that could be administered in about 45 minutes. The interview contained eight sections: (a) demographic background and prior housing; (b) sleeping arrangements; (c) economic and survival resources; (d) military service, justice system encounters, and victimization; (e) physical health; (f) mental health; (g) social resources; and (h) open-ended responses about happy, sad, and frustrating events. Most questions in the first three sections were developed by Douglass et al. (1988) to survey Detroit's elderly homeless population. Although these items have not been used extensively, several were also used by Rossi, Fisher, and Willis (1986) in their Chicago study of the elderly homeless.

The remaining sections (with the exception of the open-ended questions) were derived from the Duke Multidimensional Functional Assessment: OARS Methodology (Fillenbaum, 1988) and the Duke–UNC Health Profile (Parkerson et al., 1981). The items have been used extensively with elderly community samples and have been demonstrated to be adequate in terms of reliability and validity evidence. The open-ended questions focused on the respondents' perceptions of their transition to homelessness and the kinds of services they needed.

Results

Sleeping Arrangements

The majority of respondents (71%) stayed 6 months or less in the shelter in which the interview took place. Eighteen percent reported being in the current shelter fewer than 7 days, and 37% reported fewer than 30 days. However, in the preceding week, 40% had slept in the streets, 11% having done this more than three times; 8% slept in an empty building; 14% slept in a public building such as a bus station or airport one or more times; and 84% reported never sleeping in someone's home.

Fifty percent of the respondents indicated a need to rest during both day and night, and about 29% revealed that they had to sleep in places other than the shelter. Many of the shelters in which the interviews were conducted closed during the day, often forcing people to leave buildings by 5:30 or 6 a.m., regardless of weather conditions. A frequent comment by older people referred to their inability to find places to rest during the day or to get comfortable when they were not feeling well or during extreme weather conditions.

One man reported having had many nights when he could not find an available bed in a shelter and having to sleep "behind some bushes." He expressed his fear and discomfort. In particular, he stated that he had rickets as a child, leaving him with a great deal of discomfort in one of his legs and making it difficult to crouch and sleep in unconventional locations. He said that his family had always been poor and never had money to get him help. He went on to say that currently he had shoes with inadequate soles and supports, so his feet got wet easily and hurt him as the day proceeded with no place to rest or sleep. He stated that he felt like a "real person on the inside" but knew that to others he was "a bum." Tears were in his eyes as he related this.

Financial Resources, Employment Status, and Income in Past Month

The majority of respondents earned less than $200 per year and received little outside assistance. For example, only 41.0% received food stamps, 9.8% received help from Medicaid, and 9.7% received SSI or Social Security retirement benefits. Also, only 9.5% turned to families for financial help, and 11.1% received help from friends. Only 6.3% received Veterans Administration (VA) retirement benefits, and 3.2% received VA disability payments, although 54% reported having served in the military. In the "other" category, 38% of the respondents reported having received money for plasma donations, and others worked at odd jobs on a daily basis.

Almost 13% of the respondents were working for pay at the time they were interviewed. Of those who were not working, 60% were either temporarily laid off because of illness or were unemployed and looking for work. Only 13% reported being permanently disabled, and 13% reported being retired.

Military Service, Justice System Record, and Victimization

Over half (54.0%) of the respondents reported having served in the military, 33.3% had served time in a state or federal prison, 65.1% had served time in a city or county jail, and 42.9% had been placed on probation.

More than half of the respondents (58.7%) reported that no crimes had been committed against them during the time they had had no permanent residence; 41.3% indicated the opposite. Twenty people (31.7%) had been robbed; 12 (19.0%), beaten; 10 (15.9%), deprived of their legal rights; and

2 (3.2%), raped; 3 (4.8%) indicated other kinds of victimizations. Most of those interviewed (87.1%) indicated feeling safe in the shelter.

Physical Health

About 18% of respondents reported being in an alcohol detoxification program, and 67% indicated that their health problems presented impediments to daily life.

Respondents rated their health as excellent (11.1%), good (28.6%), fair (38.1%), or poor (22.2%). These results are comparable to the Detroit study, which looked at homeless people 50 and over. Compared to health ratings of a general community population 65 and over, a much lower percentage of homeless older adults perceived their health as excellent; 11.1% (homeless) versus 36.1% (community) (Markides, 1989). The perceptions of homeless older adults were more in accordance with a sample of young and old adults below the poverty line, who perceived their health as poor. Health was rated as poor more often by the homeless (20%) and the poor (21%), compared to the general community sample of people 65 years and older (10%) (Markides, 1989).

Respondents indicated having an average of 4.3 disease conditions out of a possible 25 on the instrument. The top 10 conditions were arthritis, rheumatism, or bursitis (54.0%); circulation problems in arms and legs (49.2%); dental problems (46.0%); high blood pressure (33.9%); heart problems (30.6%); irregular heartbeat (30.2%); emphysema or chronic bronchitis (25.4%); trouble holding urine (22.2%); fractured or broken bones (20.6%); kidney disease (14.3%); and asthma (14.3%).

Because it was expected that people might not have received medical care and might therefore be without diagnoses, respondents were also asked about specific symptoms that they had experienced during the past week. Of 28 symptoms, respondents indicated that they had suffered an average of 6.1. They had had some or a lot of trouble with vision (50.8%), felt depressed or sad (46.1%), got tired easily (43.5%), hurt or ached in a part of the body (42.9%), felt nervous (39.7%), had a hard time sleeping (34.9%), experienced headaches (34.9%), had difficulty walking (33.9%), had difficulty hearing (28.5%), had weakness in a part of the body (27.0%), had difficulty chewing (25.4%), had indigestion (22.3%), experienced poor memory (22.2%), had aching teeth or gums (19.0%), and had difficulty moving bowels (12.7%). Forty-four percent indicated that they had a problem with their health because of drinking, and 54.0% indicated that they smoked. The mean number of cigarettes smoked was 18.9 per day.

Several questions were asked regarding recent use of the health care system. When asked about use of hospital emergency rooms in the past year, 42.9% reported having used this care with a frequency of one to nine times, 34.9% indicated needing health care beyond what they currently receive, and 23.8% indicated needing health care in the past year but not being able to obtain it.

Mental Health

When asked about being a patient in a mental hospital or community mental health facility in the year preceding the date of interview, 12.7% responded "yes"; of the remaining group, 17.0% indicated that they had been patients in the past. These results were similar to the Detroit study, in which about one third of the sample was found to have had previous institutional mental health experience (Douglass et al., 1988). In our study, 15 (23.8%) of the respondents indicated a need for treatment or counseling for personal, family, nervous, or emotional problems, and only 6 (9.5%) were receiving help. When asked about the symptoms of depression and nervousness in the past week, 46.1% reported feeling sad and depressed, and 39.7% reported feeling nervous. Analyses of scores on the Center for Epidemiological Studies–Depression Scale (CES-D) showed that 48.4% reported feeling depressed, 44.0% reported feeling sad, and approximately 35.0% had CES-D scores in the clinically depressed range (Radloff, 1977).

Social Resources and Important People

We also asked respondents to name people in their lives who were important to them, whether or not they liked them, but to name only those with whom they had had contact in the past month. An average of 2.5 people were named, with 12 (19.0%) listing no one. Respondents rated each of the individuals they named for the degree to which each person was helpful and/or upsetting, and for the most part, respondents had found these people helpful and not at all upsetting. Respondents were also asked about whether they felt they had certain social support.

Whereas 68% of the respondents reported having someone in whom they trusted and confided, 32.0% reported having no one, 22.6% reported feeling lonely quite often, and 36.5% reported feeling lonely sometimes. Thirty-five percent of respondents indicated that there was no one who could provide help for as long as needed if the respondent were sick, 14% had no one who could provide help for a "short time" of a few weeks to 6 months, and 15% had no one to help even "now and then," such as driving them to a medical appointment or fixing a meal for them.

Family

Most respondents (61.9%) reported having adult children, siblings, or other relatives, and most lived within an hour's drive. Less than half of the respondents had phoned, written, or had personal contact with these family members in the past 2 months. For those people who reported having relatives in the area, the large majority (85.7%) were opposed to living with them, yet they were less likely to think that the relatives would be opposed to having the respondents move in (50.0%). The same pattern occurred when the referents were adult children.

Discussion

In our interviews of 63 homeless older adults, we attempted to document and understand the daily experiences and conditions of homelessness in this group. Our findings provide strong evidence that such individuals are especially vulnerable across a number of domains, including physical health, mental health, financial resources and possibility for resources, and availability and quality of social networks. The expected life changes that emerge from growing old are exacerbated by the condition of homelessness, and this condition brings on a set of additional physical and psychological difficulties for these individuals to endure.

The study presents a portrait of homeless older adults who have physical and mental problems that are difficult to cope with under impoverished and homeless circumstances. For example, we found in our interviews that the medical and physical problems that homeless older adults reported were substantial. Problems such as arthritis, inadequate circulation, and emphysema are difficult to manage under the best circumstances. In addition, symptoms such as poor vision, dental problems, trouble holding urine, and getting tired easily do not mesh well with the harshness of street and shelter life. Further, medical treatment for these problems was minimal and/or perceived to be unavailable to these individuals, despite the mechanisms that exist in legislation that would permit some degree of medical treatment. Efforts should be concentrated on ensuring that available resources are made accessible to these individuals through outreach.

The mental health profiles that we obtained in our sample showed highly elevated depression levels, a finding that is not particularly surprising given the reality in which these individuals are living. Almost 30% reported being in a mental hospital or community mental health facility in the past, but the more disturbing finding was that approximately 35% of the sample could be classified as falling in the clinically depressed range and that nearly half of the sample felt sad and depressed. This finding underscores the necessity for readily available mental health services and aggressive outreach to these individuals.

Though available, the support networks seemed weak. Even though respondents identified an average of 2.5 people in their social network, 32.0% admitted having no one in whom to confide. In addition, though most had relatives living nearby, less than half had any kind of personal contact within a 2-month period. Thus, during this time of great stress and need, family support seemed inaccessible. With little hope of finding a job that would pay them enough to pay rent and purchase food, their circumstances appeared dismal. The majority of them were not receiving government assistance that could augment their income, enable them to purchase food, or enable them to get health care. Sadly, 41.3% were victims of crime. Older homeless adults should be provided separate facilities, to feel safe, be able to rest day and night, manage chronic and acute illnesses, help to regain their sense of self-respect, and develop a system of positive social interactions.

Our cross-sectional study speaks only to the experiences and health of older homeless adults at one slice in time. Although this methodology provides a good description of several of the physical and psychosocial issues that affect the daily lives of these individuals, it cannot address the broader and richer questions of the extent to which these problems and conditions exist over time and how conditions at early stages of homelessness affect later stages and maintenance of homelessness. We suggest that a longitudinal approach will more adequately track the progression of deleterious health and social support conditions for older homeless adults and the migration patterns of these individuals. By following homeless older adults over time, we may more clearly understand the precursors of problems and identify those factors that do and do not appear to contribute to long-term homelessness. Moreover, a longitudinal design can address directly a sampling issue that was mentioned earlier. That is, the design can address for how long these individuals stay homeless and to what extent they move in and out of homelessness. This sampling issue cannot be determined from a slice-of-time approach, which tends to oversample individuals who have been homeless for longer periods rather than those who are temporarily homeless. Because these two classes of situations may have very different precursors and effects, it is important that such distinctions be made unambiguously.

Implications of Study: What Can Be Done

Sack (1994) reported that while Andrew Cuomo was head of the homeless commission for the Dinkins administration in New York City, he believed that the homeless needed more than homes. Cuomo recommended that the city develop a "continuum of care" (p. 42) that would enable people to progress toward independence. This innovative plan was called HELP—Housing Enterprise for the Less Privileged. Beginning in 1988, Cuomo worked as head of HELP until he became assistant secretary to Henry Cisneros, secretary of HUD. Seven HELP complexes are in operation in New York City, housing about 4,000 people, mostly families with children. Cuomo envisions similar housing nationally. Residents receive mandatory counseling and social services and are assisted in finding homes so that their stay is limited to 6 to 8 months. Ninety-five percent of residents in this program remain self-sufficient. Cisneros and Cuomo have won White House and Congressional approval for an increase in this year's homeless budget, from $571 million to $823 million, and President Clinton has proposed doubling this figure to $1.6 billion for the next fiscal year. Cuomo points out that it is ironic that recently the government provided emergency housing for 10,000 displaced earthquake victims within a week's time, yet it is unable to mobilize to provide housing for people who have been suffering without homes for longer periods of time (Sack, 1994).

Many elderly homeless people avoid shelters; they fear the aggressiveness of younger people and do not like the staff's insensitivity to their needs (Cohen & Sokolovsky, 1989). It therefore stands to reason that older adults would benefit from shelters geared specifically to meet their needs. Cohen, Onserud, and Monaco (1992) initiated a separate service program for older homeless persons in the Bowery section of lower Manhattan. Originally held in an existing structure that offered a senior lunch program, it later expanded to a larger space nearby. The service program, Project Rescue, was set up to address "ameliorable problems" (p. 466) identified through a prior research study of Cohen and Sokolovsky (1989). Although the project did not include a separate shelter, it operated between 9 a.m. and 5 p.m., providing older people with a safe place to rest and to meet with service workers, who eventually helped them with the kinds of services needed. Three years after individuals began the program, an evaluation was done to determine outcomes on specific measures. Ninety-three percent of the sample had two or more favorable outcomes, and 53% had three or more. The strongest predictors of outcomes included number of service encounters, perceived level of social support, and type of presenting problem. The researchers were encouraged by the project's outcomes.

If health care professionals could identify homeless older adults in emergency rooms and mental health clinics or as inpatients, definitive steps could be taken to refer them to the department of social service. Identification of these adults could be facilitated by asking a few, very straightforward questions at intake and by training nursing staff to be particularly aware of the type of medical problems and background circumstances that may be indicators of recent homelessness. This step could at least begin the complex process of evaluating their status for entitlements and eligibility for housing options. Many individuals, homeless or not, benefit from the help of a counselor or advocate in working through the application process for government programs. In our study, veterans in particular were unaware of their benefits; several had been waiting for weeks to determine whether or not health care could be received at a VA hospital. Often, individuals are ashamed to state that they are homeless and provide the address of the local shelter as their own. Health care professionals should become familiar with the shelter address in their community so that they can identify homeless clients and be sensitive regarding treatment and follow-up plans.

Because of the lack of research into the kinds of programs that facilitate recuperation from impoverished circumstances and reincorporation into the community, creative strategies of coordination and cooperation within community agencies must be attempted. For example, within each shelter, case management teams can be formed, involving nurse practitioners, psychologists, community health nurses, physicians, social workers, and community advocates who can work together to formulate model plans for particular types of residents. An in-depth interview with each older adult staying in the shelter should include the resident's perceived health and social problems. This intake interview will help the team determine the nature of the referrals needed. A physical assessment, including blood pressure, dental, and vision screening, can help identify problems that cause daily problems and develop a triage system for dealing with them. Community health nurses should consider including the community shelters in their case loads.

Kiesler (1991) argued that public policy priorities for the homeless should be stable housing, income enhancement and stabilization, and attention to physical health. He specifically stated that services provided within the realm of alcohol and drug problems and mental illness should not be among the top three priorities because they do not get at basic solutions and prevention approaches. Rather, many alcohol, drug, and mental illness symptoms emerge from the conditions of homelessness, and such symptoms would be substantially reduced if his recommended priorities were addressed.

As we attempt to find long-term solutions to homelessness, there is a pressing need to design and implement innovative strategies and outreach programs to help meet the needs of homeless older adults. In addition to these programs, we also need rigorous evaluation studies that will help us understand the effectiveness of these program and intervention efforts. Studies such as the one that we have reported here represent preliminary descriptive steps in identifying the types of everyday hardships and challenges (psychological, social, financial, medical, physical) that face older adults as they navigate through streets without permanent shelter. Our findings suggest a number of possible directions for outreach and program design. For instance, our data on receipt of government services and on the need for reliable social connections provide support for programs in which willing and trained advocates would be matched with older homeless adults who present at shelters. In such a program, the advocate would be available to assist in the application and completion of often complicated and not easily accessible government benefit forms and to provide social support from time to time. In addition, the older homeless adult's need for rest, day and night, underscores the necessity for shelters to make resting areas available throughout the day, possibly creating separate quarters for older residents. The cross-sectional nature of the study, although informative, limits our description to one slice in time. Longitudinal research is critical to track individuals moving in and out of homeless circumstances and to provide necessary data to help service providers understand and design programs targeted to the long-term functioning needs of these individuals.

REFERENCES

Auslander, G. K. (1988). Social networks and the functional health status of the poor: A secondary analysis of data from the national survey of personal health practices and consequences. *Journal of Community Health, 13*(4), 197–209.

Boondas, J. (1985). The despair of the homeless aged. *Journal of Gerontological Nursing, 36,* 9–12.

Brickner, P. W., Filardo, T., Iseman, M., Green, R., Conanan, B., & Elvy, A. (1984). Medical aspects of homelessness. In H. R. Lamb (Ed.), *The homeless mentally ill.* Washington, DC: American Psychiatric Association.

Burt, M., & Cohen, B. (1989). *America's homeless: Numbers, characteristics, and programs that serve them* (Urban Institute Report 89-3). Washington, DC: Urban Institute Press.

Chen, Y-P. (1991). Improving the economic security of minority persons as they enter old age. *Minority elders: Longevity, economics, and health.* Washington, DC: Gerontological Society.

Coalition for the Homeless. (1984). *Crowded out: Homelessness and the elderly poor in New York City.* New York: Author.

Cohen, C. I., Onserud, H., & Monaco, C. (1992). Project Rescue: Serving the homeless and marginally housed elderly. *The Gerontologist, 32,* 466–471.

Cohen, C. I., & Sokolovsky, J. (1989). *Old men of the Bowery.* New York: Guilford.

Cohen, C. I., Teresi, J., & Holmes, D. (1988a). The mental health of older homeless adults. *Journal of the American Geriatrics Society, 36,* 492–501.

Cohen, C. I., Teresi, J., & Holmes, D. (1988b). The physical well-being of old homeless men. *Journals of Gerontology, 43,* 121–128.

Cohen, C. I., Teresi, J., Holmes, D., & Roth, D. (1988). Survival strategies of homeless men. *The Gerontologist, 28,* 58–64.

Commonwealth Fund Commission on Elderly Living Alone. (1988). *Aging alone: Profiles and projections.* Baltimore: Author.

Congressional Budget Office. (1990). *Preliminary cost estimate for the homeless outreach act of 1990.* Unpublished manuscript. (Available from Maria Foscarinis, National Law Center on Homelessness and Poverty, 918 F Street NW, Washington, DC.)

Dennis, D. L., Buckner, J. C., Lipton, F. R., Levine, I. (1991). A decade of research and services for homeless mentally ill persons. *American Psychologist, 46,* 1129–1138.

DeParle, J. (1990, July 1). Federal cash for the homeless: It's there but tough to get. *New York Times,* p. 14.

DeParle, J. (1994, February 17). Report to Clinton sees vast extent of homelessness. *New York Times,* pp. 1, 20.

Division of Aging and CARES. (1991). *North Carolina Aging Services Plan: A guide for successful aging in the 1990s: Vol. 3. A full report.* Raleigh: North Carolina Department of Human Resources.

Doolin, J. (1986). Planning for the special needs of the homeless elderly. *The Gerontologist, 26,* 229–241.

Dorwart, R. A. (1988). A ten-year follow-up study of the effects of deinstitutionalization. *Hospital Community Psychiatry, 39,* 287–291.

Douglass, R. L., Atchison, B. J., Lofton, W. J., Hodgkins, B. J., Kotowski, K., Morris, J., Lenk, K., & Singer, L. (1988). *Aged, adrift and alone: Detroit's elderly homeless. Final report to the Detroit Area Agency on Aging, October 1988.* Ypsilanti, MI: Department of Associated Health Professions.

Fillenbaum, G. G. (1988). *Multidimensional functional assessment of older adults: The Duke Older Americans Resources and Services procedures.* Hillsdale, NJ: Erlbaum.

First, R. J., Rife, J. C., & Toomey, B. G. (1994). Homelessness in rural areas: Causes, patterns, and trends. *Social Work, 39,* 98–108.

Foscarinis, M. (1991). The politics of homelessness: A call to action. *American Psychologist, 46,* 1232–1238.

Goetcheus, J. (1990). *Hearing before the subcommittee on health and the environment of the committee on energy and commerce* (House, Serial No. 101-176). Washington, DC: U.S. Government Printing Office.

Goodman, L., Saxe, L., & Harvey, M. (1991). Homelessness as psychological trauma. *American Psychologist, 46,* 1219–1225.

Hodgkins, B. J., Douglass, R .L., & Lam, H. (1990, November). *Determinants of self-reported health status among the homeless elderly in Detroit: A preliminary analysis.* Paper presented at the 43rd Annual Scientific Meeting of the Gerontological Society of America, Boston.

Hooyman, N. R., & Kiyak, H. A. (1993). *Social gerontology* (3rd ed.). Boston: Allyn & Bacon.

Housing Assistance Council, Inc. (1991, March). *Addressing homelessness in rural communities.* Washington, DC: Author.

The invisible parade [Editorial]. (1994, February 20). *New York Times,* p. 12, section 4.

Jackson, K. T. (1987). The Bowery: From residential street to skid row. In R. Beard (Ed.), *On being homeless: Historical perspectives* (pp. 68–79). New York: Museum of the City of New York.

Jordan, M. (1988, August 19). In '87, 83% in N. Va. shelters were employed, study says. *Washington Post,* pp. D1, D4.

Keigher, S. M. (1991). *Housing risks and homelessness among the urban elderly.* New York: Haworth Press.

Keigher, S. M., Berman, R. H., & Greenblatt, S. T. (1991). Overview of the Chicago study of elderly persons at housing risk. In S. M. Keigher (Ed.), *Housing risks and homelessness among the urban elderly* (pp. 19–25). New York: Haworth Press.

Kiesler, C. A. (1991). Homelessness and public policy priorities. *American Psychologist, 46,* 1245–1252.

Kondratas, A. (1991). Ending homelessness: Policy challenges. *American Psychologist, 46,* 1226–1231.

Kusmer, K. (1987). The underclass in historical perspective: Tramps and vagrants in urban America, 1870–1930. In R. Beard (Ed.), *On being homeless: Historical perspectives* (pp. 20–31). New York: Museum of the City of New York.

Kutza, E., & Keigher, S. (1991). The elderly "new homeless": An emerging population at risk. *Social Work, 36,* 288–293.

Lindsey, A. M. (1989). Health care for the homeless. *Nursing Outlook, 37,* 78–81.

MacDonald, R. R. (1987). Introduction. In R. Beard (Ed.), *On being homeless: Historical perspectives* (pp. 7–8). New York: Museum of the City of New York.

Markides, K. S. (1989). *Aging and health: Perspectives on gender, race, ethnicity, and class.* Newbury Park, CA: Sage.

Martin, M. A. (1987). Homeless women: An historical perspective. In R. Beard (Ed.), *On being homeless: Historical perspectives* (pp. 32–41). New York: Museum of the City of New York.

National Coalition for the Homeless. (1987). *Rural homelessnesss in America: Appalachia and the South.* New York: Author.

National Coalition for the Homeless. (1991). *Fatally flawed: The Census Bureau's count of homeless people.* Washington, DC: Author.

National Institute of Mental Health. (1991). *Additions and resident patients at end of year, state and county hospitals, by age and diagnosis, by state, United States, 1989.* Rockville, MD: Author.

National Resource Center for Rural Elderly. (1992). *Housing programs and services for elders in rural America.* Kansas City: University of Missouri.

North Carolina Division of Community Assistance. (1988). *Estimate of the homeless population of North Carolina, July 1988.* Author.

Ovrebo, B., Minkler, M., & Liljestrand, P. (1991). No room in the inn: The disappearance of SRO housing in the United States. In S. M. Keigher (Ed.), *Housing risks and homelessness among the urban elderly* (pp. 77–93). New York: Haworth Press.

Parkerson, G. R., Gehlbach, S. H., Wagner, E. H., James, S. A., Clapp, N. E., & Muhlbaier, L. H. (1981). The Duke-UNC health profile: An adult health status instrument for primary care. *Medical Care, 19*(8), 806–828.

Persily, N. A., & Albury, S. R. (1991). The growing elderly population and utilization. In N. A. Persily (Ed.), *Eldercare* (pp. 11–31). Chicago: American Hospital Association Publishing.

President. (1993). Federal plan to break the cycle of homelessness (Executive Order 12848). *Federal Register, 58,* No. 96.

Quigley, E. (1992). The homeless. *Congressional Quarterly Review, 2,* 665–687.

Radloff, L. S. (1977). The CES-D Scale: A self-report depression scale for research in the general population. *Applied Psychological Measurement, 1,* 385–401.

Rossi, P. (1989). *Down and out in America.* Chicago: University of Chicago Press.

Rossi, P. H. (1990). The old homelessness and the new homelessness in historical perspective. *American Psychologist, 45,* 954–959.

Rossi, P. H., Fisher, G., & Willis, G. (1986). *The condition of the homeless in Chicago.* Chicago: National Opinion Research Center.

Rossi, P. H., Wright, J. D., Fisher, G. A., & Willis, G. (1987). The urban homeless: Estimating composition and size. *Science, 235,* 1336–1341.

Roth, D., & Bean, G. (1986). New perspectives on homelessness: Findings from a statewide epidemiological study. *Hospital and Community Psychiatry, 37,* 712–719.

Roth, D., Toomey, B. G., & First, R. J. (1992). Gender, racial, and age variations among homeless persons. In M. J. Robertson & M. Greenblatt (Eds.), *Homelessness: A national perspective* (pp. 191–211). New York: Plenum Press.

Rothman, D. J. (1987). The first shelters: The contemporary relevance of the almshouse. In R. Beard (Ed.), *On being homeless: Historical perspectives.* New York: Museum of the City of New York.

Sack, K. (1994, March 27). Andrew Cuomo. *New York Times Magazine,* pp. 40–43.

Shapiro, I. (1989). *Laboring for less.* Washington, DC: Center on Budget and Policy Priorities.

Shinn, M., Knickerman, J. R., & Weitzman, B. C. (1991). Social relationships and vulnerability to becoming homeless among poor families. *American Psychologist, 46,* 1180–1187.

Tessler, R. C., & Dennis, D. (1989). *A synthesis of NIMH-funded research concerning persons who are homeless and mentally ill.* Rockville, MD: National Institute of Mental Health.

Toomey, B. G., First, R. J., Greenlee, R., & Cummins, L. (1990). *Counting the rural homeless: Political and methodological dilemmas.* Columbus, OH: Department of Mental Health.

U.S. Department of Health and Human Services, Public Health Service. (1990). *Healthy people 2000: National health promotion and diseases prevention objectives* (DHHS Publication No. 91-50212). Washington, DC: U.S. Government Printing Office.

U.S. Department of Health and Human Services, Public Health Service. (1992). *Outcasts on Main Street: Report of the federal task force on homelessness and severe mental illness.* Washington, DC: DHHS, in cooperation with the Interagency Council on the Homeless and the Task Force on Homelessness and Severe Mental Illness.

U.S. Department of Housing and Urban Development. (1984). *A report to the secretary on the homeless and emergency shelters.* Washington, DC: U.S. Government Printing Office.

U.S. Department of Housing and Urban Development. (1994). *A priority: Home! The federal plan to break the cycle of homelessness* (HUD-1454-CPD). Washington, DC: U.S. Government Printing Office.

Wallsten, S. M., & Panter, A. T. (1995). *Homeless older adults in five North Carolina counties.* Manuscript submitted for publication.

Wassem, R. E. (1993, February 25). *Emergency food and shelter program for homeless people* (CRS Report for Congress No. 93-261 EPW). Washington, DC: Library of Congress, Congressional Research Service.

Wassem, R. E., & Robinson, D. H. (1993, December 30). *Homeless assistance: Programs and funding issues* (CRS Report for Congress No. 94-3 EPW). Washington, DC: Library of Congress, Congressional Research Service.

Waxman, L. D., & Reyes, L. (1990). *A status report on hunger and homelessness in America's cities.* Washington, DC: U.S. Conference of Mayors.

Wilkerson, I. (1989, May 2). As farms falter, rural homelessness grows. *New York Times,* p. A1.

Williams, L., Sobol, L., Alker, J., & Lozier, J. (1991). *Mourning in America: Health problems, mortality, and homelessness.* Washington, DC: National Coalition for the Homeless.

Wright, J. (1990). *Hearing before the subcommittee on health and the environment of the committee on energy and commerce* (House, Serial No. 101-176). Washington, DC: U.S. Government Printing Office.

CHAPTER 9

The Psychosocial Care of Older Persons: The Pioneering Work of Dr. Irene Burnside

Linda J. Garand and Kathleen C. Buckwalter

Idealists . . . foolish enough to throw caution to the winds . . . have
advanced mankind and have enriched the world.—*Emma Goldman,
1869–1940*

W ho more fitting to highlight in the inaugural issue of this
Advances in Gerontological Nursing than Dr. Irene Mortenson
Burnside, a true leader in geropsychiatric nursing over the
past 50 years and into the present. Dr. Burnside is a nurse, philosopher,
and scholar who began advocating for psychosocial care of older persons
at a time when many older adults in our society resided in convalescent
hospitals and asylums and received, at best, only custodial care. The
humanity, vision, imagination, and personal commitment she has devoted
to the psychosocial care of older persons as her career evolved has helped

Author notes. The authors wish to thank the following individuals for their contributions
to this article: Madeline Speery for clerical support; Dr. Kathryn Kavanagh and Dr. Toni
Tripp-Reimer for guidance in shaping questions for Dr. Burnside; Ruth Garand for creative ideas; Dr. Patricia Donahue and Mary Anders for editorial comments; and last, Dr.
Irene Burnside for her willingness to share aspects of her life and career with fellow nurses.

213

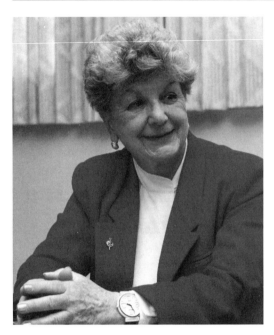

FIGURE 9.1   Irene Burnside.

set the stage for the recognition of geropsychiatric nursing as a respected
and much needed subspecialty in psychiatric nursing (Figure 9.1).

The following tribute attempts to capture the forward movement of
geropsychiatric nursing history as seen through the eyes of one of its
greatest pioneers. Recollections of Dr. Burnside's childhood years are set
forth, along with an account of her increasing interest in and devotion to
the field of geropsychiatric nursing. The chapter concludes with a partial
list of significant contributions made by Dr. Burnside during her career
that shed light on the evolution of psychosocial nursing care of the elderly
in America over the past 50 years.

EARLY YEARS

Born in 1923 in the tiny town of Grove City, Minnesota, Irene Burnside
had a turbulent childhood, as did many children who grew up during the
Great Depression. Innumerable families had to struggle on a daily basis
just to feed and clothe their members. At the age of 5, Irene was sent to
live with relatives (her grandfather, his cousin, two aunts, and one uncle)
because her mother was ill and her father was unable to care for her and

her sister. Separated from her immediate family, Irene started a new life on a farm in central Minnesota. Those early years had a profound impact on shaping Irene's interests and her determination.

When Irene first arrived at the family farm, the family discussed the contributions she would make toward maintaining the farm. Her uncle, commenting on her stature, stated, "She's too skinny, she won't be able to milk a cow, and I don't know if she's big enough or smart enough to drive a tractor" (Burnside, personal communication, November 22, 1993). Irene quickly learned how to milk a cow and drive a tractor in an effort to avoid a destiny as the family dishwasher.

In her younger years, Irene, who obtained her elementary education in a one-room country school, aspired to be a teacher. Having no siblings to play with, she set up a schoolroom in the closet under a staircase, which housed the sweeper and cleaning rags. Sometimes she would "teach" piano lessons to imaginary students, using her uncle's accordion, turned on its side, to simulate a piano. Or she would sit on a stool and surround herself with books. "I was a little kid in this closet, emulating a teacher. The nurse was on one side [of me] and the teacher on the other. I would make exams and grade the papers. Relatives would let me have one shelf in the closet as my desk. It was a world I created for myself, a type of escape" (Burnside, personal communication, November 23, 1993).

During Irene's growing-up years, two women in particular served as her role models. One was a teacher: Abigail Quigley McCarthy, former wife of Eugene McCarthy, who taught Irene in high school and instilled in her the importance of writing well (Burnside, 1991). The other was a nurse: her aunt, the only person in the family who had finished high school. Irene describes her aunt as a very special woman. "I always had her to look up to. When I was ill with childhood diseases, she gave me complete bed baths with soothing back rubs. I thought, if she got out of this environment and finished high school when nobody else did, I'm not only going to finish high school, I'm going to college" (Burnside, personal communication, November 22, 1993). In addition to allowing Irene to set up an imaginary classroom, her aunt would take her for long walks outdoors, where Irene developed a love for nature. In a time when money and material items were scarce, her aunt found a special cabinet with shelves and a glass front for Irene to store "treasures" she found as they hiked together.

Speaking about her childhood, Irene has commented, "You know it shapes you, it does something to you" (Burnside, personal communication, November 23, 1993). The love and respect Irene received from her aunt laid the foundation for Irene's career as a nurse and nurse educator and fostered her sensitivity to and respect for the environment. Irene's childhood experiences thus etched their impressions into her life history, permanently altering its course.

NURSES' TRAINING

When Irene graduated from high school in the spring of 1941, her career choices seemed limited: most women became either homemakers, secretaries, teachers, or nurses. Limited finances prohibited Irene from entering a 4-year academic program to pursue a career as an educator. Admiration for her aunt (who "always knew what to do when someone was ill or injured") led to Irene's decision to pursue a career in nursing (Burnside, personal communication, November 23, 1993). In the fall of 1941, at the age of 17, Irene entered a 3-year program at the Ancker Hospital School of Nursing in St. Paul, Minnesota, on borrowed money (of which she paid back every penny).

Numerous historical accounts describe the conditions in which nurses were trained from the days of Florence Nightingale onward (Baer, 1985; Hegge, 1990; Rush, 1992; Shea, 1990; Spellbring, 1991). During the 1940s, when Irene was a student, nurses' training was fraught with such issues as lack of privacy, disrespect, inflexibility, and lack of sleep or comfort for the trainees. Nurses were expected to carry out menial housekeeping chores while they engaged in the physical (i.e., custodial) care of patients (Burnside, personal communication, November 23, 1993).

Despite these issues, the nursing students developed a strong respect for the traditions of nursing and the commitment it required. For example, Irene recalls:

> Students were on probation (or "probies") for the first six months of training. Probies were bused to the University of Minnesota, where they studied anatomy, physiology, and other basic sciences. If students successfully completed their six month probationary period, they went through a capping ceremony. The capping ceremony was a symbolic celebration of entree into nurses' training, where the probies walked down the aisle with candles, like Florence Nightingale, and your big sister, a senior, put your cap on. (Burnside, personal communication, November 23, 1993)

Irene's class wore white stockings, white shoes, long blue-and-white pinstripe uniforms with large white aprons and organdy caps. The uniforms were so heavily starched that Irene wore a washcloth around her collar to prevent skin irritation. Hair could not touch the collar of the uniform, and cologne, nail polish, rings, and earrings were not allowed. Students who did not cut their hair short had to wear hairnets.

Nurses' training was very hierarchical in the early 1940s, even in the trainees' home, where the trainees moved to a higher floor in the home after each year of successfully completing their studies. "Probies" were housed in the basement with bars over the windows, juniors lived on the second floor, and seniors lived on the third floor. In spite of the hierarchical structure of the trainees' home, there was a tremendous sense of camaraderie among fellow students. (In fact, Irene's class celebrated its 50th graduation anniversary with a Mexican cruise in February 1994.)

Another aspect of nurses' training that Irene recalls was the "total lack of privacy and the numerous house rules" (Burnside, personal communication, November 23, 1993). As president of the student government, Irene was required to report fellow nurses who broke house rules. Student nurses were not allowed to be married. "We knew that one of our fellow nurses was married; we were scared they would find out and kick her out" (Burnside, personal communication, November 23, 1993). Trainees had to be in their rooms by ten o'clock every night, except for one night a week, when they were allowed to stay out until midnight. If someone failed to return to the nurses' home by curfew, the student government had to decide on a punishment. Trainees were allowed to go home one weekend a month, but most could not afford the expense of going home at all. If the trainees were sick, they had to "pay back every day" they were sick once their training was completed. When trainees paid back that last day, the other students ripped their uniform off them as a symbol of completing the training (Burnside, personal communication, November 23, 1993).

Because of the shortage of nurses during World War II, the student nurses were often in charge of entire wards very early in their training. "We went through the polio epidemic and cared for patients in iron lungs, but we also cared for people with scarlet fever and diphtheria" (Burnside, 1991, p. 19). As Irene recalls, "My contagion supervisor was not pleased when two of us [trainees] contracted scabies" (Burnside, personal communication, March 29, 1994).

Trainees often worked split shifts, starting with morning care at seven o'clock, taking a break for school at ten o'clock, and returning to work at four o'clock to finish the day with the evening care. "There was always someone to call if something went wrong, but we were basically in charge of a ward while in training" (Burnside, personal communication, November 23, 1993).

Even though trainees were responsible for the care given on an entire ward, they had very little authoritative power. Irene remembers "having to always write that the patient appeared to not be breathing when we knew damn well he was dead." When a physician, resident, or chaplain was in a nurse's presence, the nurse had to stand up and offer her chair or move to the side to allow them to enter the elevator first, even if the student had been working for hours (Burnside, personal communication, November 24, 1993).

In 1944, in her last 3 months of nurses' training, Irene elected to do a rotation in the field of psychiatric nursing. During that rotation, which occurred at the Rochester State Hospital in Rochester, Minnesota, Irene gained a better understanding of mental illness and the effects it had on individuals and their families. At the time, psychotropic drugs had not yet been developed, and camisoles and leather restraints were still common forms of psychiatric treatment. In the 1940s the field of psychiatric care was still in its infancy.

> Patients were wrapped in full-body canvas restraints and cold hydrotherapy was one prevalent treatment. Patients were taken out of leather and canvas restraints to dance or play baseball with the nursing students. Student nurses helped provide recreation for the patients, but it was very hard to dance polka to waltz music. (Burnside, personal communication, March 14, 1994)

Irene's experiences on "these back wards, filled with demented old ladies," made her aware for the first time of the field of geropsychiatric nursing, and they had a major impact on her future academic pursuits (Burnside, personal communication, November 24, 1993).

ARMY NURSING DAYS

In 1942, during her second year at Ancker, Irene joined the Army Cadet Nurse Corps, which had just been launched by Lucille Leone Petry.

Irene's participation in the corps helped her remain in nursing school by paying for her final 2 years of training. "The Cadet Corps was a godsend. It provided a uniform (which reduced the need for clothes), a monthly stipend, and paid for books. In the 1940s, having ten dollars a month meant that we were living high on the hog" (Burnside, personal communication, November 23, 1993).

Irene graduated from nurses' training in 1944, when she was 20 years old—1 year too young to be eligible to take state boards to practice as a nurse. While she waited for her 21st birthday, she studied for the state board examination and worked at a very reduced salary. After successfully passing the state board exams, Irene began her active service with the Army Nurse Corps. She was sent to the South Pacific to serve with the occupation troops in Okinawa, Japan; shortly after, VJ (Victory over Japan) Day occurred.

By the age of 22, Irene had been promoted to first lieutenant and had "tremendous responsibilities" as head nurse of a 100-bed ward of medically ill soldiers in Osaka, Japan. Irene believes that she learned a lot from that experience.

> The discipline of nurses' training and the discipline in the Army, doing push-ups in the snow at Fort Carson in Colorado and long twenty-mile marches helped me. I could be disciplined back then because it was a time in my life where I had to [be disciplined] if I wanted to stay where I was in the Army or in nurses' training. I could not afford to be a maverick. I can now be disciplined about doing a book and meeting deadlines. (Burnside, personal communication, November 23, 1993)

Irene is grateful to the army for several other reasons as well. For instance, it afforded her an opportunity to travel. For another, she met her future husband while stationed with the corps in Japan. Finally, her stint in the army allowed Irene to receive GI Bill benefits, which would eventually enable her to return to school and pursue further studies.

BACHELOR OF FINE ARTS DEGREE

When World War II was over, Irene and her fiancé, Dean Burnside, returned to the United States. They were married in Colorado, where Irene held positions as a staff nurse and an industrial nurse from 1948 to

1953. In 1953, Irene became disenchanted with the nursing profession, stating "My disenchantment was never caused by nursing, itself. Newly hired nurses were poorly paid ($1.25/hour and my baby-sitter cost 75 cents/hour), had to work evening or night shifts, and nearly always worked weekends" (Burnside, 1991, p. 20). The stress of living a fragmented life and constantly having to work undesirable shifts led Irene to the decision to enter school full-time.

Although nurses' training had given Irene an appreciation for the sciences, she felt she did not know enough about the aesthetic aspect of life, for example, art, poetry, and architecture. Working on her bachelor of fine arts (BFA) degree at the University of Denver, Irene focused her studies on interior design. When asked about the influence of the BFA on her career, Irene credits her design studies with giving her an extra sensitivity to the physical environment in which the elderly are cared for. In one of her writings, Irene poignantly describes the environment in which she conducted one-to-one therapy with an elderly client. The therapy was held

> . . . in a fish-bowl of a day room. The distraction of other patients, and the sounds of a television that was on constantly were difficult to tune out. Although my concentration and hearing was impaired (by environmental influences), the client didn't appear to be bothered, for he was used to it. (Burnside, 1971, p. 105)

Irene's interest in the impact of physical surroundings has persisted throughout her career, as she continues to note the importance of "realizing how profoundly all of us are affected by the environment in which we must live, especially if it is one we did not choose, would never have chosen and know that we will not be able to leave" (Burnside, 1993, p. 12).

But despite the benefits of her training in interior design (the BFA degree was also helpful when Irene and her husband were building a new home), Irene soon realized that she was not cut out for a career in interior design. She returned to nursing.

MASTER OF SCIENCE, ADULT PSYCHIATRIC NURSING

From 1957 to 1963, Irene held positions as staff nurse and home health nurse while living in Martinez, California. In 1964 she enrolled full-time at the University of California, San Francisco (UCSF), to obtain a master of science degree in adult psychiatric nursing. Although Irene had a diploma in nursing and a BFA degree, she was required to complete a year of course work before she could enter the master's degree program. She describes that first year of graduate school as "horrendous"; she took 21 credits one semester.

As part of her clinical practicum in graduate school, Irene began to work at the Napa State Hospital in central California. At the hospital, Irene was assigned to care for a man who was diagnosed as catatonic schizophrenic.

> He had been isolated in a back ward, restrained in a camisole for at least three years. One day I took him out to my car and let him sit in it. He had never seen a stick shift; he didn't know anything about the inside of a car. The introduction of psychotropic medication had enabled this man to come out of isolation, to sit in my car and tell me about his life. (Burnside, personal communication, November 22, 1993)

Irene's sensitivity to this man's isolation and her love for nature set the stage for her later willingness to take her elderly patients outside the care environment, for walks or just smelling the spring air.

The master's degree program in adult psychiatric nursing at UCSF was 36 credit hours of course work plus a practicum. Irene finished the program in one year, graduating in 1966. "It was very intense; for example, driving 50 miles to a state hospital two times a week for practicum" (Burnside, personal communication, November 22, 1993).

POST–MASTER'S CERTIFICATE, ADULT PSYCHIATRIC NURSING

Even with a master's degree in psychiatric nursing, Irene felt as though she still did not have the necessary experience or education for therapeutic one-to-one or group interactions, so she entered the post–master's program in adult psychiatric nursing at UCSF. During the 1-year preparation for the post–master's certificate, Irene focused her education on group interactions and the relationship between the nurse leader and patients, which would lay the theoretical groundwork for the remainder of her group work with the elderly.

As a post–master's student, Irene would often "trek off to the back wards of a state hospital to do one-to-one therapy with a 79 year old man" (Burnside, 1971, p. 103). This man, whom Irene later referred to as "Mr. Weston" in her writings, had been delivered to the state psychiatric hospital by the police after he was found sleeping in a stranger's car. He had a diagnosis of "organic brain syndrome," as many elderly patients did in the days before various types of dementia were recognized. "Interspersed with the delusional content of his speech were meaningful bits and pieces of his prior life" (Burnside, 1971, p. 103).

Irene identified several important themes emerging from her work with Mr. Weston: "(1) the ability to conceal anxiety; (2) living in memories—the importance of past life; (3) living in a fantasy world, which I felt was necessary to enable him to survive his environment; and (4) the importance of touch" (Burnside, 1971, p. 105). Irene accepted the fact that she would not influence Mr. Weston's delusional thought patterns. She eventually came to understand the delusions "as a defense against a bleak environment. If he were to give up even part of his delusions, what could I replace them with?" (Burnside, 1971, p. 105).

The theoretical framework Irene used when working with Mr. Weston was that of Goldfarb (1955, 1958). Goldfarb was a psychiatrist who saw patients for a maximum of 15 minutes, and "his aim in each session was to provide emotional gratification for the patient and to increase his self-esteem" (Burnside, 1971, p. 108). Other theorists who influenced Irene's work were "Robert Butler and Erik Erikson in life review and reminiscence, Dorothy Orem's self-care theory, Harry Stack Sullivan's ideas on threats to self-esteem, and Hildegard Peplau's interpersonal process" (Burnside, personal communication, November 23, 1993).

While she was still working on her post–master's certificate, Irene was invited by her mentor, Marion Kalkman, to be a lecturer for the Department of Nursing at UCSF in 1967. That invitation marked the beginning of Irene's career as an educator in nursing. It also helped to launch her on her career as a pioneering group therapist and scholar.

GROUP WORK WITH OLDER PERSONS

Year chases year, decay pursues decay,
Still drops some joy from with'ring life away—*Samuel Johnson*

The words of Samuel Johnson describe how Irene Burnside felt when she began group work with the elderly over 25 years ago (Burnside, 1969). Soon after Irene completed her post–master's certificate in adult psychiatric nursing in 1967, she visited a neighbor who was residing in a convalescent hospital following a leg amputation. The neighbor informed Irene, "I'll go batty if I don't get out of here. I'll be like the rest of these poor souls in here. There's no one to talk to" (Burnside, personal communication, November 23, 1993). Looking at the environment, Irene understood what he meant and decided she could do something to alleviate the problem.

As early as 1944 (while working in the back wards during nurses' training), Irene had been struck by the isolation and withdrawal of patients who resided in state institutions and convalescent hospitals, which were comparable to nursing homes today. "Psychosocial care of older persons (at that time) consisted of making paper flowers and having Mitch Miller sing-alongs. They didn't have activity directors in those days" (Burnside, personal communication, November 23, 1993). But Irene's previous practicum experience with patients such as Mr. Weston during her master's and post–master's education had convinced her that older persons could benefit from psychosocial nursing care.

Irene decided to start doing group work on a volunteer basis at a nearby nursing home. Simply gaining entrée into the nursing home was the first of many obstacles she faced. The nursing home administrator canceled three appointments that Irene made to discuss her desire to volunteer as a group leader. She obviously did not want this volunteer effort in her nursing home. Irene shared her frustrations with a physician with whom she was working on a suicide hot line. It turned out that he had many residents at the nursing home, and he told Irene she could work with his patients.

With the encouragement and assistance of the physician and the staff (to whom she had brought brownies during her earlier visits), Irene selected six patients who met the four criteria she had established for group membership. The participants were to be (a) mobile (including wheelchair bound), (b) verbal (she did include one man who was aphasic but who could shake his head to communicate), (c) coherent, and (d) able to tolerate sitting in a group for 45 minutes once a week (Burnside, 1969).

The agenda Irene developed for the group was simple. She would "include a generous amount of 'laying on of the hands,' I would provide sweet things to eat, keep the patients in a small circle, and pace myself (both verbally and intellectually) to the patients' speed" (Burnside, 1969, p. 69). As a theoretical base for the group work, Irene initially used the Fundamental Interpersonal Relations Orientation (FIRO), a method designed to enhance communication and diminish the group members' sense of isolation and pattern of withdrawal (Burnside, 1969).

It wasn't long before Irene observed four themes emerging from this group experience: limited mobility, inability to engage in self-care, physical and psychological isolation, and diminished sensory acuity and dexterity (along with incontinence). Furthermore, although Irene had started the group therapy sessions with every intention of using a "here and now" approach whenever she could, she soon came to realize that "there and then" was what her elderly patients wanted to discuss.

> At first, they complained about the living conditions and food at the institution. Eventually, they talked about being immigrants to the United States, the bootlegging days, and they talked about their parents and what it was like to grow up when they did. I would see them blossom right in front of me. I would encourage them to be the authority on whatever they were telling me. I empowered them. They were in charge, it was their life. (Burnside, personal communication, November 23, 1993)

As Irene became intrigued by her patients' sense of history and by the possibilities of allowing *them* to teach *her* about a world she had never known, she quickly abandoned her original agenda of here-and-now for the naturally evolving themes of reminiscence.

> When joyously led, the people forget their burdens; in wrestling joyous with difficulties, they even forget that they must die. Joy's greatest quality is in the encouragement it affords the people (*I Ching*, 1989).

Irene continued to be a group therapy leader with these patients for 2 years. "They taught me almost everything I know about aging. There was not much work being done in gerontological nursing at that time, so I learned from them about aging, nursing homes, illness, disability, blindness, about heartache. I learned so much from those residents" (Burnside, personal communication, November 23, 1994). In effect, Irene had learned firsthand the meaning of Erik Erikson's phrase, "to be–through having been"—a phrase that became the theoretical foundation of her subsequent work with the elderly (cited in Burnside, 1969).

Although Irene felt rewarded by her work with the patients, she felt frustrated by the nursing staff's general lack of interest toward group therapy. The staff seemed to view her as an "egghead from the university" because she had a master's degree and was on the faculty at UCSF. The nurses apparently were not interested in learning, and they exhibited some resentment toward Irene and her desire to educate them about what she was learning.

After 2 years of witnessing Irene meeting with her group once a week (1968–1970), the nursing staff eventually got used to seeing her. They didn't quite understand why she brought her pet dog in for the blind man to hold (maybe Irene was one of the first pet therapists), and they definitely didn't understand why a nurse would want to do group therapy, as most staff members considered that the domain of psychologists and social workers.

One nursing assistant, however, was very supportive of the work Irene was doing with the patients. Irene tried to teach this aide (in addition to being a group therapist, educator, activity director, and pet therapist, she was also a mentor) to run the therapy group, but when the aide became ill soon after Irene left the nursing home, the group work stopped.

Irene's face lights up when she discusses the long-term effects of her group work with the elderly patients at the nursing home. Even though the formal group therapy sessions were discontinued shortly after her departure,

> by the time I left the nursing home, the effect was long range. They were meeting in subgroups after I left. The woman who was losing her vision went to the blind man to find out where he got talking books. The man from Cornell University, who could get around, asked to be moved in with the wheelchair-bound blind man so that they could help each other. All of my hard work did have positive results for these residents. (Burnside, personal communication, November 23, 1993).

PIONEERING GERONTOLOGICAL NURSING SCHOLAR

Irene's persistent desire to address the psychosocial needs of elderly patients living in the nursing home set the stage not only for her pioneering group therapy work with older persons, but also for her growth as a gerontological nursing scholar. Irene had started doing group work with nursing home residents in 1968, a time when nursing care of the elderly was barely palliative and no nurses were doing therapy with the aged. Indeed, no particular nurse leader from 1900 to 1968 had focused specifically on work with the elderly (Wells, 1979). Interestingly, it was not until 1967—only 1 year prior to Irene's group therapy experience—that the American Nurses Association (ANA) presented a position paper on psychiatric nursing, endorsing the role of the clinical specialist as therapist in individual, group, family, and milieu therapies (Murray & Huelskoetter, 1984). Furthermore, it was not to be until 1973 that gerontological nurses would be granted certification through the ANA (Burnside, 1988).

As Irene's group work progressed, she felt "a real need to get other perspectives about working with the aged" (Burnside, personal communication, November 24, 1993). She sought all the education she could regarding older persons, although there were few published articles related to the care of the elderly. Journal articles prior to 1960 focused on the general care of the aged (Adams, 1939; Gelbach, 1943; Holbrow, 1931; Merritt, 1952); geriatric eye, ear, nose, and throat clinics (Buckner, 1948); orthopedic issues (Newton, 1948); care of the aged in state mental institutions (Nace, 1951); care of the aged surgical patient (Sholtis, 1951); and foster care (Cryan, 1954). By 1971, extensive literature searches revealed a total of only 296 published articles related to gerontology, with 21.3% of the total publications for that year on geriatric nursing (Brimmer, 1979).

In an attempt to gain a more thorough understanding of the psychosocial needs of older persons, Irene began studying during the summers of 1970, 1971, and 1972 at the Ethel Percy Andrus Gerontology Center, located at the University of Southern California in Los Angeles. There Irene studied under such well-known gerontologists as Robert Butler, Eric Pfeiffer, Alvin Goldfarb, Ethel Shanas, Bernice Neugarten, Jack Weinberg, James Birren, and Isadore Rossman. Irene noted, "I took classes from these non-nurses because there were no nurses teaching geropsychiatric nursing in 1970" (Burnside, personal communication, November 22, 1993). However, the "one person" in gerontological nursing who did influence Irene was Dorothy Moses. Dorothy, thought to be the first nursing instructor to put students in a geropsychiatric setting, was the first nurse to teach at the Andrus Gerontology Center (Irene became the second nurse to teach there). Dorothy was also the first female president of the Western Gerontological Society, which is known today as the American Society on Aging (Burnside, personal communication, November 23, 1993).

Within a few years, Irene had acquired sufficient practical experiences and scholarly expertise to start publishing accounts of the impact group interaction had on older persons. Her book, *Psychosocial Nursing Care of the Aged* (1973), was one of the first texts in nursing to address psychosocial issues with older people.

But she knew she could not be content to stop there. As early as 1971, Irene had observed,

> It has been my experience as an instructor in psychiatric nursing for the past four years, that nursing students are reluctant to choose an elderly person for one-to-one relationship therapy. Our youth-oriented culture is certainly made explicit by the choice of patients when students are placed in the clinical arena. Students, if and when they can be motivated and encouraged to work with the aged, can effect great change. (Burnside, 1971, p. 108)

In the face of this observed lack of motivation among students, Irene felt even more driven to write. Since 1968, she has made significant scholarly contributions to the field of geropsychiatric nursing: she has published widely in professional journals, has written more than 20 book chapters, and has edited 10 books pertaining to psychosocial and nursing care of elders (see Appendix).

Gerontological nursing leaders have used and continue to use many strategies—including confrontation, coalition formation, arbitration, and exchange—to ensure desirable outcomes regarding the health and well-being of the elderly (Harrington & Cruise, 1984). Irene is regarded as a nursing leader not only because she influenced the behavior of others but also because she focused on making structural changes in the field of nursing and publishing accounts of those changes. The combination of her pioneering actions and her scholarship eventually helped lead to the recognition that nurses are in a key position to address the psychosocial needs of elderly patients.

NURSE EDUCATOR

The position Irene had taken in 1968 as lecturer for the Department of Nursing at UCSF helped her begin to realize her childhood dream of becoming an educator. But in 1969, while Irene was still teaching at UCSF and conducting her group therapy sessions at the nursing home, her husband was diagnosed as having amyotrophic lateral sclerosis (Lou Gehrig's disease). He died in December 1970. Widowed at age 47, Irene remained at UCSF until 1972, when her youngest child graduated from high school. At that time, she decided that teaching gerontological nursing to classes of only five or six students was less than fulfilling, and she moved to Los Angeles to join the staff of the Andrus Gerontology Center at the University of Southern California.

From 1972 to 1976, Irene served as coordinator of nursing education at the center. From 1976 to 1979, she was an author, lecturer, and consultant in gerontological nursing across the United States and abroad, including Canada, Norway, Sweden, Finland, Malaysia, and Australia. It is interesting to note that Irene began educating students about the psychosocial care of older adults before the ANA House of Delegates had approved resolutions concerning the educational preparation of gerontological nurses in 1978 (Burnside, 1988).

In 1979, Irene joined San Jose State University in California as a lecturer. There she became first an assistant professor and later a tenured associate professor in gerontological nursing. In the summer of 1990, Irene was a visiting fellow at the Phillip Institute in Melbourne, Australia, and a visiting professor at the Medical University of South Carolina in Charleston in the summers of 1991 and 1992. Irene's most recent educational position is adjunct professor, San Diego State University. In all of these academic positions, she has taught gerontological nursing courses.

PHD IN GERONTOLOGICAL NURSING

Irene's decision to pursue a doctorate in gerontological nursing was due in part to her association with other gerontological researchers. Dr. James Birren, who was director of the Andrus Gerontology Center when Irene was there, had a particularly strong influence on her. Dr. Birren's example helped Irene to see the importance of theory development and research in gerontology.

Eventually, Irene decided to pursue her lifelong interest in reminiscence, first kindled during her 1968 group experiences in the nursing home. She began working on her PhD in gerontological nursing at the University of Texas in Austin during the summer months, beginning in

1982, while continuing to teach at San Jose State University during the regular academic year. In 1985, Irene was diagnosed with cancer, and it became apparent to her that she needed to take time off from her studies and teaching responsibilities to pursue treatment.

Irene was eventually able to resume her studies on a full-time basis at the University of Texas. Her dissertation, based on her study of reminiscence in community-based older women, was titled "The Effects of Reminiscence Groups on Fatigue, Affect, and Life Satisfaction in Older Women" (Burnside, 1990). She received her PhD in gerontological nursing in 1990.

> To be in the class of 1990 at the University of Texas at Austin meant that President Bush was my commencement speaker. That was exciting in itself, but when he singled out three students for special recognition and I was one of them, I was beside myself! I decided there that it pays to be old [she was sixty-six years old at the time] and that perhaps I really am chronologically-gifted. (Burnside, 1991, p. 20)

Irene believes that the PhD in gerontological nursing gave her "credibility" and that furthering her education secured her place in the field of gerontological academe.

GEROPSYCHIATRIC NURSING CARE IN OTHER COUNTRIES

Of the many factors that are known to determine health beliefs and behaviors, culture is the most influential variable (Harwood, 1981). When discussing nursing care of the elderly in other countries, Irene underscores the importance of the ability to be sensitive to cultural traditions. "In the United States we have lost sight of the individual patient's cultural heritage" (Burnside, personal communication, November 23, 1993).

Irene believes that many of the problems seen in long-term care settings in the United States have their counterparts in other countries.

> For instance, when I was in Norway in the 1970s, they asked me if confused and alert patients should be segregated. In Australia, they were struggling with the overuse of restraints in long-term care. Greece and Malaysia had not even developed an interest in the care of their aged when I was there. Malaysia was still combating com-

municable diseases such as anthrax. In Greece, the elderly were usually cared for by family members and had not become a national priority yet. (Burnside, personal communication, November 23, 1993)

Irene has observed with pleasure, however, the extent to which the
Scandinavian countries have developed a sensitivity for the aged. She recalls
visiting a nursing home in Scandinavia at which a female architect had
designed a sauna that accommodated wheelchairs. In Finland,

> there were long balconies outside of the rooms. In the springtime,
> bed-bound patients would be wheeled out on the balconies (bed and
> all) so they could hear the first cuckoo of spring. In Sweden, when
> May Day arrived, the residents were wheeled onto the balcony to see
> the children dance around the May Pole. (Burnside, personal com-
> munication, November 23, 1993)

Interestingly, Irene's pioneering work with the elderly has not passed
unnoticed in other countries. Dr. Jan-Erik Ruth, a professor at the Center
for Gerontological Training and Research in Östersundom, Finland, has
noted that one of the center's doctoral students was doing a dissertation
on group therapy with the elderly and found Irene to be the "originator
of psychosocial group work with older persons" (J. Ruth, personal communication, March 4, 1994).

GEROPSYCHIATRIC NURSING IN THE FUTURE

Irene believes that gerontological nursing today continues to lack adequate attention in nursing curricula at all levels. She has asserted that a
major issue facing the field of gerontological nursing today is education.
"I'm afraid we don't have enough qualified and motivated instructors.
We have nurses who aren't interested in the aged but have to teach
gerontology classes and it shows" (Burnside, personal communication,
November 23, 1993). When asked how this issue may be resolved, Irene
replied,

> I think there have to be more rewards in taking care of older people.
> Another helpful solution would be to include test questions about
> care of the aged on nursing board exams. Once instructors find out
> they need to be more than one step ahead of their students when

teaching gerontological nursing, they will learn more and hopefully will get "hooked" on some of the many issues facing our elderly today. (Burnside, personal communication, November 23, 1993)

In Irene's view, one of the most significant changes in nursing care of the aged during her career is the rise of the gerontological advanced practice nurse.

The Geriatric Nurse Practitioner was something unheard of early in my career. I think it is exciting that nurses are now carrying their own case loads and nursing is being recognized as an important entity in the delivery of health care [see Masse, 1994, per Burnside]. Nurses are being recognized as specialists in gerontological nursing today. For example, Thelma Wells has studied incontinence in older persons, Neville Strumpf and Lois Evans [are recognized experts] in the use of restraints, and Kathleen Buckwalter and Geri Hall in the care of persons with Alzheimer's disease. (Burnside, personal communication, November 23, 1993)

Irene continued, "I also have been happy to know that nurses are considered psychotherapists with the elderly. In the 1940s, nurses had one-to-one interactions, but they were not considered psychotherapists" (Burnside, personal communication, November 23, 1993).

ACHIEVEMENTS AND AWARDS

According to Irene, one of the most satisfying aspects of her career has been "all the years of nursing that I did as a home health nurse, an industrial nurse, medical nurse, and a psychiatric nurse. I was given the privilege of being with people at the most private and personal times of their lives (birth, illness, and dying)" (Burnside, personal communication, November 22, 1993). A second source of satisfaction for her has been "the power of the pen. You can reach a lot of people (by writing) whom you can't reach by talking. Writing appears to have a rippling effect similar to water when a rock is thrown in it" (Burnside, personal communication, November 22, 1993). The "rippling effect" Irene refers to has been demonstrated by the impact her books have had on the nursing care of the aged over the past 50 years.

Irene's many achievements have frequently been recognized and applauded, not only by the nursing community but beyond as well. She has received such honors as the Gerontological Nurse of the Year award from the ANA in 1990; the Joseph C. Valley Gerontological Professional of the Year award from the University of Texas Health Science Center, School of Nursing, in 1988; the First Long-Term award from the National League for Nursing in 1981; the *American Journal of Nursing* Book of the Year award, twice (*Psychosocial Caring throughout the Life Span* [Burnside, Ebersole, & Monea, 1979] in 1980 and *Working with the Elderly: Group Process and Techniques,* in 1979), the Lulu Hassenplug award from the California Nurses' Association, 1977; the American Writer's Association AMMY award (Best Book of the Year by Non-Physician for a book on a medical subject, *Nursing and the Aged*) in 1977; and the Meritorious Service award from the American Association of Homes for Aging in 1976. She has been listed in *Who's Who in American Nursing* (1975), *Who's Who in International Women* (1977), *Notable Women (*1976, 1977), and *Who's Who of American Women* (1976, 1977, 1978, 1979). She also was named Fellow in Gerontological Society of America (1985) and Fellow in American Academy of Nursing (1981) and holds a Standard Teaching Credential (awarded for life) from the state of California.

Irene's most recent honor came in May 1993, when she was asked to deliver the Commemorative Address for the Army Cadet Nurse Corps as it celebrated its 50th anniversary in Bethesda, Maryland. In a letter inviting Irene to deliver the address, Assistant Surgeon General Julia R. Plotnik wrote, "As one of the most distinguished Cadet Corps graduates, it would be a great honor for us to have you address the group" (Plotnik, personal communication, February 1994).

When asked about awards, Irene has commented that

> all of the awards gave me honor, but I'd have to say that the Geronting Award [from the Andrus Gerontology Center in 1975] made me feel honored because it came from a Center on Aging and it was recognition from a multidisciplinary group interested in improving the care of our aged. (Burnside, personal communication, November 23, 1993)

The Founder's Award, Excellence in Creativity, from Sigma Theta Tau in 1991 is also very special to Irene because Dr. James Birren wrote a wonderful letter of support, noting the work she had done with groups of cognitively impaired older persons 20 years previously.

CONCLUSIONS

"On a clear day you can see as far as you can look." The quotation is from a man in Irene's first therapeutic group almost 30 years ago (Burnside, 1991). Being a true visionary and idealist, she has incorporated this man's words into thoughts and actions that have guided her life and career. Irene Burnside's career spans the past 50 years of American nursing history. She pioneered the practice of nurses conducting therapeutic group work with older persons. Although she is interested in all group modalities with older persons, she continues to pursue her particular interest in furthering reminiscence group therapy and group therapy with cognitively impaired elderly.

If nursing is viewed as more than an encounter between individuals, during which the nurse attempts to foster the well-being of the individual client, then in a broader perspective, the nurse is one who attempts to improve the well-being of entire groups of clients in society. Irene's work with the elderly has set the stage for more attentive and effective psychosocial nursing care of the aged for many generations to come.

REFERENCES

Adams, Y. (1939). My elderly patient. *American Journal of Nursing, 39,* 302.

Baer, E. D. (1985). Nursing's divided house: An historical view . . . the last third of the 19th century. *Nursing Research, 34*(1), 32–38.

Brimmer, P. F. (1979). Past, present and future in gerontological nursing research. *Journal of Gerontological Nursing, 5*(6), 27–34.

Buckner, B. (1948). A geriatric EEBT client. *American Journal of Nursing, 48,* 557–559.

Burnside, I. M. (1969). Group work among the aged. *Nursing Outlook, 17*(6), 68–72.

Burnside, I. M. (1971). Gerontion: A case study. *Perspectives in Psychiatric Care, 9*(3), 103–108.

Burnside, I. M. (1973). *Psychosocial nursing care of the aged.* New York: McGraw-Hill.

Burnside, I. M. (Ed.). (1988). *Nursing and the aged* (3rd ed.). St. Louis: C. V. Mosby.

Burnside, I. M. (1990). *The effects of reminiscence groups on fatigue, affect and life satisfaction in older women.* Unpublished doctoral dissertation, University of Texas, School of Nursing, Austin.

Burnside, I. M. (1991, Winter). From one who is chronologically gifted: Aging well. *Generations, 15*(1), 19–20.

Burnside, I. M. (1993). Healthy older women—in spite of it all. *Journal of Women and Aging, 5*(3/4), 9–24.

Burnside, I. M., Ebersole, P., & Monea, H. (1979). *Psychosocial caring throughout the life span.* New York: McGraw-Hill.
Cryan, E. (1954). Foster home care for older people. *American Journal of Nursing, 54,* 954–956.
Gelbach, S. (1943). Nursing care of the aged. *American Journal of Nursing, 43,* 1112–1114.
Goldfarb, A. I. (1955). Psychotherapy of aged persons. *Psychoanalytic Review, 42,* 2.
Goldfarb, A. I. (1958). Psychotherapy of the aged. *Psychoanalytic Review, 43,* 1.
Harrington, C., & Cruise, M. (1984). Leadership in gerontological nursing. *Gerontology and Geriatric Education. 43*(3), 99–111.
Harwood, A. (1981). *Ethnicity and medical care.* Cambridge, MA: Harvard University Press.
Hegge, M. (1990). In the footsteps of Florence Nightingale: Rediscovering the roots of nursing. *Imprint, 37*(2), 74–77.
Holbrow, J. (1931). Some problems in nursing and aged patient. *American Journal of Nursing, 30,* 174–175.
I Ching (Blofeld ed.) (1989). In P. L. Berman (Ed.), *The courage to grow old* (p. 42). New York: Ballantine Books.
Masse, H. (1994). APNs talk about their practice. *California Nurse, 90*(3), 9.
Merritt, L. (1952). Young ideas for elderly patients. *American Journal of Nursing, 52,* 713.
Murray, R. B., & Huelskoetter, M. M. (1984). *Psychiatric/mental health nursing: Giving emotional care.* Norwalk, CT: Appleton & Lange.
Nace, F. (1951). The care of the aged in a state mental hospital. *American Journal of Nursing, 51,* 366–369.
Newton, K. (1948). Orthopedic problems of older people. *American Journal of Nursing, 48,* 508–511.
Rush, S. L. (1992). Nursing education in the United States, 1898–1910: A time of auspicious beginnings. *Journal of Nursing Education, 31*(9), 409–414.
Shea, C. A. (1990). Feminism: A failure in nursing? In J. McCloskey & H. Grace (Eds.), *Current issues in nursing* (pp. 448–454). St. Louis: C. V. Mosby.
Sholtis, L. (1951). Nursing the elderly surgical patient. *American Journal of Nursing, 51,* 726–729.
Spellbring, A. M. (1991). Nursing role in health promotion: An overview. *Nursing Clinics of North America, 26,* 805–814.
Wells, T. (1979). Nursing committed to the elderly. In A. Reinhardt & M. Quinn (Eds.), *Current practice in gerontological nursing* (pp. 187–196). St. Louis: C. V. Mosby.

APPENDIX: SELECTED BIBLIOGRAPHY OF BURNSIDE PUBLICATIONS

Books

Burnside, I. M. (1973, 1st ed.; 1980, 2nd ed.). *Psychosocial nursing care of the aged.* New York: McGraw-Hill.

Burnside, I. M. (1973). *Films on aging.* Los Angeles: Andrus Gerontology Center.

Burnside, I. M. (1974). *Sexuality and aging.* Los Angeles: Andrus Gerontology Center.

Burnside, I. M. (1976, 1st ed.; 1981, 2nd ed.). *Nursing and the aged.* New York: McGraw-Hill.

Burnside, I. M. (Ed.). (1978, 1st ed.; 1984, 2nd ed.). *Working with the elderly: Group processes and techniques.* Boston: Jones & Bartlett.

Burnside, I. M. (1988). *Nursing and the aged: A self-care approach* (3rd ed.). St. Louis: Mosby Year Book.

Burnside, I. M., Ebersole, P., & Monea, H. (Eds.). (1979). *Psychosocial caring throughout the life span.* New York: McGraw-Hill.

Burnside, I. M., & Schmidt, M. G. (Eds.). (1989). *Working with older persons: Group process and techniques* (3rd ed.). Boston: Jones & Bartlett.

Chapters in Books

Burnside, I. M. (1990). Conducting groups with people with Alzheimer's disease. In *Conference proceedings of the Alzheimer's Association.* Perth, Australia: Promaco Conventions Pty. Ltd.

Burnside, I. M. (1992). Incorporating curriculum. In *Successful aging . . . beyond illness: Conference proceedings of the Southern Regional Education Board.* Atlanta, GA.

Burnside, I. M. (1993). Healthy older women in spite of it all. In J. D. Garner & A. A. Young (Eds.), *Women and healthy aging: Living productively in spite of it all* (pp. 1–23). New York: Haworth Press.

Burnside, I. M. (1995). Reminiscence and life review in nursing practice. In J. E. Birren, G. M. Kenyon, H. Schroots, T. Svenson, J. Ruth, & R. Heikkenen (Eds.), *Aging and biography.* New York: Springer Publishing Co.

Burnside, I. M. (1995). Themes and props: Adjuncts for reminiscence therapy groups. In B. Haight & J. Webster (Eds.), *The art and science of reminiscing: Theory, research, methods, and application.* Washington, DC: Taylor & Francis.

Burnside, I. M. (in press). Reminiscence. In J. E. Birren (Editor-in-chief), *Encyclopedia of gerontology.* New York: Academic Press.

Recent Refereed Journal Articles

Burnside, I. M. (1990). Reminiscence as an independent nursing intervention for the elderly. *Issues in Mental Health Nursing, 11*(1), 33–48.

Burnside, I. M. (1990). The frail elderly: Those 85 and over. *Nursing Administration Quarterly, 14*(2), 37–41.

Burnside, I. M. (1991, Winter). From one who is chronologically gifted: Aging well. *Generations, 15*(1), 19–20.

Burnside, I. M. (1991). A scarce professional: The geropsychiatric clinical nurse specialist. *Clinical Nurse Specialist, 4*(3), 122–127.

Burnside, I. M. (1993). Healthy older women—in spite of it all. *Journal of Women and Aging, 5*(3/4), 9–24.

Burnside, I. M. (1993). Themes in reminiscence groups with older women. *International Journal of Aging and Human Development, 37*(3), 177–189.

Burnside, I. M. (1994). Group work with older persons. *Journal of Gerontological Nursing, 20*(1), 43–45.

Burnside, I. M., & Haight, B. (1992). Reminiscence and life review: Analyzing each concept. *Journal of Advanced Nursing, 17,* 855–862.

Burnside, I. M., & Haight, B. (1992). Reminiscence and life review: Conducting the processes. *Journal of Gerontological Nursing, 18*(2), 39–42.

Burnside, I. M., & Haight, B. (1994). Reminiscence and life review: Therapeutic interventions for older people. *Nurse Practitioner, 19*(4), 55–61.

Burnside, I. M., & Newbern, V. (1994). Needs of older persons in the emergency department. *Journal of Gerontological Nursing, 20*(7), 54–56.

Burnside, I. M., & Preski, S. (1992). Clinical research with community-based older women. *Journal of Gerontological Nursing, 18*(6), 13–18.

Burnside, I. M., Bowsher, J., Bramlett, M., & Gueldner, S. H. (1993). Methodological considerations in the study of frail elderly people. *Journal of Advanced Nursing, 18,* 873–879.

CHAPTER 10

Epilogue—Gazing Through the Crystal Ball: Gerontological Nursing Issues and Challenges for the 21st Century

Meridean L. Maas and Kathleen C. Buckwalter

D r. Whall's introductory chapter highlighted many of the current and future education and practice needs of gerontological nursing. She challenged nurses to address these needs, lest we abandon the future of elder care. In this epilogue we build on her remarks and other content presented in this inaugural volume, as we attempt to forecast selected changes with which nursing education, practice, and research will have to contend in the coming years. As the title suggests, we will endeavor to identify and briefly discuss how the projected changes in sociodemographics and the health care and service delivery systems will affect nursing care in the next century.

IMPLICATIONS OF CHANGING DEMOGRAPHICS FOR LONG-TERM CARE

An accurate gaze into the future for gerontological nursing begins with a description of the changing demographics of the elderly population.

Planning for the human and financial resources that will be required to meet the needs of the elderly in the 21st century must be based on predictions about the number of elderly in the population and the health and functional care needs of various elderly cohorts.

Prediction: Clinicians, policymakers, economists, community developers, and researchers will be forced to pay attention to those who are 85 and older and to their family caregivers.

Current data indicate that the elderly population in the United States will continue its rapid growth beyond the year 2020. The rate of growth of the elderly population, however, will vary among its three cohorts: the young-old (ages 65–75), the old (ages 75–85), and the oldest-old (age 85 and older). The number of elderly who are age 85 and older is expected to more than double, from 2.39 million in 1980 to 5.16 million by the year 2000 (Rosenwaike, 1985). The young-old will increase most rapidly from 2000 to 2020 as post–World War II "babies" pass age 65, and the oldest-old will increase most rapidly from 2020 to 2080 as they celebrate their 85th birthdays and beyond (U.S. Department of Health and Human Services, 1987). The size of elderly cohorts will be influenced by changes in life expectancy, which are expected to exceed a median age of 85 for both males and females. As life expectancy is extended, there will be rapid increases, particularly in the number of elderly black males and the number of white females ages 85 and older.

Those passing age 65 in the next century can be expected to have a greater average number of years of education, paralleled by increased economic resources and improved quality of life. Among whites, however, families will be smaller, providing fewer informal care resources. Conversely, blacks will continue to experience a poorer economic status, but they will have larger families, providing greater opportunities for informal care.

The availability of family caregivers will be limited by (a) the existence of family members able to provide care, (b) the ability of those members to provide all the care needed, and (c) the caregivers' ability to tolerate burdens associated with care, which is a predictor of institutionalization. Other factors will limit the traditional availability of family caregivers who are women (wives, daughters, and daughters-in-law): (a) declines in marriage and childbearing over the past few decades, (b) declines in remarriage rates among divorced elderly, (c) more women in the work force unwilling to leave their jobs to provide care, and (d) delays in childbearing age into the 30s, resulting in daughters in their 50s who are in the work force and still have demands from children in their 20s, at the same time they have parents in their 80s who require care.

Thus, given projected demographic changes, fewer elders in the next century are likely to have family caregivers available. The issue of how much can be fairly expected of family caregivers will undoubtedly become a policy issue in the next few decades. Obviously, when formal care replaces informal care, costs to the public will rise.

The effects of morbidity and disability on the elderly in the 21st century are difficult to predict, particularly because they depend on the success of primary and secondary interventions—both curative and preventive—during the next decade. Based on current medical data on the oldest-old, many of the conditions projected to be most common in this cohort result in chronic disabilities that are amenable to rehabilitation (National Center for Health Statistics [NCHS], 1985), whereas others are responsive to primary and secondary interventions of a preventive nature. However, the projected large increases in conditions such as hip fractures and dementia among the oldest-old up to 2050 will have a great impact on the functional impairment of this rapidly growing segment of the population (Brody, 1984).

For every person currently in institutional care, there are an estimated four more persons in the community who require some form of long-term care. By the year 2000, about 18% of the elderly (over 5 million) are projected to have some impairment that requires the help of others. Although 1.75 million of these impaired elderly will be in nursing homes or other institutions, a staggering 3.5 million needing long-term care will not be institutionalized. This unmet need will be compounded by the lack of family caregivers. Furthermore, about 75% of the disabled elderly currently living outside institutions rely solely on informal care. This number of dependent elders is expected to grow as the proportion of elderly, especially those over age 75, in the U.S. population increases (Griffin, Leftwich, & Smith, 1989; Strumpf & Knibbe, 1990). Dependencies for assistance range from instrumental activities of daily living (IADLs), such as cooking, shopping, and cleaning, to personal care activities of daily living (ADLs), such as toileting, dressing, bathing, transfer, ambulation, and eating.

Eighty percent (80%) of the oldest-old do not have spouses, and 52% of the oldest-old who live in the community live alone—facts that have implications for both the health care system and the housing/service industry (Harris & Associates, 1986). Economic problems are prevalent among the oldest-old, who have the highest percentage of persons living in poverty of any age group (Bould, Sanborn, & Reif, 1989). Twenty-three percent of the oldest-old live in rural areas, and rural residence poses especially difficult problems for cost-effective program development (Bould et al., 1989). The rural oldest-old, especially minorities, are poorer than their urban counterparts (Wentowski, 1981).

Recent estimates indicate that one half of the women and almost one third of the men who turned 65 in 1990 will require nursing home care during their lifetimes (Sheridan, White, & Fairchild, 1992). As the result of an aging population and increasing life expectancy, the number of elderly residents in nursing homes could nearly double by the year 2020 (Kemper & Murtaugh, 1991). Based on current disability and institutionalization rates (NCHS, 1985), the number of frail and institutionalized elderly will increase from 5.7 million in 1980 to 8.9 million in 2000, to 12.2 million in 2020, and to 17.8 million in 2040. Even if these projections are altered to reflect expected decreases in morbidity and disability rates, the demand for trained health care personnel and community-based services will continue to be great. The need for formal services to replace current informal care services is expected to increase, because of the trend toward smaller families and the lack of available family caregivers.

Prediction: There will be increased demand for more, better-trained, better-paid, and more diverse workers in the long-term care industry.

By 2030 the elderly will constitute 20% of the population and use 30% of health care resources. To provide adequate health care, at least 36,000 geriatricians and more than 1.1 million registered nurses (RNs) will be required (Select Committee on Aging, 1992). The total need for full-time equivalent (FTE) RNs by 2020 is forecast to be 1,126,000 (72% of available supply), compared to 584,000 working with elderly in 1990 (41% of available supply). Table 10.1 contains projections of the numbers of nursing personnel FTEs that will be needed to meet the needs of the elderly in nursing homes in 2020 compared to the number available in 1990 (Select Committee on Aging, 1992). Nursing staff representing more diverse racial and ethnic origins also will be needed to optimize the quality of care.

The projected demand for nursing home care has sparked debate over costs and the adequacy of nursing homes to deliver quality care. Although there will certainly be a need to increase the number of FTE RNs in long-term care, it may not provide the whole solution for quality in nursing homes. Nurses in the next century, including gerontological nurses, will

TABLE 10.1 Nursing FTEs Needed in Nursing Homes in 2020 Compared to 1990

Nursing Personnel	Year 2020	Year 1990
Registered nurses (RNs)	223,900	94,900
Licensed practical nurses (LPNs)	167,000	112,100
Nursing assistants (NAs)	671,100	421,900

be required to have more advanced skills and competencies (Valanis, 1994). Gerontological nurses in particular will need more primary care skills and skills that will enable them to manage the care of elders over an extended period and across care settings. There also is a need to examine closely the role that nursing homes should play in providing long-term care and how these homes can be effectively managed (Kane & Kane, 1991).

Profits in nursing homes will be determined by how well employees' skills are used to improve productivity. Staff will have to be "cross-trained" to do several different jobs, with flexible boundaries between nursing assistants (NAs), and dietary and housekeeping workers (Fogel, 1994). Continuous quality improvement (CQI)–type programs will become more important, with a focus on resident outcomes. Nursing homes will have to be administered so that all personnel will "work smarter" in a resource-scarce environment that emphasizes quality outcomes at the least cost.

There will be more demand for RNs, licensed practical nurses (LPNs), and nursing assistants (NAs) in community settings where the emphasis is on health promotion, prevention of illness, and the maximizing of functional independence. Nurses will have a strategic role in supporting family caregivers, providing the appropriate amount of respite care, and determining the amount of formal services that are needed to care for elders.

CHANGES IN HEALTH CARE AND SERVICE DELIVERY SYSTEMS

The implementation of hospital cost containment, which has contributed to increasing numbers of patients being discharged "quicker and sicker," has fueled the growth of the home health care industry and has escalated the need for all posthospital services (Wood, 1986). The total number of home health agencies has more than doubled since 1981, when Medicare and Medicaid made home care benefits more liberal (Reif, 1984). Capitated reimbursement systems, which pay a fixed amount for the care of individual patients, will promote managed care and primary care with an emphasis on prevention and early detection.

Prediction: The move from inpatient to community-based care will continue in the 21st century.

Both the long-term-care industry and hospitals are diversifying by expanding: into subacute care on the high end of the health care continuum and into assisted living on the low end (Stahl, 1994). Service integration will permeate the health care delivery system, with many skilled nursing facilities becoming one of several "spoke" services.

Lamb (1994) recently suggested that the shape of new health care delivery systems will be defined by four key goals: (a) achieving satisfactory quality outcomes at acceptable costs, (b) using professional resources as effectively and efficiently as possible, (c) providing services in the most appropriate setting for the least cost, and (d) finding financial and other incentives for all players to work toward common goals.

Hospitals will downsize, streamline, and redesign as the shift to community-based care occurs. This will mean a need for integration of acute and chronic care services. Nurses will be accountable as case managers for how their clients move through various systems. If nurses "seize the moment," we will see the rise of nursing health maintenance organizations (HMOs) (Lamb, 1994).

Thus, nursing research efforts will have to justify reimbursement and policy changes and evaluate both costs of care and outcomes in community nursing centers. In addition, sustained collaboration by interdisciplinary groups of active researchers will be essential (Kahn & Prager, 1994). For this goal to become a reality, concerted efforts must be made to educate health care professionals in a cross-disciplinary model, and academic institutions, funding sources, and publishers must acknowledge and reward multidisciplinary research and practice efforts.

In November 1994, the Long-Term Care Task Force of the Gerontological Society of America identified a number of research questions related to the building of a community-based long-term-care service system that must be addressed by nurses, other health care providers, and policymakers (Caro & Callahan, 1994). Examples of these future research issues include the following:

1. How will consumer-driven service delivery systems differ from more traditional systems in their effectiveness?
2. How can service delivery systems for the elderly be effectively adapted for the nondisabled elderly (or vice versa)?
3. How can flexibility in service delivery systems strengthen their ability to meet the needs of various age and disability groups?
4. How effectively do various service delivery systems make provisions for recruitment, training, supervision, compensation, and career opportunities for home care workers?
5. How effectively do various models of service-supported housing allow the disabled to retain significant autonomy?
6. Under what circumstances can successful state and local service delivery programs be effectively replicated?

These and other related issues will need to be systematically evaluated as our health care delivery system shifts to more community-based long-term-care opportunities.

Prediction: There will be more community-based long-term-care options for the elderly, such as assisted and independent living.

Community-based long-term care (CBLTC) is that component of comprehensive health care in which services are provided to persons and their families in the home (through respite care, day care, etc.) or in assisted living facilities in order to promote or restore health or minimize the effects of illness and disability. Services are usually planned and coordinated by an agency using employed staff or contractual arrangements. CBLTC is different from nursing home care in that services are provided to persons living at home or in a homelike environment (e.g., assisted living facility) rather than to residents of institutions (Miller, 1991).

CBLTC usually refers to services provided to frail elderly and disabled persons of all ages. The objectives of the services are to assist these individuals with basic tasks of living and/or to provide relief to their caregivers (e.g., respite services). CBLTC services cover a broad range, from skilled-level, medically related services provided by professional staff all the way to social support services provided by nonprofessionals or informal (family and friends) caregivers. Ideally, the formal (paid) community-based services should complement rather than impede those services provided by informal caregivers.

As mentioned previously, by the year 2000 about 5 million elderly will need long-term care, but only about 1.75 million will receive that care in nursing homes or other institutions. There are several possible approaches to this looming problem of having millions of elderly needing long-term care: (a) reducing the need for home care by improving the health of older people, (b) finding and paying for home care when disability and frailty preclude continued independence and self-care, and (c) providing better integration across the total continuum of care and better coordination of different care providers who subscribe to a biosocial view of health care that includes both medical and social components. Various residential care models are a response to the need to develop alternatives to the medical model currently emphasized in most long-term-care facilities. These alternatives include a range of state-licensed residential living environments such as foster care, family homes, residential care facilities, and assisted living arrangements (Brown-Wilson, 1994).

The lack of federal guidelines to standardize residential care is another element that will have to be addressed in the coming years. At present, state regulations vary widely regarding environmental, programming, and nursing care standards; most set minimum staffing ratios at quite low levels. Although residential care settings vary in size from small private homes for up to four residents to large congregate care facilities that may care for more than 100 residents, all offer assistance/care and share with the residents the responsibilities for ADLs. Ideally, the care provided is flexible, resident- and family-oriented, and intended to optimize individual dignity, functioning, health, and well-being. The physical environment and design features of the facility should support the functioning of the impaired older adult and accommodate behaviors and diminished abilities (Alzheimer's Association, 1994). However, consumers should question residential providers about all aspects of services, including the philosophy of care, number and type of staff, staff training and supervision, and costs to determine if resident and family needs will be met. Assisted living is a model of supportive housing that will continue to grow rapidly because of consumer preferences and costs associated with traditional models of long-term care (Brown-Wilson, 1994). In summary, assisted living issues that require review in the future include changes in nursing home reimbursement that will cause some residents to move back into the community, growth of the elderly population, and availability of home- and community-based care.

Other types of facilities and services are likely to be available or expanded for the elderly in the 21st century. These facilities and services will better reflect the physical, mental and spiritual needs of residents, family, and staff and have a less "institutional feel," as well as help to establish a true continuum of care. They include, for example, (a) more sophisticated services in the home; (b) elder cottage housing to care for aging parents; (c) multigenerational habitats to enhance contact, support, cooperation, and interaction; (d) naturally occurring retirement communities; (e) planned community-based retirement and continuing care–life care facilities; (f) multipurpose or mixed-use facilities; (g) innovative congregate living facilities; (h) board-and-care or small group homes; (i) respite care facilities for short-stay or overnight care; (j) specialized facilities and services, such as those for patients with dementia or chronic mental illness, ventilator-dependent patients, and those in need of rehabilitation; (k) hospice and palliative care services in both institutions and the community; and (l) increasingly skilled nursing care in both the community and institutions (Mann, 1994).

Prediction: More nursing homes will be built, federal and state subsidies will be tighter, and more union organizing efforts will surround long-term care.

Currently 32,000 nursing homes care for 2.2 million elderly (Goodfellow, 1994). The long-term-care industry will need to build 200,000 new beds by 1995 to maintain current levels of care at a projected cost of $7 billion, which will come from public sale of securities.

However, nursing homes are facing an inexorable economic squeeze, caught between rises in labor costs, cost-control legislation and regulations, and mandated ceilings on reimbursement. Yet consumer demands and federal regulations pressure these facilities and their administrators to increase levels of care. Because of this dilemma, major nursing homes are adopting interim strategies to attract private-pay residents, who at present contribute only 40% of nursing home revenues. Nursing homes will continue to seek higher levels of reimbursement and will develop various marketing strategies to improve their ability to provide needed care (Goodfellow, 1994).

Nursing homes will continue to admit persons who are more acutely ill and who need close monitoring and special therapies. Further, nursing homes will have to continue to compete with hospitals for some of the same personnel, although hospitals receive more Medicare payments for comparable patients and can afford to pay higher salaries (Goodfellow, 1994). For RNs, the highest hourly rate was $18.91 in hospitals, followed by $16.82 in home care and $15.26 in nursing homes, according to the 1994–1995 Home Care Salary and Benefits Report (Hospital and Healthcare Compensation Service, 1994). Labor in nursing homes averages about 60%–70% of operating costs, so any increases in labor costs will affect profit margins (Goodfellow, 1994). Policymakers must consider higher reimbursement rates, particularly for more acutely ill patients who are admitted to long-term care but are not eligible for reimbursement, in order for the needed RNs to be recruited and quality care to be achieved.

If older patients use health care facilities more for shorter stays, as predicted, then patient turnover rates will increase; with higher patient turnover rates, the need for professional and service workers, especially nurses, will increase. Although hospitals are downsizing, new legislation may mandate a minimum number of staff members per patient, a movement that is likely to be supported by organized labor unions. Nursing home administrators can move to avoid unionization by better meeting employees' needs and increasing staff morale. High turnover among nursing home staff will continue to be a critical problem. Increasing communication between staff and management, establishing effective grievance procedures, and providing good orientation programs for new employees, in addition to more competitive wages, are some of the recommended actions to increase job satisfaction and retention (Goodfellow, 1994).

Thus, the outlook for the next century is for more nursing home beds, tighter control of federal and state subsidies, stricter accounting of nursing home revenues and costs, limitations of return on nursing home investment, and more widespread unionization of nursing homes and hospitals.

Prediction: New skills will be required for nurses who manage the care of patients in the 21st century in order to enact more autonomous roles and to confront more complex ethical issues.

Valanis (1994) describes several competencies she believes will be critical for nurses in the future. Nurses should be able to (a) practice independently and evaluate their own performance; (b) identify gaps in knowledge and initiate professional development activities to keep current with changes in practice and to solve practice problems; (c) assess patient needs from the patient's point of view and empower patients/families to participate actively in the care to the extent that they are able; (d) manage care across facility boundaries, providing patients/families with continuity; (e) synthesize knowledge and skills of nursing with those of public health science to promote the health of the community; (f) ensure cost-effective quality care; (g) differentiate nursing functions from those of other professional and nonprofessional health disciplines, articulate nursing functions clearly to others, and participate in collaborative practice; (h) exert leadership in ensuring nursing's unique contribution to policy concerning the prevention and remedial aspects of illness, cooperating with other professions in planning for positive health on community, state, national, and international levels; and (i) support peers in improving existing nursing skills and in developing new skills.

Nurse-managed care of elderly persons will challenge the competencies of gerontological nurses. The gerontological nurse will need to be an advocate who emphasizes health promotion and prevention of illness in order to assist the elderly to maintain optimum function and control over their lives. The gerontological nurse also will need to foster personal control and autonomy and ensure that elders, even the cognitively and physically impaired, participate in decision-making processes and retain their right to make choices. Enabling elders to participate and make choices will be difficult but no less essential when some of their choices, such as pursuing an unhealthy life-style, opting for withholding treatment, requesting physician-assisted suicide, or selecting advance directives (living wills), conflict with the nurse's personal values. As Dr. Whall notes in the introductory chapter in this volume, these nursing competencies, especially as they relate to the care of the elderly, must be emphasized in educational curricula, research, and practice settings if nursing is to have a future in elder care in the next century.

CONCLUSIONS

In summary, the themes and predictions presented in this epilogue highlight the need for nursing leadership in elder care in the next century. Nurses must work to create the professional and political will to avoid a crisis in long-term care. We must work to create models of care that are appropriate for the elderly and their families; pursue adequate funding and reimbursement for programming and services; support the preparation and retention of adequate numbers of qualified nursing providers; increase our research to assess the effectiveness of care strategies; increase our emphasis on health promotion, community-based services, and continuity of care; and strengthen the gerontological and professional ethics content of our curricula. If we in the nursing community can focus our concerted efforts on these most critical areas, gerontological nursing will be well prepared to thrive in the 21st century.

REFERENCES

Alzheimer's Association. (1994). *Residential settings: An examination of Alzheimer issues.* Chicago: Author.

Bould, S., Sanborn, B., & Reif, L. (1989). *Eighty-five plus: The oldest-old.* Belmont, CA: Wadsworth.

Brody, J. A. (1984). The best times/the worst times: Aging and dependency in the 21st century. In S. R. Ingman & I. R. Lawson (Eds.), *Ethical dimensions of geriatric care: Value conflicts of the 21st century* (pp. 3–22). Dordrecht, Holland: D. Reidel. (Philosophy and Medicine Series, No. 25).

Brown-Wilson, K. B. (1994, August 15). Long-term care in the 21st century: Assisted living: Model program may signify the future. *Brown University Long-Term Care Quality Letter,* pp. 1–4.

Caro, F. G., & Callahan, J. (1994, November). *Toward improved federal support for research on delivery of home and community based long-term care.* Paper presented at the meeting of the Gerontological Society of America, Atlanta.

Fogel, B. S. (1994, April 25). Involvement, cross-training are keys to good labor force. *Brown University Long-Term Care Quality Letter,* p. 3.

Goodfellow, M. (1994, April 25). Long-term care in the 21st century: Nursing home labor needs, problems call for proactive measures. *Brown University Long-Term Care Quality Letter,* pp. 1–3.

Griffin, K. M., Leftwich, R. A., & Smith, M. S. (1989). Current forces shaping long-term care in the 1990s. *Journal of Long-Term Care Administration, 17*(3), 8–11.

Harris & Associates. (1986). *Problems facing elderly Americans living alone.* New York: Author.

Hospital and Healthcare Compensation Service. (1994). *The 1994–1995 home care salary and benefits report.* Oakland, NJ: Author.

Kahn, R. L., & Prager, D. J. (1994). Interdisciplinary collaborations are a scientific and social imperative. *Scientist, 8*(14), 12.

Kane, R. L., & Kane, R. A. (1991). A nursing home in your future? *New England Journal of Medicine, 324*(9), 627–628.

Kemper, P., & Murtaugh, C. M. (1991). Lifetime use of nursing home care. *New England Journal of Medicine, 324*(9), 595–601.

Lamb, G. S. (1994, October). *New delivery systems: The call to community.* Paper presented at a meeting of the American Academy of Nursing, Phoenix, AZ.

Mann, G. J. (1994, March 14). Long-term care in the 21st century: Facilities for the elderly in the 21st century. *Brown University Long-Term Care Quality Letter,* pp. 1–4.

Miller, J. A. (1991). *Community-based long-term care: Innovative models.* Newbury Park, CA: Sage.

National Center for Health Statistics. (1985). *National Nursing Home Survey.* Hyattsville, MD: U.S. Public Health Service.

Reif, L. (1984). Making dollars and sense of home health policy. *Nursing Economics, 2,* 382–390.

Rosenwaike, I. (1985). *The extreme aged in America*. Westport, CT: Greenwood Press.

Sheridan, J., White, J., & Fairchild, T. J. (1992). Ineffective staff, ineffective supervision, or ineffective administration? Why some nursing homes fail to provide adequate care. *The Gerontologist, 32,* 334–341.

Stahl, D. A. (1994). Development of subacute care services. *Nursing Management, 25*(11), 32–34.

Strumpf, N. E., & Knibbe, K. K. (1990). Long-term care: Fulfilling promises to the old among us. In J. C. McCloskey & H. K. Grace (Eds.), *Current issues in nursing* (pp. 217–225). St. Louis: C. V. Mosby.

U.S. Department of Health and Human Services. (1987). *Report to Congress: Personnel for health needs of the elderly through year 2020*. Bethesda, MD: National Institute on Aging.

U.S. House Select Committee on Aging (102nd Cong., 2nd sess.). (1992). *Report by the chairman*. Washington, DC: U.S. Government Printing Office.

Valanis, B. (1994, October). *Skills and competencies of the future nursing workforce*. Paper presented at a meeting of the American Academy of Nursing, Phoenix, AZ.

Wentowski, G. J. (1981). Reciprocity and the coping strategies of older people: Cultural dimensions of network building. *The Gerontologist, 21,* 600–609.

Wood, J. B. (1986). The effects of cost containment on home health agencies. *Home Health Care Services Quarterly, 6*(4), 59–78.

Index

A

Abuse, as poor-quality care, 149
Academic health centers, collaboration
    with health professionals, 2
Access
    to care for ethnic elders, 37, 168–169
    to health information, 72
    to mental health services in rural areas,
      67
    problems for older adults in rural areas,
      58, 64–67, 69
    and transportation, 168
Activities of daily living (ADLs), 31, 38,
      42, 109, 115, 117, 119, 124, 140,
      146, 239, 244; *see also* Basic
      activities of daily living (BADLs);
      Instrumental activities of daily
      living (IADLs)
Activity directors, 223
Activity theory, in gerontology, 13
Actual diagnoses, 40
Acute care
    conversion of rural facilities to nursing
      home services, 63
    as division of nursing curricula, 7
Adaptation, and caregiving, 135
Adult day care (ADC),
    and ethnic elderly, 172–173
    and respite care, 138, 172–173
    in rural areas, 65, 66
Advanced directives, 247
Advanced nurse practitioners (ANPs), 63,
      71
Advice lines, telephone, 142, 143–144
Affective or personality losses, in cogni-
    tively impaired elders, 109

African-American elders; *see also* Amish
    elders; Asian-American elders;
    Hispanic elders; Italian-American
    elders; Latino elders; Native-
    American elders; Polish-American
    elders
African-American caregivers' systems
    of care, 149
demographics of, 82, 238
and family support, 171
and homelessness, 190
perceptions of health profile, 61
and use of adult day care centers,
    172–173
Age-grading theory, in gerontology, 12
Age stratification, as theory in gerontology,
    14
Ageism, 36
Aging
    biomedicalization of, 22
    positive and negative views of, 22
    rates of biological, 23–24
    trajectories of decline in, 104
Aging Health Policy Center, 188
Aging policies, *see* Policy issues
Aging process, impact of social and
    physical environments on, 38, 57
Agitation, *see* Stress
Aid to Families with Dependent
    Children, 185
AIDS, and homelessness, 184
Alaskan Native elders, 82
Alcohol consumption, and retirement, 27
Alcoholism, and homelessness, 182, 185,
    186, 201, 203, 206
Almshouses, 178, 179, 180
Alzheimer's disease (AD)

Alzheimer's disease (AD) *(continued)*
  cognitive stimulation of patients with, 140–141
  individualized music therapy, 118
  Partners in Care program, 151
  respite care for caregivers of patients with, 139
  social support through ComputerLink project, 71
  study of, by gerontological nurse researchers, 107, 110, 231
  support groups for caregivers of persons with, 144
  symptoms and signs of, 109, 110
  "whole disease care planning," 107
Ambulatory care, outreach programs and, 70–71
American Academy of Nurse Practitioners, 63
American Academy of Nursing, 232
  Expert Panel on Rural Populations, 57
American Association of Colleges of Nursing, 3
American Association of Homes for the Aging, 232
American Association of Retired Persons, 91
American Diabetes Association, 94
American Nurses Association, 7, 58, 63, 72, 86, 226, 232
  House of Delegates, 228
  Rural/Frontier Health Task Force, 57
American Society on Aging, 227
American Writers' Association, 232
Amish elders, 59, 168, 172
Amyotrophic lateral sclerosis (Lou Gehrig's disease), 228
Analytic, theory in gerontology, 14
Ancker Hospital School of Nursing, 216, 218
Andrus Gerontology Center, 226, 228, 232
Anemia, and homeless elders, 192
Anger, felt by family caregiver, 136, 137
Antagonistic pleiotropy theory, in gerontology, 19

Anthropology, and theories in gerontology, 12–13, 33
Anticipatory caregiving, 147
Anxiety
  disorders, and homelessness, 186
  among family caregivers, 137, 141
  and retirement, 27
  and stress thresholds, 110–111, 118
Approach behaviors, and health promotion, 84
Area Agencies on Aging (AAAs), 66
Area Health Education Centers (AHECs), 69, 72
Army Cadet Nurse Corps, 218, 219, 232
Arthritis, chronic, 24, 33, 70, 192, 202
Arthritis Self-Care Project, 70
Asian-American elders, 82
Assisted living facilities, 242, 243, 244
Association for Gerontology in Higher Education, 3
Asthma, and homeless elders, 192, 200
Autonomy
  definition of, for elders, 38
  and housing needs of elders, 38
  parental, and caregiving activities, 147
Avoidance behaviors, and health promotion, 84

B

Baccalaureate programs, and gerontological nursing curriculum, 3
Basic activities of daily living (BADLs), 31
Bathing, intervention strategies for cognitively impaired elders, 119–120
Beck Dressing Performance Scale, 121
Behavior; *see also* Approach behaviors; Avoidance behaviors, Risk behaviors
  of caregivers vs. care recipients, 118–119, 122–123
  patterns, beliefs, and values of older adults, 36
  problems, 141, 148

Behavioral intervention, 119
Behavioral losses, in cognitively impaired
    elders, 109–110
Behavioral management, 106
Belgium Ministry of Public Health and
    the Environment, 103
Beliefs
    of ethnic elders, 157, 161, 169, 173
    of nurses, in shared responsibility for
        care, 173
    of older adults, 36
Biological aging, rates of, 23–24
Biological markers, 24
Biology, and theories in gerontology,
    17–19
Biomarkers, *see* Biological markers
Black elders, *see* African-American elders
Board-and-care homes, 245
Body transcendence, 26
Bowery, New York, 179, 187, 195, 205
Breast screening exams
    effectiveness of self-examinations, 43
    and rural elders, 61
Bronchitis, and homeless elders, 192, 200
Buddhist philosophy, and late-life
    transitions, 22
Burden of care
    for family caregiver, 137, 145, 149
    in home care, 238
    objective vs. subjective, 144
    respite care as form of relief for, 138
Bureau of Health Professionals
    and agenda for health professions
        reform, 2, 5–6, 8
    White Paper Panel of, 1
Burnside, Irene, 213–233; *see also*
        Psychosocial nursing care
    achievements and awards, 231–232
    army nursing days, 218–219
    childhood, 214–216
    college education, 219–222, 228–229
    group work with older adults, 222–225
    international experiences, 229–230
    nurse educator, 227–228, 230–231
    nurse scholar, 225–227, 228–229
    nurses' training, 216–218

C

California Nurses' Association, 232
Cancer, treatment of, and shifting
        caregiver roles, 150
Capitated reimbursement systems, 242
Capping ceremony, 216
Cardiac surgery, and caregiver role, 150
Care
    access to, *see* Access
    acute, *see* Acute care
    burden of, and institutionalization, 238
    of cognitively impaired older adults,
        103–129
    continuum of, 65
    of ethnic elderly, 157–173
    formal vs. informal, 239, 240
    goal-directed, 110
    home, *see* Home care
    individual ethnic biases and, 169–170
    multidisciplinary, 111–113
    nursing home, *see* Nursing home care
    of older adults in the 21st century, 1
    plans, ethnic values and behaviors,
        173
    psychosocial, *see* Psychosocial nursing
        care
    quality of, *see* Quality of care
    shared responsibility for, 173
    universal vs. individual needs, 173
Care planning and management, 142
Care receiver, acute care utilization by,
        and family caregiving, 134
Caregiver burden; *see also* Burden of care
    subjective, experienced by family
        caregivers, 137, 138
    in home care, 238
Caregiver(s); *see also* Family caregiving;
        Home health care; Respite care
    African-American, 148, 149, 172–173
    anger, feelings of, 136, 137, 138
    anger response to incontinence, 138
    anxiety, feelings of, 137, 141
    assessment of health of, 141
    behavior, and impact on care receiver,
        118–119, 122–123

Caregiver(s) *(continued)*
  burden, *see* Burden of care; Caregiver
    burden
  competence, feelings of, 136
  control, sense of, 141, 142
  depression, feelings of, 136, 137, 141,
    145, 149
  emotional distress, disphoria, 137,
    138
  emotional needs, 152
  ethnicity and assessment of, 170
  hostility, feelings of, 137
  individualized education of, 141
  morale of, 144
  mutuality, 142
  negative affect, 137, 138
  nurses as, 146
  problem-solving skills, 136, 145
  quality of life, 141
  respite care, 141, 145
  role of, *see* Caregiving role
  role strain, 142
  social skills, 136
  strain, feelings of, 136, 137, 149
  stress, feelings of, 136, 140, 152
  support program, 141–142
  telephone support for, 143–144
  well-being, 144
Caregiver Load Scale, 147
Caregiver support nurses (CSNs), 141
Caregiving
  abuse, as poor-quality care, 149
  activities, *see* Caregiving activities
  amount of, *see* Caregiving activities
  anticipatory, 147
  conceptual approach to the study of,
    135
  effects on family, 134
  enhancement of, 148
  ethnic biases and, 169–170, 172–173
  for frail older people, 135
  formal care replacing informal care,
    239, 240
  hands-on, 147
  negative response to problems of, 136
  neglect, as poor-quality care, 149

  nurses' contributions to knowledge of,
    135
  nursing interventions related to,
    136–146
  preventive, 147
  processes of, 133, 135
  protective, 147
  quality of care in, 146, 148–149
  research on, 135–136
  role, *see* Caregiving role
  rewards of, 142, 149
  supervisory, 147
  systems of care, 149
  theories related to, 135
  training program, in rural setting, 70
  transitions in care provided, 146,
    149–150
Caregiving activities
  and caregiving role, 146
  categories of, 146–148
  disease progression and transitions in,
    150
  research on, 146–147
  type and amount of, 146–147
Caregiving families; *see also* Family
    caregiver
  nursing support of, 135
Caregiving role
  changes in, 149–150
  experience of, in late life, 29
  meanings of, 147
  nature of, 146, 148
  research on, 146–151
Carondelet St. Mary's Health
    Maintenance Organization, 88
Case management, 67, 140
Case management teams, for homeless
    elders, 206
Case manager(s), 88, 242
Cellular biology, and theories in
    gerontology, 18
Center for Epidemiological Studies-
    Depression Scale (CES-D), 201
Center for Gerontological Training and
    Research, 230
Cerebrovascular disease, 24

Certification of gerontological nurses, 72–73
Certified registered nurse anesthetists (CRNAs), 63
Children, ties with rural elders, 60
Chronic care, as division of nursing curricula, 7
Chronic disabilities in elders
  and costs of health care, 134
  and rehabilitation, 239
Chronic diseases
  of homeless elders, 191, 192
  incidence among poor ethnic elderly, 167
  progression of, and transitions in caregiving, 150
  resource materials for living with, 91
  and self-care, 33
Chronic illness, and family caregivers, 151
Chronological age, 24
Chronologically gifted, 229
Circulatory problems, and homeless elders, 192, 200, 202
Classism, 36
Coalition for the Homeless, 185, 188
Codon fidelity theory, in gerontology, 18
Cognition, and nursing care, 108–110
Cognitive assessment, 105
Cognitive-behavioral therapy, 126–127
Cognitive decline, 108; *see also* Cognitive impairment; Cognitively impaired elders
Cognitive developmental transitions, 22, 25–27
Cognitive disorders
  nursing interventions for older adults with, 103–129
  study of, in nursing curriculum, 3–4
Cognitive functions, improvements in, 104, 108–110, 127, 128, 141
Cognitive impairment, 103
  symptom clusters associated with, 108–109, 110
Cognitive interventions
  with impaired elders, 124–128, 140–141; *see also* Cognitively impaired elders; Interventions

Cognitive psychology, and theories in gerontology, 16–17
Cognitive stimulation, of patients with Alzheimer's disease, 140–141
Cognitively impaired elders
  bathing interventions, 119–120
  cognitive interventions, 124–128, 140–141
  communication strategies with, 113–115
  conceptual foundations of interventions for, 106–111
  context of nursing care for, 107–108
  difficulties in making choices, 109, 117
  dressing interventions, 120–123
  goal-directed care, 110
  group therapy with, 233
  multidisciplinary care for, 111–113
  and nursing care, 103–129
  nursing interventions for, 113–124, 124–128
  nursing research on, 68, 105–106, 128–129
  nutrition and feeding interventions, 115–119
  and peer group support from "health ministers," 71
  physical interventions, 115
  premises governing care of, 107
  progressively lowered stress threshold model (PLST), 106, 110–111, 118
  and relation to network of family and friends, 34
  role of gerontological nurse with, 112, 247
  sleep interventions, 123–124
  and stress thresholds, 110–111, 118
  and trajectories of decline, 104
  and use of quality of life indicators, 34
Collaboration
  between academic health centers and health care providers, 2
  with family caregivers, 151
  among health professionals in home care team, 140

Collaboration *(continued)*
  among interdisciplinary groups of
    active researchers, 242
  among multidisciplinary care team
    members, 113
Comfort measures, in caregiving, 147
Committee on Health Promotion and
    Disease Prevention for the Second
    Fifty, 83
Common sense model (CSM), 33
Communication, intervention strategies
    for cognitively impaired elders,
    113–115, 120
Community-based care
  and homeless elders, 206
  projected growth of, and impact on
    hospitals, 242
  projected need for, in 21st century, 240
  research issues, 242–243
  use of community volunteers in, 70
Community-based long-term care
    (CBLTC); *see also* Community-
    based care; Long-term care
  compared to nursing home care, 243
  as complement to informal caregiving,
    243
  definition of, 243
Community health nurses, 206
Community Mental Health Center Act,
    189
Community nursing centers, 242
Community resources
  of cognitively impaired elders, 107
  of ethnic elderly, 170–173
  mobilization of, 71–72
  Pew Health Professions Commission
    report and, 6
  in rural areas, 66
  use of volunteers, 70
  utilization of, 2, 66
Compensatory skill acquisition theory, in
    gerontology, 17
Competence
  of family caregivers, 136, 141
  and housing satisfaction among elders, 37
  of older adults, 96

Competencies
  critical for nurses, 246
  of gerontological nurses, 247
Computer communication technologies
  and nurses, 68–69
  and support for rural elders, 70–71
ComputerLink, Alzheimer's disease
    patients and, 70
Conative or planning losses, in cognitively
    impaired elders, 109
Conceptual intervention, 119
Congregate living facilities, 245
Congregate meals, in rural areas, 65, 66
Content areas, vital, 3–4
Continuing care—life care facilities, 245
Continuity, as theory in gerontology, 15
Continuous quality improvement (CQI)
    programs, 241
Continuum of care, 65, 69, 204, 242, 244,
    245
Control
  and autonomy, 38
  sense of, among caregivers, 141
Coping, 27
Cornell University, 225
Cost effectiveness
  of health promotion programs, 93
  rural areas, program development, and
    problems of, 240
  and use of complex technology, 6
Costs
  of health care for older people, 134
  of health care, and family caregiving,
    134
  for health promotion programs, 91–94
  of home care, 143, 239
  increases in, due to loss of informal
    care systems, 239
  nursing research on, 242
  in PREP study, 143
Cottage housing, for aging parents, 245
Counseling, as part of posthospital
    support program, 140
County farms, 178
Critical gerontology theory, 12
Cross-linking theory, in gerontology, 18

Cross-training, 241
Crystallized vs. fluid intelligence, as
    theory in gerontology, 16
Cultural affiliation, providing context for
    nursing, 36
Cultural dimension
    as construct of model of environmental
        sphere, 36–37
    and nurses' lack of awareness about
        impact of, 37, 43
    reasons for considering, in gerontologi-
        cal nursing, 36–37
Cultural factors, and definition and status
    of elderly, 36
Cultural heritage, 37, 229
Cultural sensitivity, and Triandis model,
    164
Cultural traditions, sensitivity to, 229
Customary routines, to enhance
    caregiving, 148
Curriculum, *see* Gerontological nursing
    curriculum

D

Day care, adult, *see* Adult day care
Decision making, for ethnic elderly,
    169–170
    subjectivity in clinical assessment and,
        169
Decline, natural trajectories of, 104
Deinstitutionalization, and homelessness,
    185, 189
Demented elders; *see also* Mental health;
    Mental illness
    cognitive stimulation programs with,
        140–141
    and use of quality of life indicators, 34
Dementia
    and family caregiving study, 137
    managing behavior problems in, 148
    and organic brain syndrome, 222
    projections of, among oldest-old, 238
    stages of, and choice of nursing inter-
        ventions, 107–108, 110–111
Demographic trends and projections

changes in, and implications for long-
    term nursing care, 237–241
of frail and institutionalized elderly,
    240
of numbers of older adults, 59–60, 82,
    238
of RNs, 62–63
of rural elders, 59–60
of rural RNs, 62–63
Dental care, annual checkups and rural
    elders, 61
Dental problems, and homeless elders,
    192, 200, 202
Dental screenings, 88
Denver Free-Net, 72
Department of Health and Human
    Services, 2, 103
Department of Housing and Urban
    Development, 181, 182, 185, 188,
    204
Department of Social Service, 188
Dependency, *see* Functional dependency
Depression
    in family caregiving, 136, 137, 141,
        142, 145, 149
    and homelessness, 186–187, 201, 203
    and retirement, 27
    in rural elders, 61
Developmental
    issues in aging, 25–27
    perspective on aging, 26
    responses to late-life transitions, 31
Dexterity in older adults, diminished, 224
Diabetes, 24, 191, 192
Diagnoses
    in context of late-life transitions, 41
    definition of, 40
    as knowledge domain in model of nurs-
        ing sphere, 20, 40–41
    as one of three categories of nursing,
        40
    sociocultural variables influencing,
        169–170
Diagnosis related groupings (DRGs), 140
Dialectical gerontology theory, 12
Diet, *see* Nutrition

Diets, high-fiber and low-fat, among rural elders, 61
Dimensions in model of environmental sphere, 35–40; *see also* Social dimension; Cultural dimension; Physical dimension; Spiritual dimension
Diphtheria, 217
Disability
  chronic, and rehabilitation, 239
  effects of, on elderly, 239
  functional status as measure of, 31
  incidence among poor ethnic elderly, 167
Disabled elders
  and community-based long-term care, 243
  and reliance on informal care, 239
Disease prevention
  as distinguished from disease prevention, 84
  as division of nursing curricula, 7
  and homelessness, 191
  increased emphasis on, and demand for nursing professionals, 241
  in Pew Health Professions Commission report, 6
  priorities for, 84–85
  and self-care, 32–33
Disengagement theory, in gerontology, 13, 25
Disorders, *see* Cognitive disorders; Psychiatric disorders
Divergent thinking decline, as theory in gerontology, 17
Double jeopardy hypothesis, in gerontology, 13
Dressing, intervention strategies for cognitively impaired elders, 120–123
Drinking problems, *see* Alcoholism
Drug abuse, and homelessness, 182, 185, 186, 206
Duke Multidimensional Functional Assessment: OARS Methodology, 198
Duke-UNC Health Profile, 198

Duke University, 4
Dysdifferentiation theory, in gerontology, 18

E

East Tennessee State University, 71
Education, among rural elders, 60
Ego development in late life, 25
Ego transcendence, as late-life phenomenon, 25
Elder abuse, Phillips and Rempusheski's model for, 165
Elder care
  and cognitive impairment, 103–129
  competence, right of self-determination and, 96
  continuum of care, 65
  cost of, 134
  development of nursing curricular content regarding, 4, 7, 8
  ethnic identity as issue in, 157
  facilities for, 245
  family as major provider of, 134
  family values and effect on, 172
  interdisciplinary education for, 3
  issues and challenges for the 21st century, 237–247
  nurses' strategic role in, 241
  skin color as variable influencing, 166
  state board examinations and, 3
  telephone support in, 143–144
  use of informal resources, 65
  use of wellness/health promotion center, 94–96
  viewed as phase in continuum of life, 8
Elder sphere, in Iowa conceptual model, 20, 22–35
Elderly; *see also* Demographic trends and projections; Disabled elders; Female elders; Frail elders; Homeless elders; Impaired elders; Minority elders; Poor elders; Rural elders; *and specific nationalities*
  common health problems of, 192

cost of health care for, 134
who do not want to be well, 95–96
Emergency Food and Shelter Program,
181, 182
Emergency medical technicians (EMTs),
72
Emotional disorders; *see also* Mental
health; Mental illness
homelessness as risk factor for, 186
Emotional support, 29; *see also* Social
support
Emphysema, and homeless elders, 192,
200, 202
Enculturation, 36
Enrichment processes, in caregiving, 148
Environment; *see also* Physical environment; Social environment
controlled, for cognitively impaired
elders, 108, 110–111
impact of, on health, 35
impact of, on meal-taking, 116–117,
118
and processes of gerotranscendence, 37
Environmental safety and elders, *see*
Safety
Environmental sphere, in Iowa conceptual
model, 20, 35–40
Ergonomic design, and functional
capacity in elders, 38
Error (catastrophe) theory, in gerontology,
19
Ethel Percy Andrus Gerontology Center,
226; *see also* Andrus Gerontology
Center
Ethical tradition, and competent adults,
96
Ethnic affiliation, of elders, 36
Ethnic background vs. race, 166
Ethnic bias, in clinical decision making,
169
Ethnic elderly
access to care and , 168–169
beliefs, values, and impact on care,
169–170, 170–173
and care issues, 157, 167–173
decision making and, 169–170

and disparities in health care, 168–169,
169–170
family and community support for,
170–173
gaps in care for, 172
and health care services, 37
influence of personal perceptions on
study of, 164
and poverty, 167
problems in comparing studies of, 162,
165–167
state of knowledge about, 162–167
Ethnic groups, vs. term "race," 159
Ethnic identity
definition of, 157
and elder care 157, 165
maintenance of, among elders, 160
Ethnicity
in clinical decision making, 1669–170
confounding aspects of comparing
"ethnic" studies, 165–167
definition of, 158, 161–162
elder care issues related to, 157–158,
165
in gerontological research, 157–173
Identificational Ethnicity Scale (IES),
158, 161–162
inconsistency in use of term, 157–158,
165
in relation to definition of health and
wellness, 83
self-declared, 157
symbolic, 162
Examinations, *see* Physical examinations
and screenings; State board
examinations
Exchange theory, in gerontology, 12
Exercise; *see also* Physical activity
and health self-care behavior of elders,
33
marketing of, to older adults, 97
promotion, as nursing intervention, 42
and retirement, 27
among rural elders, 61
Expanded home health nursing intervention, PREP, 142

Expert schema theory, in gerontology, 17
Explanatory model (EM), 33

F

Facilities for elder care, 245
Faculty, *see* Nursing faculty
Families
  and care of cognitively impaired
    elderly, 107
  and care of ethnic elderly, 170–173
  caregiving and, 70, 133–152, 238
  size of, and formal care services, 240
Family caregiver; *see also* Caregiver(s);
    Caregiving; Families
  availability of, 238–239
  and community-based long-term care,
    243
  and cost of health care for elders, 134
  and delivery of care, 146
  estimates of level of assistance of, 134
  ethnicity and, 170–173
  health services interventions, 139–140,
    145
  and homeless elders, 194–195, 202, 203
  in-home nursing interventions,
    140–143, 143–145
  interaction with nurses, 133
  nurses' support of, 152, 241
  nursing interventions with, 133,
    136–146
  partnerships with, 151
  preparation of, 134
  psychoeducational interventions,
    136–138, 145
  respite care intervention, 138–139, 145
  satisfaction of, as outcome variable,
    139, 140
  stress, 140
  support group intervention, 144, 145
  telephone interventions, 143–144, 145
  tolerance of burden of care and institu-
    tionalization, 238
  transitional care intervention, 143, 145
Family caregiving; *see also* Caregiving
  families

  as major source of long-term care for
    older people, 134
  nature of role of, 133–152
  processes, 133
Family consultant, 139
Family homes, 244
Family network, 30
Family roles, changes in, 27, 28–29
Family support systems, 173; *see also*
    Caregiving families; Ethnic elderly;
    Family caregiver; Social support
Family ties, rural elders and, 60
Fatigue, effect of reminiscence groups on,
    229
Federal Emergency Management Agency
    (FEMA), 181, 182
Female elders
  functional dependency, 31–32
  and homelessness, 190, 194
  reminiscence group work with, 229
  and retirement, 27–29
Feminist theory, and caregiving, 135
Flophouses, 180, 187
Formal care, *see* Care; Caregiver(s);
    Caregiving; Informal care
Foster care of the elderly, 226, 244
Frail elders
  caregiving for, 135, 151
  and community-based long-term care,
    243
  and peer support from "health
    ministers," 71
  projected number of, 240
  use of telephone support systems with,
    143–144
Free-radical accumulation theory, in
    gerontology, 18
Friends network, 30
Functional ability
  and late-life illness, 24
  and nursing outcomes, 44
  in relation to definition of health and
    wellness, 83
  of rural elders, 60
Functional capability (or capacity)
  biomarkers as predictors of, 24

and changes in social role, 29
and choice of nursing interventions, 107
effect of environmental forces on, 36–37
effect of physical environment on, 37–38
ergonomic design and reduced, 38
maintenance of, as goal for health care of elderly, 83, 85
and normative biological involution, 23
Functional dependency
distribution and determinants of, 32
duration of, 31
prevalence of, 31
rates of, for women, 31–32
Functional health, definition of, 31
Functional impairment
projections of, among oldest-old, 239
Functional independence, 38, 85, 241
Functional reserve, 23
Functional status
and health, 20, 31–32
as measure of disability, 31
as nursing outcome variable, 43, 139
Fundamental Interpersonal Relations Orientation (FIRO) method, 224
Future, of gerontological nursing, 1–9, 230–231

G

Gender; *see also* Female elders
and differences in social role experiences, 27
Generalized slowing hypothesis, as theory in gerontology, 16
Generativity, 26
Genetic clock, *see* Hayflick limit
Geriatric care, delivery in the community, 3
Geriatric nurse practitioner, *see* Gerontololological nurse practitioner
Geriatric scholarship, summary of early, 226
Gerontic nursing institutes, 98–99

Gerontological clinical specialist (GCS), 88
Gerontological nurse practitioner (GNP)
and ANA resolutions regarding educational preparation of, 228
certification topics for, 72–73
competencies of, 247
nurse-managed care of elderly persons, 247
and opportunities in wellness/health promotion center, 88
primary care skills needed by, 240
projected demand for, 240–241
recommendations of Pew Health Professions Commission, 2, 6
rise of, 231
training for care of rural elders, 71–72
and use of theory in nursing care, 20
Gerontological nursing
enrollment problems in, 4–5, 6–7
future for, 1–9, 230–231
graduate education in, 4–5
Iowa conceptual model of, 11–44
issues and challenges for 21st century, 237–247
and provision of primary care, 3
scope of, 20
Gerontological nursing curriculum
at baccalaureate level, 3, 7–8
consequences of past and present educational practices, 4–5
critical competencies to be stressed, 267–247
and effect on care of older adults, 3
gerontic nursing institutes and, 98
gerontological curricular thread, 8
at graduate level, 4
implications of increased demand for long-term care, 240
lack of prepared faculty to teach, 3, 4, 5, 230
lack of support for inclusion of, 4
national standards for, 3, 4
recommended changes in, 6–8
research regarding, 4–5
rural health practicums, 72

Gerontological nursing curriculum
    (continued)
    rural issues, 69
    teaching strategies for, 3, 6
    vital content areas in, 3–4
Gerontological nursing leaders, strategies
        used by, 227
Gerontological nursing research; *see also*
        Nursing research
    gerontic nursing institutes and, 98
    in health promotion, 96–97
    quality and quantity of, 5
    review of, 4–5
    and rural issues, 67–69
    and scarcity of graduate programs, 4–5
    summary of early, 226
    theory development in, 11
    theory-based, 11, 20
Gerontological Society of America, 232,
        242
Gerontology, major theoretical
        perspectives in, 11–20
Gerontology-prepared faculty
    as resource persons, 8
    service on state board agencies, 8
    shortage of, 2, 3, 4, 5, 7, 230
    team teaching and, 8
    training of, 7
    and training of future researchers, 3, 4, 5
Geropsychiatric nursing, 213, 214, 218,
        227
Gerotranscendence
    effect of environmental forces on, 37
    facilitating in elders through life review,
        42
    as late-life phenomenon, 25–27
GI Bill, 219
Glaucoma, and homeless elders, 192
Government Printing Office, and
        resources for health promotion
        programs, 91
Great Depression, 179, 214
Group homes, 245
Group work with the elderly, *see*
        Psychosocial nursing care;
        Psychosocial interventions

H

Hands-on caregiving, 147
Happiness, as indicator of quality of life,
        34
Hartford Foundation, John A., 103
Hayflick limit (genetic clock) theory, in
        gerontology, 19
Health
    as construct in model of elder sphere,
        30–35
    definition of, 82–83
    of ethnic elderly, and poverty, 167
    functional, definition of, 31
    impact of environment on, 35
    mental, *see* Mental health
    as part of wellness, 82–83
    as process and outcome, in elder
        sphere, 30–35
    rural conceptualizations of, 61–62
    and social support, 29–30
Health behavior, 20, 32–33, 43, 167
Health care; *see also* Care; Rural health
        care
    access problems, 58, 64
    changes in, and implications for
        nursing care, 241–247
    delivery, *see* Health care delivery
        systems
    disparities in, 168
    impact of oldest-old on, 239
    new focus of, 58
    reform of, *see* Health care reform
    reimbursement issues, 64, 91
    self-care, 32–33
    service integration, 242
    telephone support in, 143–144
    use of informal resources, 65
Health care costs, *see* Costs
Health care delivery systems
    changes in, 58, 242
    goals of, 242
Health Care for the Homeless Project,
        191
Health care professionals
    as multidisciplinary team, 111–113

projected needs for, in 21st century, 1, 2, 5–6, 240
Health care reform; *see also* Reform
  and family caregivers, 151
  and financing of health promotion, 98
  implications for nursing care, 241–247
  issues related to, 98
Health care utilization
  among ethnic elders, 37
  as outcome variable, 139
Health education, 84
Health habits, 33
Health maintenance organizations (HMOs)
  Carondelet St. Mary's Health Maintenance Organization, 88
  nursing health maintenance organizations, 242
Health maintenance services, 86, 88
  cost-effectiveness of, 93
Health ministers, 71
Health outcomes, *see* Outcomes
Health potential, 84
Health practices, frequency among elders of positive, 61
Health profile, differences between rural and urban elders, 60–61
Health promotion; *see also* Disease prevention; Health; Wellness; Wellness program services
  definition of, 84
  in definition of health and wellness, 83
  as distinguished from disease prevention, 84
  as division of nursing curricula, 7
  gerontic nursing institutes and, 98–99
  gerontological nurse and, 247
  and homelessness, 191
  increased emphasis on, and demand for nursing professionals, 241
  marketing of, 97
  Pew Health Professions Commission report and, 6
  and preventive health, 97
  priorities for, 84–85
  reimbursement systems and, 91

research in, 96–97
resources materials for, 91–92
role in enhancing health of older adults, 81–99
and self-care, 32–33
Health promotion programs, for older adults
  calendar of, 94, 95
  cost-effectiveness of, 93
  costs of, 91–94
  elements of, 84–85
  models of, 85–86
  personnel needs for, 88, 90, 92
  priorities of, 86–87
  services offered, 87–88, 89
  strategies for organization of, 86–87
  types of, 88, 89, 94
  use of, by older adults, 94–96
  wellness services in, 89
Health promotion strategies, marketing of, 97
Health screening/health protection services, 33, 42, 87–88
Health self-care, 32–33
Health services interventions with caregiving families, 139–140, 145
Healthwise Program, 86
Healthy Lifestyles for Seniors program, 33, 86
Hearing
  impairment, and late-life illness, 24
  screenings, 88
Heart
  disease, and late-life illness, 24
  problems, and homeless elders, 192, 200
Hermeneutic gerontology theory, 12
High blood pressure, and homeless elders, 191, 200
Hispanic elders, 59, 82, 171, 190
HIV-related illness, and homelessness, 184
Home Health Agencies, 242
Home health care
  community-based long-term care, 243
  increasing need for, 241–242, 244
  reducing need for, 244

Home health care *(continued)*
  residential care models, 244
  rural vs. urban use of home-based
    services, 66
  transition from hospital, 149–150
  use of community volunteers in, 70
Home health nurses, and family care-
    givers, 134, 142–143
Home health nursing intervention, PREP,
    142
Home ownership, rural elders and, 60
Home-based services, *see* Home health
    care
Homeless elders
  average age of death, 191
  emergency rooms and identification of,
    205
  health care professionals' sensitivity to,
    205, 206
  health problems of, 191–193, 200–201
  housing options, 203–207
  interventions with, 203–207
  numbers of, 188–189
  profile of, 189–191
  in rural communities, 193–194
  social supports and, 194–195, 201–202
  use of single room occupancy (SRO)
    hotels, 180
Homeless persons
  definition of, 183–184, 187
  demographics of, 184–187
  mental illness among, 186–187
  from rural areas, 187–188
  social relationships among, 195
Homelessness
  estimated extent of, 185–186
  factors contributing to, 185, 189, 190,
    203–204
  history of, 178–183
  Interagency Council of the Homeless,
    181
  McKinney Homeless Assistance Act, 181
  and mental illness, 182, 184, 186–187,
    189, 190, 196, 201, 203, 206
  methodological issues in studying,
    187–188, 203–204

as risk factor for emotional disorder,
    186–187
  and social support, 180, 181, 185, 189,
    190, 192, 193, 194–195, 196,
    201–202, 205
  solutions to, 204–207
  vulnerability to, 184–185
Hospice and palliative care services, 245
Hospitals
  closures, 67, 189
  conversion to nursing homes, 63
  cost containment measures of, and
    resulting growth of home health care,
    241–242
  discharges and days of care in, for
    elderly, 30, 134
  and homelessness, 189
  impact of increased community-based
    care on, 242
  integration of acute and chronic
    services, 242
  in rural communities, 66–67
  space for wellness centers for elders,
    92
Hospitalization
  availability of social support on
    duration of, 30
  after in-home health services, 139
  transition to home health care, 149–150
Hostility, among family caregivers, 137
House Subcommittee on Health and the
    Environment, 190, 191
Housing
  emergency or temporary shelters as,
    204–205
  facilities for elder care, 245
  impact on function and well-being in
    late life, 37–38
  lack of affordable, and homelessness,
    184, 185, 189
  objective vs. subjective reasons for
    elders to remain in home, 38
  in rural communities and homelessness,
    193–194
  satisfaction, in elders, 37–38
  shelters, for homeless adults, 204–207

Housing Assistance Council (HAC), 187, 193
Housing Enterprise for the Less Privileged (HELP), 204
Housing Risks of the Elderly Project, 190
HUD, *see* Department of Housing and Urban Development
Human factors method, 38
Hydrotherapy, 218
Hypertension, 24, 192

I

Identificational Ethnicity Scale (IES), 158, 161–162
Illness behaviors, 33
Illness representation models, 33
Immunologic theory, in gerontology, 18
Immunizations, 88
Impaired elders
  caregiving of, 133
  categories of caregiving activities for, 147
  numbers of, 239
Incentives for being well, lack of, 91
Income, differences among rural and urban elders, 60
Incompetence
  parental, and caregiving activities, 147
  and right of self-determination, 95
Incontinence
  among homeless elders, 200, 202
  and management of anger response in family caregiver, 138
  study of, by gerontological nurse researchers, 231
Individualized caregiver education, 141
Informal care, reliance of disabled elderly on, 239
Informal resources, of elder care, 65, 238
Information and referral services, 65
Information loss model, in gerontology, 16
Information technology
  ComputerLink project and Alzheimer's disease patients, 71

Denver Free-Net and access to health information, 72
Medical College of Georgia Telemedicine Project, 72
in nursing education, 6, 72
and professional competence, 6, 72
use by rural health professionals, 68–69
In-home care, 65, 70; *see also* Home care
In-home nursing, 140–143
In-home nursing interventions, with caregiving families, 140–143, 145
In-home respite, 138
Injury, ergonomic design and reduced functional ability, 38
Innovative routine breakers, to enhance caregiving, 148
Institute of Medicine, and definitions of health and wellness, 83
Institutionalization of elderly adults
  caregiver's tolerance of burden of care and, 238
  in ethnic communities, 172
  projections regarding, 240
Instrumental activities of daily living (IADLs), 31, 140, 146, 239
Instrumental care, 147
Insurance, effect of lack of, 67, 168, 190
Intellectual losses, in cognitively impaired elders, 109
Interagency Council of the Homeless, 181
Interdisciplinary home care team, 139
Intermediate care facilities (ICFs), in rural areas, 67
Interventions
  areas of, 42–43
  behavioral, 119
  with caregiving families, 133, 136–146, 150
  with cognitively impaired elders, 113–124, 124–128
  conceptual, 119
  distinctions among several interventions, 145–146
  home-based, 140–143
  with homeless older adults, 204–207

Interventions *(continued)*
  individual vs. group, with family caregivers, 137–138
  late-life transitions, well-being and, 20
  and nursing diagnoses, 40
  as nursing knowledge domain in model of nursing sphere, 40, 41–43
  and nursing outcomes, 41
  in nursing sphere, 20, 40, 41–43, 44
  primary and secondary, and older adults, 239
  progressively lowered stress threshold model (PLST), 106, 110–111, 118
  settings of care and, 107, 112
  sociocultural variables influencing, 169–170
  and trajectories of decline, 104
  during transitions in caregiving, 150
Introjectivity, 26
Iowa conceptual model, of gerontological nursing, 11–44
Iron lungs, 217
Isolation
  and late-life illness, 24–25
  physical and psychiatric, 224
  of psychiatric patients, 223, 224
  and social support transitions, 29
  and telecommunication technologies, 68–69
Italian-American elders, 158, 163, 163

K

Keep-in-Touch system, 142
Kellogg Foundation, 4, 103
Kidney disease, and homeless elders, 200

L

Late-life development
  and cultural dimension of environmental sphere, 36
  and physical dimension of environmental sphere, 37–38
  and social dimension of environmental sphere, 36

Late-life events, as transitions, 22
Late-life illness and comorbidity, 22, 24–25
Late-life phenomena, ego transcendence as, 25
Late-life transitions, 20
  categories of, 22–23
  as construct in model of elder sphere, 22–30
  health as developmental response to, 30–31
  and nursing diagnoses, 41
  nursing interventions for, 42
  and nursing-sensitive client outcomes, 43–44
Latino elders, 171
LaVeist model, of race, 164
Legal tradition, and competent adults, 96
Leisure activity, as source of identity in late life, 28
Levels of processing model, in gerontology, 17
Licensed practical nurses (LPNs), 241
Life course
  as interpretation of biopsychosocial phenomena, 20
  as theory in gerontology, 14, 20
Life satisfaction
  effect of reminiscence groups on, 229
  and gerotranscendence, 25
  and health, 20
  as indicator of quality of life, 34
  and retirement, 27
Life-span transitions, as theory in gerontology, 15
Lifestyle
  elderly who do not want to be well, 95–96, 247
  focus on, rather than disease, 95
  health practices, self-esteem, and social support, 86
  and health promotion, 32–33, 84, 87, 88, 98
  of homeless elders, 191, 192
  impact of social and physical environments on, 57

legal and ethical traditions related to, 96

and nursing interventions, 42

policy issues, health promotion and, 99

and quality of life for older adults, 83

teaching of, at senior nutrition centers, 86

unhealthy, 247

Lipofuscin (age pigment) accumulation theory, in gerontology, 18

Long-term care; *see also* Community-based care

assisted living, 242

in continuum of care, 65

counterparts in other countries, 229–230

factors related to effective services in rural communities, 64–65

marketing strategies for, 245

projections regarding need for, 239–241

reimbursement issues, 245

research issues, 242–243

residential care model, 244

service integration, 242

subacute care, 242

Long-term care facilities (LTCs)

and care of cognitively impaired elders, 106

and ethnic elderly, 172

and space for wellness centers for elderly, 92

Losses, in cognitively impaired elders, 108–110

Lou Gehrig's disease, 228

M

Mammograms

reimbursement for, through Medicare, 91

and rural elders, 61

waiver of fees for, 91

Mammography, 88

Managed care, 151, 242

Management of pain, *see* Pain

Marketing

of health promotion strategies, 97

to improve provision of long-term care, 245

McKinney Homeless Assistance Act, 181, 182

McKinney programs, 182

Meals-on-Wheels, 65

Medicaid, 172, 173, 189, 190, 191, 199, 242

Medical College of Georgia Telemedicine Project, 72

Medical University of South Carolina, 228

Medicare, 91, 242, 245, 134

Mental health

access to services in rural areas, 67

and curriculum content areas, 3–4

dementia, 222

and health promotion services, 88, 89

Ohio Department of Mental Health study, 193

organic brain syndrome, 222

problems, and late-life illness, 24–25

psychiatric treatment during the 1940s, 218, 223

and retirement, 27

of rural elders, 61, 68

services in wellness program, 89

themes of behavioral responses to, 222

Mental illness

and almshouses, 179, 180

and homelessness, *see* Homelessness

Mental status, 140

Mentally disabled, and entitlements, 189

Mentally ill, and shelters, 180

Methodological issues, in studying homelessness, 187–188

Minority, definition of, 158, 160–161

Minority elders

confusion related to group classification of, 166

definition of, 161

demographic projections of, 82

and effects of inequality and discrimination, 161

and ethnic neighborhoods, 160

Minority elders *(continued)*
  health promotion research regarding, 97
  and homelessness, 190, 194
  and maintenance of ethnic identity, 160
  need for health care providers for, 6
  rural residency and poverty among, 240
Minority nurses, need for increased numbers of, 2, 6, 240
Mobility in older adults, limited, 224
Models
  of gerontological nursing, 21
  of health promotion programs, 85–86
  of residential care facilities, 244
  of wellness, health promotion centers, 85–86
Modernization theory, in gerontology, 12
Modified Mini-Mental State Exam, 126
Molecular/genetic biology, and theories in gerontology, 18–19
Monitoring, of transitions, 145
Montana State University, 72
Moral reasoning, as theory in gerontology, 15
Morale of caregivers, 144
Morale, as indicator of quality of life, 34
Morbidity, effects of, on elderly, 239
Multidisciplinary care, 111–113
Multigenerational habitats, 245
Multipurpose or mixed-use facilities, 245
Musculoskeletal impairment, and late-life illness, 24, 42
Museum of the City of New York, 178
Mutality, 142

N

Napa State Hospital, 221
National Institute on Aging, 2, 6
National Institutes of Health, 2
National League for Nursing, 232
  and gerontological nursing curricular standards, 4, 8
National Resource Center for Rural Elderly, 189
National Rural Health Association, 69

National Survey of Personal Health Practices and Consequences, 195
Native-American elders, 82
Neglect, as poor-quality care, 149
Neo-Freudian social theorists, in gerontology, 14
Network
  family vs. friends, 30
  qualitative dimensions of, 29
  quantitative dimensions of, 29
  social, *see* Social network
Networking, by and among rural health care providers, 62, 64, 68–69
Neuroendocrine theory, in gerontology, 17
New Deal reforms, and homeless people, 180
New Mexico Statewide Health Promotion with Elders project, 33, 86
New York Bowery, *see* Bowery
Nonmetropolitan, *see* Rural
Normative biological involution, 22, 23–24
North American Nursing Diagnosis Association, 41
Nurse anesthetists, *see* Certified registered nurse anesthetists
Nurse educator, Irene Burnside as, 216, 227–228
Nurse practitioners; *see also* Gerontological nurse practitioner
  need for increased numbers of, 2–3
  role in rural health care, 63
Nurse researchers; *see also* Nursing research
  contributions to knowledge about caregiving, 135
Nurse scientists
  mentor programs, 69
  and rural health and nursing practice, 62, 67–69
  scholarship of Irene Burnside 213, 225–227
Nurse-managed care, 247
Nurse-managed clinics, in rural communities, 69

Nurses; *see also* Gerontological nurse practitioners; Licensed practical nurses; Registered nurses
and care of ethnic elderly, 173
as case managers, 242
critical competencies of, 246
as part of multidisciplinary team, 111–113
as skilled caregivers, 146
Nurses' training
capping ceremony, 216
during 1940s, 216–218
Nursing, geropsychiatric, *see* Geropsychiatric nursing
Nursing Approaches to Quality Care for the Elderly module series, 72–73
Nursing assistants (NAs), 241
Nursing centers, 69; *see also* Nurse-managed clinics
Nursing curriculum, *see* Gerontological nursing curriculum; Nursing education
Nursing diagnosis, *see* Diagnoses
Nursing education; *see also* Gerontological nursing curriculum
consequences of past and present practices, 4–5
critical competencies to be stressed, 267–247
implications of increased demand for long-term care, 241
recommendations for changes in, 2, 3, 5–6, 6–8
for rural nurses, 62–63
stimulating interest in health care of elders, 227, 230–231, 247
stimulating interest in health care of rural elders, 69
structure of nursing curricula, 7–8
Nursing faculty; *see also* Gerontology-prepared faculty
collaboration among, 7, 8
new models of practice for, 71
Nursing health maintenance organizations, 242
Nursing history, geropsychiatric, 214

Nursing home admissions, after in-home health services, 139
Nursing home care, 65
compared to community-based long-term care, 243
family caregivers as partners with nursing staff, 151
geropsychiatric, 223–225, 226
and health promotion strategies, 96
projected number of elderly needing, 240
projections regarding demand for, 240
nurse practitioners and, 240–241
resident outcomes and quality of, 241
Nursing homes
availability of beds in rural areas, 66–67
caregiving roles in, 151
and convalescent hospitals, 223
job satisfaction and retention in, 246
labor costs in, 245
number of, 245
numbers of impaired elderly in, 239, 245
patient turnover, 246
productivity, profits, and cross-training, 241
projected personnel needs, 240–241
reimbursement and its effect on, 245
reimbursement issues and growth of alternative care facilities, 244
rural, 66–67
staff, and family caregivers relationship to, 151
staff diversity, 240
staff turnover, 246
unionization in, 246
Nursing interventions, *see* Interventions
Nursing outcomes, *see* Outcomes
Nursing research
on caregiving activities, 146–148
of caregiving for older people, 135–136, 146–151
of caregiving role, 146–151
on cognitively impaired elders, 68, 105–106, 108–109, 110–111, 128–129

Nursing research *(continued)*
of community-based long-term care
service systems, 242–243
in geropsychiatry, 225–228
in health promotion for older adults,
96–97
on homelessness, 187–188, 196–207
on impact of environmental forces on
elders, 35, 37, 38, 43
and interdisciplinary collaboration, 242
on policy issues, 242
qualitative and quantitative methods, 30
of reimbursement issues and practices,
242
on rural gerontological nursing practice,
67–69
on self-care of elders, 32–33
on social support, 29–30
on stress thresholds, 110–111, 118
Nursing sphere
in Iowa conceptual model, 20, 40–44
three nursing knowledge domains of, 40
Nursing systems
counseling, as nursing intervention, 42
as division of nursing curricula, 7
and gerontology-prepared nursing
faculty, 7, 8
and health self-care behavior of elders,
33
nutrition centers for seniors, 86
risk behaviors and, 85
among rural elders, 61
Nutrition
aging and altered metabolic
requirements, 115
centers, for seniors, 86
and feeding interventions, 115–119
and feeding problems, 116
Santa Monica City Senior Nutrition
and Recreation Program, 86
teaching of, and lifestyle, 86

O

Objective burden, *see* Burden of care;
Caregiver burden

Objective functional status, and
definitions of health for elders, 31
Ohio Coalition for the Homeless, 193
Ohio Department of Mental Health
study, 193
Older homeless adult, *see* Homeless elders
Oldest-old
demographic projections of, 82, 238
health promotion research regarding, 97
and homelessness, 191
impact of numbers of, on health care
system, 239–240
projections regarding functional
impairment among, 239
in rural areas, compared to urban, 60
Omnibus Budget Reconciliation Acts of
1987 (OBRA '87), 96
On Lok Senior Health Services, 85
On-call help, 140
One-to-one therapy, *see* Psychosocial
nursing care
Organic brain syndrome, 222
Outcomes
as domain of nursing knowledge in
model of nursing sphere, 20, 40,
43–44
elders' beliefs and values in relation to,
168
functional status, health behavior, and
well-being, 43
of interventions with cognitively
impaired elders, 128–129
and late-life transitions, 43–44
nursing-sensitive, 43
Outreach programs, for rural elders, 71
Outpatient visits, after in-home health
services, 140

P

Pain,
decreases in, 70
management of, 148
Parkinson's disease
assistance in moving in, 148
Denver Free-Net and, 72

Parkinson's Spouses Study, 150
Partners in Care, 151
Partnerships, with family caregivers, 151
Patient functioning, 140
Patients
    with chronic mental illness, and
        homelessness, 189
    cognitive stimulation of, 140–141
    early discharge of, and home health
        care, 241
    isolation and withdrawal, 223, 224
    psychiatric treatment during 1940s, 218,
        223
    sense of history, 224
    sensitivity to cultural heritage and
        traditions, 229
    turnover rates in health care facilities,
        246
Person–environment
    interactions, 22
    phenomena, 20
Person/environment fit, in gerontology,
    13, 37
Personality development, and theories in
    gerontology, 14–15
Personality dimensions, and theories in
    gerontology, 15–16
    traits, 15–16
    types, 16
Pew Health Professions Commission
    assessment of need for primary care
        nurse practitioners, 2
    recommendations regarding nursing in
        the 21st century, 6, 8
Phillip Institute, 228
Philosophy, and theories in gerontology,
    12
Physical activity; *see also* Exercise
    as key ingredient to healthy aging, 85
Physical care, interventions, 115
Physical dimension, as construct of
        model of environmental sphere,
        37–38
Physical environment
    in definition of health promotion, 84
    design of, and functional capacity, 38

elders' need for autonomy vs. need for
        security, 38
    and health maintenance/promotion
        services, 88, 89
    impact on function and well-being in
        late life, 37
    impact on rural elders, 57
    modifying, by caregivers, 150
    and nurses' lack of awareness about
        impact of, 37, 43
    as part of treatment, 221
    of residential care facilities, 244
    respect for, Burnside and, 216, 220
Physical examinations and screenings
    gender-specific services, 89
    and health promotion services, 42,
        87–88, 89
    among rural elders, 61
Physical fitness; *see also* Exercise;
        Functional ability
    marketing of, to older adults, 97
Physically impaired elders, role of
        gerontological nurse with, 247
Physician-assisted suicide, 247
Plan of care, and ethnic values, 173
Policy issues, related to care of older adults
    with cognitive impairment, 103–129
    ethnic elderly and, 166–167
    health promotion research and, 99
    homelessness and, 206
    life trajectories and, 36
    replacement of informal care by formal
        care, 239
    research on, 242
    wellness, 98
Policy making
    and care of cognitively impaired older
        adults, 104
    legislation empowering nurses to fulfill
        responsibilities, 112
    and wellness issues of older adults, 98,
        99
Policymakers; *see also* Policy issues
    family caregiving, health care costs and,
        134
    and homelessness, 180

Polio epidemic, 217
Polish-American elders, 158, 163, 171
Poor elders, 60, 189, 190, 195; *see also*
    Homeless elders
  use of single room occupancy (SRO)
    hotels, 180
Poorhouses, 178
Population increases, among older adults,
    see Demographic trends and
    projections
Posthospital support program, 140
Poverty
  confounding effects on older adults, 67
  ethnic elderly and, 167
  and homelessness, 178, 180, 182, 184,
    185, 189, 190, 193, 195
  and oldest-old, 240
  and rural minority elders, 240
  and rural residency, 240
Practitioner programs, call for increased
    numbers of, 2
PREP pilot study, 142
PREP system of nursing interventions,
    142–143
Preparedness, Enrichment, and
    Predictability (PREP) in caregiving
    situations, 142
Prevention; *see also* Disease prevention
  capitated reimbursement systems and,
    242
  health screenings and health promotion
    services, 87–88
  preventive caregiving, 147
  primary and secondary interventions
    for, 239
Preventive caregiving, 147
Problem-solving skills, *see* Caregiver
Protective caregiving, 147
Prime Time Seniors, 86
Primary care centers, and need for geron-
    tologically prepared nurses, 3
Primary care nursing programs
  and gerontological nursing content, 7
  recommendations for changes in, 6–8
Primary care nursing workforce, recom-
    mendations for changes in, 2, 6

Primary care services
  capitated reimbursement systems and,
    242
  as objective in health promotion
    programs, 86
Primary care skills, needed by GNPs, 241
Privacy, and older adults, 121
Probies, 216, 217
Problem-solving skills, of family
    caregivers, 136
Processing deficit model, in gerontology,
    17
Productivity, and cross-training in nursing
    homes, 241
Progressively lowered stress threshold
    model (PLST), 106, 110–111, 118
Project Rescue, 205
Psychiatric disorders
  study of, in nursing curriculum, 3–4
  treatment of, during the 1940s, 218
Psychiatric nursing
  American Nurses Association position
    paper on, 226
  during the 1940s, 218
Psychoeducational nursing interventions,
    145
Psychology, and theories in gerontology,
    14–17, 33
Psychosocial care, *see* Psychosocial
    nursing care
Psychosocial group work, 230; *see also*
    Psychosocial nursing care
Psychosocial interventions
  with caregiving families, 136–138
  during the 1940s, 218
  psychotropic drugs, 218, 221
  and support groups, 144
Psychosocial nursing care, Irene Burnside
    and
  comparison with other countries,
    229–230
  criteria for group membership, 223
  Fundamental Interpersonal Relations
    Orientation (FIRO) method, 224
  group work, 221, 222–225
  of older adults, 213

one-to-one therapy, 220, 222, 227
pet therapy, 225
physical environment and impact on, 220, 221
reminiscence therapy, 224, 228–229
themes emerging from Burnside's work, 222, 224
theoretical framework, 222, 224
treatment activities, 223–224
Psychotherapists, nurses as, 231
Public health, rural health care delivery and, 63
Public policy, *see* Policy issues

Q

Qualitative dimensions, of network, 29
Quality of care
for cognitively impaired older adults, 104, 105
Continuous Quality Improvement (CQI) programs, 241
in family caregiving, 146, 148–149
and legislative empowerment of nurses to assure, 112
in relation to health and wellness, 83
resident outcomes, 241
Quality of family care, 149
Quality of life, for older adults
contrasted to concept of well-being, 34
definitions and measures of, 34
for family caregivers, 141
gerontological nursing research on, 97
and health promotion strategies, 96
and late-life illness, 24
in relation to health and well-being, 33–34
Quality outcomes, 242
Quantitative dimensions, of network, 29

R

Race
definition of, 158–160
and disparities in health care, 168–169

hereditary traits vs. socially acquired traits, 159
LaVeist conceptual model of, 164
myth of, 159
in relation to definition of health and wellness, 83
science of, 158–159
vs. term "ethnic groups," 159
Race classification, descriptors for, 159–160
Racism; *see also* Race
homelessness and, 182
Reciprocity, as payment issue among rural elders, 70
Recovery from illness, and availability of social support, 30
Recreation, as form of psychiatric treatment in 1940s, 218, 223
Referrals, as part of posthospital support program, 140
Reform; *see also* Health care reform
expanding use of advanced practice nurses, 63
for health professions, 2, 6, 8
Registered nurse (RN)
projected demand for, 240–241
salaries of, 245
Rehabilitation, and chronic disabilities in elders, 239
Rehospitalization rate, with transitional care, 143
Reimbursement
capitated systems of, 242
for family caregiving, 134
justification of, through nursing research, 242
incentives for wellness, 91
inequities between rural and urban areas, 64
for mammograms, through Medicare, 91
in nursing homes, 244, 245
reciprocity as form of payment, 70
for rural hospitals, 67
for wellness and health promotion services, 91, 93

Religion, and spirituality, 40
Relocation, 29, 37
Reminiscence therapy
　with cognitively impaired elders, 108
　to facilitate gerotranscendence, 42
　Irene Burnside and, 224, 228–229, 233
Reminiscence groups, 229
Remotivation therapy, with cognitively
　impaired elders, 125
Research, *see* Nursing research; Rural
　research
Residential care facilities; *see also* Home
　health care
　lack of federal guidelines to standardize
　　care, 244
　models of, 244
　variations in settings of, 244
Respite care
　and adult day care centers, 172–173
　with caregiving families, 138–139, 141
　and community-based long-term care,
　　243
　in ethnic families and communities, 172
　facilities, 245
　and nurses, 241
　as part of posthospital support
　　program, 140
　as relief for burden of care, 138–139,
　　145
　types of, 138
Restraints
　study of, by gerontological nurse
　　researchers, 231
　use in Australia, 229
　use in psychiatric treatment in 1940s,
　　218
Retirement
　communities, 245
　facilities, community-based, 245
　and mental health, 27
　as social role transition, 27–28
　and women, 27–29
Risk behaviors, 85
Risk diagnoses, 40
Risk reduction, for older adults, 85
Rituals, and ethnic elderly, 169–170, 173

Rochester State Hospital, 218
Role
　accumulation, 28
　experiences, and gender differences, 27
　in family, and changes in, 27, 28–29
　of family caregivers, 133–152, 145–146
　of health professionals in care of
　　homeless adults, 205, 206
　of nurses, in care of impaired older
　　people, 133
　of nurses, with family caregivers,
　　145–146
　supplementation and enhancement of,
　　for elders, 42
Role theory, and caregiving, 135
Routines, to enrich caregiving, 147
Rural caregivers, 70
Rural, definition of, 58–59
Rural elders
　access issues, 64–67
　demographics of, 59–60, 240
　increased interest in, 57
　health needs of, and nursing reform,
　　73–74
　health profile, 60–61
　health promotion research regarding, 97
　and homelessness, 193–194
　impact of social and physical
　　environments on, 57
　lack of public transportation, 60
　National Resource Center for Rural
　　Elderly, 189
　and nursing centers, 69
　and problems for cost-effective program
　　development, 240
　rate of institutionalization, 67
　regional variation of, 59
　use of services, 64–67
　utilization rates of, 65
　within-group and between-group
　　variance, 59
Rural gerontological nursing practice; *see
　also* Gerontological nursing cur-
　riculum; Gerontological nursing
　research; Rural nurses; Rural
　nursing

AD graduates as deterrent to, 73
knowledge base for, 67
Rural health care
adaptation of innovative models of,
69–70
Area Agencies on Aging, 66
crisis in, 64–65
long-term continuum of care in, 65–67
myths and realities, 57–74
nursing centers, 69
poor articulation of needs, 59
role of nurses, 62–65
use of computers in, 68–69, 70–71
Rural homelessness, among elders,
193–194
Rural nurses
associate degree (AD) graduates as, 73
computer communication technologies
and, 68–69, 71
demographics of, 62
developing programs of research, 68
role of Area Health Education Centers
(AHECs), 72
setting of practice of, 62–63
skills needed by, 71
targeting students from rural areas, 73
training of, 62, 71–72
Rural nursing, 57
heightened interest in, 57, 58
knowledge base for, 67–69
practice of, 61–64
research on, 67–69
Rural nursing homes, 66–67
Rural research, 67–69, 97

S

Safety
as nursing intervention, 42–43
and security for elders, 38
services, in wellness program, 89
San Diego State University, 228
San Jose State University, 228, 229
Santa Monica City Senior Nutrition and
Recreation Program, 86
Satisfaction of family caregiver, 139

Satisfaction of older adults; *see also* Life
satisfaction
with telephone support intervention,
139–140
Scabies, 217
Scarlet fever, 217
Schema-neural network theory, in
gerontology, 16
Schizophrenia, and homelessness, 186
Screening services, for older adults; *see
also* Physical examinations and
screenings
cost-effectiveness of, 93
types of, 89, 94
Script, theory in gerontology, 15
Security
definition of, for elders, 38
and housing needs of elders, 38
Self-care
behaviors, partnerships and, 70
diminished ability to engage in, 224
for family caregivers, 137
and health behavior, 32–33
nursing interventions to enhance, 43
as predominant form of treatment, 33
Self-concept
alterations in, 27
effect of environmental forces on, 37
Self-determination, and right to choose
lifestyle, 96
Self-esteem
and housing satisfaction in elders,
37–38
and positive lifestyle health practices,
86
and protective caregiving, 147
Self-management, 33, 70
Self-transcendence, as late-life
phenomenon, 26, 40
Senior centers, programs and activities in
rural areas, 66
Senior nutrition centers, 86
Sensory acuity in older adults, diminished,
224
Service utilization rates, among elders in
rural communities, 65

Sexism, 36
Shelter and Street Night (S-Night) operation, 185
Shelters, *see* Housing
Signal detection theory, in gerontology, 17
Single-peak creativity model, in gerontology, 17
Single room occupancy (SRO) hotels, 180
Sigma Theta Tau, 232
Skid Row, 179, 180
Skill in care, 149
Sleep
  among rural elders, 61
  intervention strategies, for cognitively impaired elders, 123–124
Sleep–wake cycle, disturbances in, 123
Smoking, among elders, 27, 201
Social competence/breakdown, in gerontology, 13
Social dimension
  as construct of model of environmental sphere, 35–36
  major components of, 35
Social environment
  in definition of health promotion, 84
  impact on rural elders, 57
  and nurses' lack of awareness about impact of, 35, 43
Social exchange theory, and caregiving, 135
Social integration, 29
Social isolation, *see* Isolation
Social network, 28, 29, 30; *see also* Social support
Social networks theory, in gerontology, 13, 29–30
Social psychology, and theories in gerontology, 13–14
Social role transitions, 22, 27–29
Social Security, and homeless people, 180, 190, 191, 199
Social Security Administration, 91
Social services, in wellness program, 89
Social status, for elders, 28
Social support
  as buffer to stress, 29

burden of, 29
and community-based long-term care, 243
through ComputerLink project, 71
for ethnic elderly, 170–173
and functional status, 32
and health, 29–30
and homelessness, *see* Homelessness
and hospitalization, 30
and lifestyle health practices, 86, 96
measurement of, 30
negative effects of, 29
nurses as offering, 111–112
research on, 29–30
and risk reduction for older adults, 85
transitions, 22, 29–30
Social support: formal/informal, as theory in gerontology, 13
Sociocultural theories in gerontology, 12–13
Sociodemographics, *see* Demographics
Sociology, and theories in gerontology, 12–13
Somatic mutation theory, in gerontology, 18
Spiritual dimension
  as construct of model of environmental sphere, 39–40
  three critical attributes of, 39
Spirituality
  definition of, 39
  in nursing, 39–40
  and religion, 40
Staff, strategies for increasing job satisfaction and retention, 246
Standards, NLN curricular, 4
State board agencies, and gerontology-prepared faculty, 8
State board examinations, and content on elder care, 3, 4, 8, 230
Status/reciprocity theory, in gerontology, 13
Strain, *see* Stress
Stress
  and agitated behaviors, among cognitively impaired elders, 118, 119, 121, 123

and coping (adaptation) theory, 135
and family caregivers, 136, 149, 152
management of, for cognitively
  impaired older adult, 110
progressively lowered stress threshold
  model of care, 106, 110–111, 118
and retirement, 27
social support as buffer to, 29
Stroke, 192
Subacute care, 242
Subculture theory, in gerontology, 12
Subjective burden, *see* Burden of care;
  Caregiver burden
Substance abuse, study of, in nursing
  curriculum, 3–4
Suicide, physician-assisted, 247
Supervisory caregiving, 147
Supplemental Security Disability
  Insurance (SSDI), 189
Supplemental Security Income (SSI), 189,
  199
Support groups, with caregiving families,
  139, 140, 141, 144, 145
Support systems; *see also* Social support
  disconnectedness from, during
  transitions, 22
Symbols, individual bias, and care of
  ethnic elderly, 169–170, 173

T

Team teaching, 8
Technology
  contribution to shift toward urban care
    centers, 64
  and costs of health care for elders, 134
  and professional competence, 6
  use of, and cost-effectiveness, 6
Telecommunications
  innovative nursing programs using, 73
  and linkage among health professionals,
    68–69
Telephone advice lines, 143–144
Telephone interventions, with caregiving
  families, 143–144, 145
Telephone monitoring, 143–144

Telephone support, 139–140
Temporal integration, 26
Terminal drop, theory in gerontology, 17
Theory of aging, 11
Therapeutic relationship, development of,
  145
Therapy; *see also* Interventions
  cognitive–behavioral, 126–127
  reminiscence, 108, 224
  remotivation, 125
  validation, 108, 124–125
  visual imagery, 126–127
Tobacco use, 85
Touch, as care need, 173
Trainees, *see* Nurses' training
Training
  of family caregivers, 134
  of NPs, *see* Gerontological nurse
    practitioners; Gerontological nursing
    curriculum
Traits, theory in gerontology, 15
Transcendence
  as late-life phenomenon, 25–27
  and spirituality, 39
Transition phenomena, 22
Transitional care intervention, with
  caregiving families, 143, 145
Transitions
  in family roles, 27, 28–29
  in late life, *see* Late-life transitions
  magnitude and frequency of, in
    caregiving, 150
  monitoring of, in caregiving, 145
  retirement, *see* Retirement
  in social role, *see* Social role transitions
Transpersonal/transcendent psychology,
  and late-life transitions, 22
Transportation
  and access to care, 168
  problems for rural elders, 60
  rural vs. urban expenditures for, 66
Treatment; *see also* Interventions
  changes in, and transitions in
    caregiving, 150
  withholding, 247
Triandis model, 164

Tuberculosis, 191
Turnover
   of patients, 246
   of staff in nursing homes, 246
Types, theory in gerontology, 16

U

Ulcers, and homeless elders, 192
Unemployment
   and homelessness, 185, 195
   and older adults, 67
Unionization, in nursing homes, 246
United Nations Educational, Scientific,
      and Cultural Organization
      (UNESCO), 159
University of California, 221
University of Colorado, 72
University of Denver, 220
University of Minnesota, 216
University of New Mexico, 73
University of Southern California, 226,
      228
University of Texas, 228, 229, 232
University of Wyoming, 73
Urinary incontinence, *see* Incontinence
U.S. Conference of Mayors, 184

V

Vaccinations, 88
Validation therapy, with cognitively
      impaired elders, 108, 124–125
Values
   of ethnic elderly, 157, 161, 169
   of ethnic family and communities and
      effect on health care, 170–173
   of older adults, 36
Veterans Administration, 199
Victory over Japan (VJ) Day, 219
Vision
   impairment, and late-life illness, 24
   problems, and homeless elders, 202
   screenings, 88
Visiting Nurse Associations, 66
Visual imagery therapy, 126–127

Volunteers
   in community-based care, 70
   and homeless elders, 177
Vulnerability, to homelessness, 184–185

W

Wallingford Wellness Project, 85
Wear and tear (rate of living) theory, in
      gerontology, 18
Weight control, 85
Well-being
   and attachment to place, 37
   of caregivers, 144
   contrasted to concept of quality of life,
      34
   definitions of, 34
   effect of environmental forces on,
      36–37
   effect of physical environment on,
      37–38
   as element of elder sphere, 31–35
   in gerontological theory, 20
   and influence of ageism, sexism, and
      classism, 36
   and normative biological involution, 23
   nursing interventions to enhance sense
      of, 41, 42, 43
   as nursing outcome variable, 43, 44
   positive and negative affects of, 34–35
   psychological, 30
   in relation to social network character-
      istics, 30
   role supplementation and enhancement
      to enhance, 42
   and social dimension of environmental
      sphere, 36
Wellness; *see also* Health; Health promotion
   barriers to, 98
   diagnoses, 40
   as distinguished from health, 33–34
   gerontic nursing institutes and, 98–99
   health as part of, 82–83
   health promotion as strategy to
      improve, 97–98
   marketing of, 97

Wellness/health promotion centers
  costs of, 91–94
  enticing elders to use, 94–95
  models of, 85–86
  personnel needs of, 88, 90
  priorities, 86–87
  services offered at, 87–88, 89
Wellness program services; *see also* Health
    maintenance services; Health
    promotion services; Wellness/
    health promotion centers
  gerontic nursing institutes and,
    98–99
  list of, 89

Western Gerontological Society, 226;
    see also American Society on Aging
Widowed elders, 29, 171
Working out systems, of care, 148
World Health Organization (WHO), 82
World War II, 171, 180, 217, 219, 238

Y

YMCAs, 86
YWCAs, 86
Young-old
  demographic projections of, 238
  and homelessness, 191

Springer Publishing Company

STRENGTHENING GERIATRIC NURSING EDUCATION
Terry Fulmer, RN, PhD, FAAN and
Marianne Matzo, PhD, RN, CS, Editors

This book is designed to promote geriatric content in the basic nursing curriculum, in order to make sure new nurse graduates are properly prepared to care for the growing numbers of elderly in the United States. Distinguished nurse educators review the current state of geriatrics and gerontology in the nursing curriculum, and make recommendations for fully incorporating it into the program of study.

STRENGTHENING
GERIATRIC
NURSING
EDUCATION

Terry Fulmer
Marianne Matzo
Editors

Partial Contents:

- Why Good Ideas Have Not Gone Far Enough: The State of Geriatric Nursing Education, *Mathy Mezey*

- Barriers in Nursing Education, *Marianne Matzo*

- Incorporating Geriatrics into the Licensure and Accreditation Process, *Terry Fulmer* and *Mary Tellis Nyack*

- Expanding Clinical Experiences, *May L. Wykle* and *Carol M. Musil*

- Student Resistance: Overcoming Ageism, *Carla Mariano*

- Normal Aging and Physiology, *Mary (Mickie) Burke* and *Susan E. Sherman*

- Psychiatric Mental Health, *Carol M. Musil and May L. Wykle*

- Elimination and Skin Problems, *Marie O'Toole*

1995   200pp   0-8261-8940-7   hardcover

536 Broadway, New York, NY 10012-3955 • (212) 431-4370 • Fax (212) 941-7842